COMMUNITY CARE

Findings from DH-Funded Research
1988–1992

Edited by
Diana Robbins

HMSO

ISBN 0 11 321567 3

Project Team:

Editor: Diana Robbins
Administration: Katie Foster
Production Editor: Alister Walters

Community Care

Findings from DH-Funded Research

1988–1992

CONTENTS

List of Figures

List of Tables

Foreword

Putting community care policy into effect presents social and health service managers with tremendous opportunities and challenges; and during the period of implementation and beyond, they will need to use all the tools at their disposal. Among the available resources are the findings of relevant research.

This document aims to draw together and summarize, in an accessible reference format, the findings of the body of research relevant to community care which has been funded by the Department of Health since 1988. More than 100 substantial research projects have been completed since then, and some important studies still in progress are flagged in the collection.

There are no simple prescriptions to be found here. Translating research findings into policy, organizational change, or improved professional practice is not straightforward. The summaries are laid out as a contribution to change, and as one small step in the creation of knowledge-based services.

The document offers the reader a number of routes around the material – by way of the introductory overview, Chapter breakdown, key words, and of course the index. It also provides interested readers with all the information they need to pursue particular studies in more detail than can be included here. This is not the kind of book which anyone will take and read through at one sitting. But I hope that managers, practitioners and researchers will turn to it again and again in the months ahead, and make full use of the range and depth of information which research has generated. Most of the important questions facing community care managers in the 1990s are reflected in the pages that follow.

HERBERT LAMING

Chief Inspector, Social Services Inspectorate
Department of Health

Reader's Guide to the Entries

The entries are grouped in Chapters, and a summary of what the Chapter contains appears at the beginning of each one. The name of the relevant Chapter is at the bottom of each right-hand page. Each Chapter has a distinctively coloured, margin-tab throughout.

Near the beginning of each entry, a number of 'key words' appear in the margin. These are not subheadings, and have not been determined by computer. They amount simply to an editorial comment on some of the themes which may be of particular interest to the reader. They do not repeat the information in the title of the entry, nor the name of the Chapter.

At the end of each entry, the names and addresses of the researchers, and a list of relevant publications (if applicable) appear. These are as up-to-date as possible, and are intended as sources of further information.

The index, which begins on page 385, provides a systematic breakdown of the material, and covers research institutions and authors, as well as the content of the research.

Abbreviations

ACA	Association for Continence Advice
ACRE	Age Care Research Europe
AIDS	Acquired Immune Deficiency Syndrome
ARC	AIDS-Related Complex
ARVAC	Association of Researchers in Voluntary Action and Community Involvement
ATC	Adult Training Centre
AWS	All-Wales Strategy
b	billion
BASSAC	British Association of Settlements and Social Action Centres
BASW	British Association for Social Workers
BIMH	British Institute of Mental Handicap
BMRU	Blind Mobility Research Unit, University of Nottingham
BRS	Behaviour Rating Scale
C	Control
CA	Citizen Advocacy
CAC	Communication Aids Centre
CAPE	Clifton Assessment Procedures for the Elderly
CCBI	Council of Churches in Britain and Ireland
CCSAP	Community Care Special Action Project
CEDR	Centre for Evaluative and Developmental Research, University of Southampton
CFI	Centrally-Funded Initiative
CHE	Centre for Health Economics, University of York
CM	Case-managed
CMHC	Community Mental Health Centre
CMHN	Community Mental Handicap Nurse
CMHT	Community Mental Health Team
CPN	Community Psychiatric Nurse
CRF	Community Residential Facility
CRSP	Centre for Research in Social Policy, University of Loughborough
CSPRD	Centre for Social Policy Research and Development, University of Wales
CSV	Community Service Volunteers
CVA	Cardio-Vascular Accident

DES	Department of Education and Science, now DFE
DFE	Department for Education, formerly DES
DH	Department of Health
DHA	District Health Authority
DHSS	Department of Health and Social Security
DMH	Darlington Memorial Hospital
DR	Direct Referral
DSS	Department of Social Security
EC	European Commission
EEC	European Economic Community
EMI	Elderly Mentally Ill
ENT	Ear, Nose and Throat
ESS	Early Signs Scale
FHSA	Family Health Services Authority
GHQ	General Health Questionnaire
GHS	General Household Survey
GP	General Practitioner
GPMH	Good Practices in Mental Health
HA	Health Authority
HARC	Hester Adrian Research Centre, University of Manchester
HB	Home-Based
HIV	Human Immuno-Deficiency Virus
HMSO	Her Majesty's Stationery Office
incl.	including
IQ	Intelligence Quotient
ISBN	International Standard Book Number
LAS	Local Autistic Society
LEA	Local Education Authority
LSE	London School of Economics
m	million
MH	Mental Handicap/Mental Health
MI	Myocardial Infarction
NACRO	National Association for the Care and Resettlement of Offenders
NALHF	National Association of Leagues of Hospital Friends
NAS	National Autistic Society
NCWP	New Commonwealth and Pakistan
NGO	Non-Governmental Organization
NHS	National Health Service
NIMROD	New Ideas for the Care of Mentally Ill/Retarded People in Ordinary Dwellings
NISW	National Institute for Social Work
No	Number
NS/ns	Not Significant

NSPCC	National Society for the Prevention of Cruelty to Children
NWRHA	North Western Regional Health Authority
OPCS	Office of Population Censuses and Surveys
OTA	Occupational Therapy Aide
p&p	postage and packing
PANT	Practitioner Assessment of Network Type
PAS-ADD	Psychiatric Assessment Schedule for Adults with a Developmental Disability
PPA	Pre-school Playgroups Association
PSE	Present State Examination
PSI	Policy Studies Institute
PSS	Personal Social Services
PSSRU	Personal Social Services Research Unit, University of Kent
QALYS	Quality of Life York Scale
RADAR	Royal Association for Disability and Rehabilitation
RDP	Research and Development in Psychiatry
REMIT	Ruddlan Elderly Mentally Infirm Team
RHA	Regional Health Authority
RIPA	Royal Institute of Public Administration
RNIB	Royal National Institute for the Blind
RNID	Royal National Institute for the Deaf
RNMH	Registered Nurse, Mental Handicap
ROP	Retinopathy of Prematurity
SAHI	Staying At Home Initiative
SC	Standard Care
SCL	Syndrome Checklist
SHA	Self-Help Alliance
SIB	Self-Injurious Behaviour
SLD	Special/Severe Learning Disabilities
SPRU	Social Policy Research Unit, University of York
SSD	Social Services Department
SSI	Social Services Inspectorate
TAPS	Team for the Assessment of Psychiatric Services
TED	Telephone Exchange for the Deaf
TR	Traditional Referral
UK	United Kingdom
USA	United States of America
VAT	Value-Added Tax
vol.	volume
vs	versus
WHO	World Health Organization
WISC	Weschler Intelligence Scale for Children
WO	Welsh Office

Introduction

THE COLLECTION

The summaries of findings in the Chapters which follow are based on research in progress in January 1988, and commissioned since then, which is relevant to planning and implementing community care policy. It has all been funded, in whole or in part, by the Department of Health, (Department of Health and Social Security until July 1988). It reflects the overriding objective of the Department's centrally-managed research programme – to provide objective information for Ministers as a basis for key policy developments – and has been tailored to answer some of the most important questions which have arisen in the debate about care in the community.

Much of the research included here has been completed, published in full, and disseminated through professional journals, newsletters, seminars and so on. But the collection has not been seen together before, and part of the purpose of this document is to present it as a whole. Taken together, the studies represent a vast amount of work – an important resource for policy-makers, managers, researchers and practitioners. The arguments developed in the body of work become clearer when project findings are juxtaposed; and the cumulative effect of some streams of research is revealed.

This publication is intended primarily as a reference document: it concentrates on providing a way into the research through brief accounts of findings, full references to other publications arising from it, and a range of signposts in the presentation, designed to show the reader around the text. It does not draw out the policy or practice implications of the research. In many cases, the researchers will have published the conclusions they draw from their own findings; and the Department has been involved in a broad range of work which has based policy or practice guidance on the results of a programme of research and development – encompassing some of the research included here.

The studies covered in this publication were all commissioned by customers within the Department with an interest in specific client groups, and this is reflected in the coverage of the collection as a whole. There is relatively little which deals with management issues which cut across all or most client groups, or which covers policy areas of importance to the development of care in the community which are outside the responsibility of the Departmental customers – housing, for example, or benefit entitlement. Because of the importance in the community care field of research on AIDS and substance misuse, a special supplement is included at the end of the collection which gives a very brief listing of relevant research projects. Links with other centrally-funded research commissioned under other Departmental headings – child-care, for example, or workforce issues – are also important, and will be clear from some of the entries which follow.

THE ENTRIES

Most of the entries represent one research study or project, which is either completed or in progress at the time of publication. The range of research represented here is very wide: reviews of literature, longitudinal studies, randomized controlled trials, small-scale, detailed case-studies, major evaluations and action research are all included. Each entry comprises the project's title, a very brief account of its objectives and research method, and a summary of the main findings if they are available. The researcher/s' names, institutions, addresses and telephone numbers are followed by a list of publications arising from each project, which has been kept as full as space will allow.

The material is broken down into six Chapters, principally by client group; and the first three are mainly, but not exclusively, concerned with elderly people. Within Chapters, entries run from broad service issues to research about particular interventions. Coloured margins show the Chapter breakdown. At the side of each entry, two or three 'key words' indicate the main issues or questions it raises; and the index provides another summary analysis of the contents. Some important client groups are not the subject of specific Chapter headings – children, for example, or minority ethnic groups – but the relevance of particular entries to their needs will be made clear by the key words, and the index.

In order to keep the collection together, and the document a reasonable length, individual accounts of the research have been kept very short – frustratingly short for some researchers, and perhaps some readers. But the other information each entry contains means that it should be possible readily to follow up any study which is of particular interest through the references to published material, or by contacting the researcher directly for the full report.

THE WORK OF THE UNITS

A feature of the centrally-commissioned programme is that a number of research units are funded by the Department, to meet Ministers' long-term needs for continuing research relevant to a core of major policy issues. Four of these have completed work which is of importance to developments in relation to community care: the Personal Social Services Research Unit (PSSRU) at the University of Kent, the National Institute for Social Work (NISW) in London, the Centre for Health Economics (CHE) and the Social Policy Research Unit (SPRU) – both at the University of York. Together, the projects completed or launched by these four units since 1988 amount to about one quarter of all the studies included here.

A major programme of evaluations of case-management schemes has been one priority at the PSSRU, incorporating work on schemes focusing on the social and health care of elderly people in Kent (see page 7), Gateshead (page 12), and Darlington (page 17), and of psychogeriatric clients in Lewisham (page 21). An overview of these schemes (page 3) draws out the implications of all the case-management experiments; and a second overview contributed by the PSSRU summarizes the main findings of the Care in the Community Demonstration Programme, which was monitored and evaluated by the unit between 1984 and 1989, (page 31).

The CHE has concentrated on studies which map current provision and identify the potential for growth in the mixed economy of care. The Centre collaborated with the PSSRU on a survey of hospices and nursing homes (page 121), and with SPRU on a survey of non-statutory nursing home provision (page 125). A further collaboration, with the Nuffield Institute of Health Services at the University of

Leeds, led to the publication of a series of studies on the implications of joint finance for inter-agency collaboration, the cost-effectiveness of services, and the participation of users and carers in the design and running of services (pages 47 and 39).

The programme of work commissioned from researchers at NISW has covered a wide range of issues of especial concern to social work professionals: services concerned with respite care (page 167), discharge from hospital (page 109), and home care (page 116) have been the subject of three studies. Broader issues such as the implications of the development of community schemes for area-based social work (page 83), and ethnic monitoring of social services (page 51) have also been tackled. Finally, at SPRU, an equally varied range of research has been completed: studies have focused in particular on the needs and circumstances of informal carers (see pages 155, 161, 164 and 151), and on the incidence and management of incontinence (pages 348, 345, 351).

Coordinated series of research projects have also been undertaken at institutions other than the units: these include the work of the Blind Mobility Research Unit (pages 365–378), and the Health Care Research Unit (pages 341, 128); the work of the Hester Adrian Research Centre in relation to learning disabilities (318, 188, 301, 271 and 275), and of the Centre for Social Policy Research and Development, at the University of Bangor, in relation to ageing and learning disabilities (pages 176, 177). Important evaluations of the All-Wales Mental Handicap Strategy have also been completed at Bangor (page 68), as well as at the Mental Handicap in Wales Applied Research Unit (pages 289–293).

SCOPE OF THE RESEARCH

It is not possible in an account of this kind to do full justice to the range and depth of work undertaken partly at the large institutions highlighted above, as well as by individual researchers working throughout England and Wales in a variety of professional contexts. It would be wrong to imply that one, neat argument emerges from the collection as a whole – it is its diversity which makes it so valuable. Nevertheless, it is possible – and useful – to identify a series of themes which have preoccupied many of the researchers represented here, and which are of central relevance to the implementation of community care policy.

At the beginning of each Chapter there is a summary of the main issues raised by the projects in that Chapter. In general, the main aim of all the research has been to illuminate how people can be cared for in the community, rather than in institutions. The research pre-dates the NHS and Community Care Act and has aims which go far wider than that Act. This is demonstrated by the summaries themselves and the chapter overviews. However, it is possible to draw from this body of research knowledge which touches on the more precise aims underlying the legislation, and the paragraphs which follow are an attempt to do this.

THEMES FROM THE RESEARCH

Cost-Effectiveness, Evaluation and Quality Assurance

Both the White Paper 'Caring for People'[1] and the policy guidance which followed it emphasized the importance of systems for monitoring the extent to which the

---

[1] 'Caring for People: Community care in the next decade and beyond', 1989, London, HMSO.

new arrangements had been successfully implemented, met existing and developing needs, and took account of the opinions of users and their carers. Every stage of the implementation process was to involve the collection of data on which rational and informed judgements about the next steps could be based.

This emphasis is repeated in the body of research funded by the Department. About half of the studies summarized here are themselves evaluations – assessments of the effectiveness of particular services or policy initiatives, judged along a range of dimensions. The most important of these also reflect the policy goals outlined in guidance: they include cost-effectiveness, the outcome and quality of life for users, and the views of users and their carers. None of these is easy to measure and the studies – as well as providing evaluations of specific initiatives – also develop models of evaluation techniques.

In an early evaluation (see page 262) of the costs and benefits of exchanging long-term residential care for care in the community, the research team based at the LSE found that a full account of costs was a complex and relatively new kind of exercise. The work of the PSSRU, already outlined above, has developed the basis for assessing costs firstly in relation to the Care in the Community Demonstration Programme, and secondly in an important series of case-studies of local case-management programmes. Costs and benefits/effectiveness have been assessed in relation to a series of community-based initiatives: psychiatric rehabilitation services (page 196), housing services for people with profound learning disabilities (page 282), care for elderly people with dementia (page 233), and Communication Aid Centres (page 338). A study which will attempt a thorough analysis of unit costs of personal social services in London is currently under way (see page 36).

Refinements in the assessment of costs have been incorporated in studies of major policy programmes: the All-Wales Mental Handicap Strategy for example, the joint finance initiative, or the European Community's HELIOS programme (page 331). Indirect costs to care staff, informal carers and users have also been analysed, (see pages 223, 161, 164).

The other half of the calculation – the benefits to users in terms of a longer or better life, to carers and to service providers – implies the need for the development of a range of performance indicators. These have been the concern of projects across all professions and client groups. Projects have developed or tested measures of quality of life (pages 112, 318 and 198). They have refined methods of data collection and analysis (pages 55, 36), and developed techniques which are of general relevance while reflecting a detailed, local situation (page 3). Work on quality assurance has been linked, in some studies, directly to the needs of service managers (page 205); others – work at the PSSRU, for example – have been directed at the broader policy scene. Practical, systematic measures of the quality of residential services is the focus of one study which is currently under way (page 282).

Value for money for the tax-payer, clarity in relation to the allocation of responsibilities, accountability, the capacity to analyse and respond to changing needs – all of these depend on the kinds of evaluative analyses which have been developed by research and which are summarized here.

Planning Services

The assessment of need and good care-management, identified as key objectives of community care policy, are reflected in the collection in a number of different ways. One project (page 259) sets out to provide a coherent basis for planning services in relation to the predicted needs of a particular client-group – people with severe learning disabilities – and has developed a guidebook for service providers from the study's findings. Other studies have used existing data sets to investigate the prevalence of incontinence (see page 345) or the extent and nature of informal care (page 151) as a means of anticipating demand.

Informed planning implies knowledge of the extent and nature of users' needs – for example, the particular needs of young people with disabilities (page 334) – and a thorough understanding of the population in a locality to be served. An important study of the ethnic monitoring undertaken by social services authorities in the United Kingdom (page 51) underlines the crucial part which monitoring must play in planning. Other projects have cleared the ground for service developments in a range of fields: through demographic studies (page 271), evaluations of service planning within Programmes (page 64), accounts of current provision for autistic children and adults (page 311) or of services for blind and partially-sighted people (page 362), and by mapping the provision of private and voluntary nursing homes (see page 125).

The transition from one service to another, or between types of care, has been investigated in several studies which are directed at the possibility of predicting relapse (pages 243, 205) or the onset of particular conditions (page 310). And one series of studies has traced the relationship between the need for services and the existence of support from informal networks, to the point where the researchers have been able to design a simple instrument to assist planners in predicting need (page 174).

Planning, care- and case-management and evaluation are the tools with which care in the community is to be built. The design of service packages which meet what users really need and want has been the preoccupation of much of the research included in this collection. The body of work specifically concerned with case-management undertaken at the PSSRU has already been mentioned. Other studies have looked at case-management in a particular context (page 354), or at the design of care packages for particular groups of users (see pages 103 and 61).

Informal Care and Informal Networks

The extent to which the activities, needs and views of informal carers are represented among the research projects in this collection is significant: the interests of carers are a central element in about 30 studies, and many more include carers among the groups to be considered in service design. Supporting carers – another key objective of community care policy – is approached from a number of different points of view in the research: financial, practical, emotional. An exploration of the financial circumstances of carers (page 161) underlines the costs of caring which must be included in the computation of the costs and benefits of policy initiatives; and other projects examine these costs in particular contexts, (page 301, for example).

'Costs' do not, of course, only involve financial losses; a number of studies are concerned with the stress experienced by carers as a result of their caring responsibilities, and with the coping strategies they develop in response to this. Analyses of the burden implied by caring for people with long-term disabilities in the community (page 207), or people with chronic schizophrenia (pages 248, 201), for children and young adults with behaviour problems (page 301) or severe learning disabilities (page 183) contribute to a fuller understanding of what providing support services will involve. Other projects have identified predictors of stress (page 180) among the carers of elderly dependants, or are concerned with preventing depression and anxiety among vulnerable groups, including carers (page 255); the ways in which carers cope with stress have been explored (see page 183), and potential conflicts of interests between service users and their informal carers identified (page 155).

What services will genuinely help carers continue their key role in maintaining their dependants at home? Evaluations of a range of family support services (see pages 158, 64, 155), respite-care services for young people with severe learning disabilities (page 325) or for elderly people (page 167, 180), of home care services (page 116), home-helps (see pages 7, 109, 230) and family-aides schemes (page 293) all help in building up a picture of the package of services which will work for carers. Some of these are directed at reducing the physical demands of caring; others will be concerned with morale.

Carers' opinions and feelings remain important once care at home is no longer feasible. A number of the studies summarized in the Chapters which follow are concerned with the views of carers about the residential options open to those dependants who continue to need their support and interest (pages 267, 321).

The people who make up the army of carers are not a single, uniform group, and their opinions and needs for support are as varied as their circumstances. The research has investigated in detail the situation of people of working age caring for spouses (page 164), parents caring for children (page 183), and people caring for elderly dependants (page 180). The functions of informal networks in supporting or replacing carers have also been investigated (pages 174–179, 106 and 109), as well as the part which can be played by volunteers (pages 158, 12 and 90), and self-help groups (page 87).

Consumer Views

A smaller, but important, group of studies is concerned with the views of service users – the extent of consumer satisfaction with innovations, the representation of their views in planning and increasing their participation in service design. Methodological issues are important here: a number of projects have been concerned to develop questionnaires and other instruments which make it possible to incorporate the views of users into the overall evaluation of service initiatives, and one has pioneered the collection of consumer satisfaction data from people who are deaf (page 359).

Some groups of users have particular difficulties in representing their own interests; for them, the development of advocacy schemes and techniques may be especially important. Projects have investigated the role of advocacy among residential care staff in promoting the interests of children with severe learning disabilities (page 321), and among citizens for adults with learning disabilities (page 284).

Participation in service planning and design is, of course, very different from simply being consulted, and involves different systems and processes. Policy guidance on the implementation of care in the community makes increased choice and participation for both users and carers an objective of the new arrangements, which will depend to a large extent on the availability of accessible information. One study is investigating the role of small, community-based action teams as catalysts for developing user-oriented services based on inter-agency collaboration (page 85).

A new emphasis on the importance of canvassing users' views is clear from the collection as a whole, over the whole range of service provision. Contexts as different as services for blind people (see page 362, young people with disabilities (page 334), people with mental health problems (pages 237, 250), and frail, elderly people are all evaluated partly by reference to the satisfaction of consumers.

The Mixed Economy of Care

Some of the parameters of a 'mixed care economy' are covered in studies which have already been mentioned: the extent of private and voluntary nursing home provision has been mapped (pages 121 and 125), and the Opportunities for Volunteering scheme evaluated (page 90) – both as a basis for future involvement and growth. The expansion of private geriatric care (page 128) and of private sector provision for elderly mentally ill people (page 230) has been investigated. One study has looked at the provision of care in the community by a range of psychiatric services for people leaving hospital, including a comparison of costs, and an analysis of the routes by which public sector finance reached the various providers (page 193).

Two projects in progress reflect the need for improved methods of assessment and quality assurance in the context of the purchaser–provider split. One will establish guidelines in relation to community nursing establishments (see page 55); the second is concerned with refining measures of the quality of residential homes for people with learning disabilities (page 282).

Analysis of the enabling role involved in managing a mixed economy (page 44) has identified some of the obstacles in the way of its development. Cultural change within local authorities had got off to a slow start, but the pace could be expected to quicken.

Collaboration, Changing the Culture, and Training

The concept of partnership is basic to community care policy. It involves partnership between users, carers and service planners and providers, and partnership between the component sectors of the mixed economy. Critically, it involves collaboration across former boundaries between statutory agencies. Many of the studies in this collection explore the potential for inter-agency collaboration and ways of achieving it. The effectiveness of liaison nurses (page 78), continence advisers (page 351), community mental handicap and mental health teams (pages 68, 250 and 219) all depend on a level of inter-agency collaboration which has not been achieved or even required in the past.

Detailed research into the organization and operation of community mental handicap teams (page 72) has provided insights into the benefits of multi-disciplinary working, and some of the barriers which have to be removed. The team framework by itself does not overcome the different and separate professional approaches represented on them. Another series of studies has looked at the influence joint finance may exert on professional cooperation, (pages 39 and 47). Once again, the researchers are able to identify progress in the development of joint working through joint finance, without underestimating the degree of cultural change involved in the joint approaches implied by future plans for care in the community.

The theme of training, and its importance in supporting innovation, appears in projects which deal with whole-service philosophies (pages 85, 289) or particular initiatives (see pages 351, 240 and 275). Professionals need to be familiar with new ways of working together and with users and carers, as well as new techniques and priorities. Projects have evaluated specific training instruments (page 348), have explored staff views of service innovations (page 264), and identified new demands on staff (page 57) which may imply an increased need for support (page 307).

Carers and consumers are also implicated in the design and implementation of new forms of care: their needs for training are not overlooked in the collection. Counselling after myocardial infarction (page 112), training patients in relaxation to help in the control of chronic pain (page 343), and training for patients and carers in the early detection of potential relapse in schizophrenia (page 207) are proposed and evaluated. Self-help techniques like these are part of the new partnership between professionals and users; full partnership depends on the development of participation described above.

Innovation

In a sense, all the projects included here are concerned with innovation. To be relevant to the implementation of community care policies – and all these studies are – each focuses on an aspect of provision which is in the process of transition to something new. Research has provided basic information for service planning; tested methods of evaluation; evaluated whole programmes of innovative care, and analysed individual initiatives. It has identified typologies, models of intervention and analysis, and instruments for research and practice. The management of innovation has been explored, as have the implications for training, team-building and collaboration.

There are some gaps of course, and some of these will be filled in the months ahead. As implementation proceeds, the development of the mixed economy will be carefully monitored, and evaluated; and the development of more effective ways of ensuring the participation of users and carers in service design and implementation remains a priority.

CONCLUSION

The policy objectives of the Department's research programme have been basically concerned to confirm that care in the community can work to the benefit of the users; and to demonstrate how it can be provided to a high standard.

The recently-completed and current research programme has underpinned these Departmental objectives by:

— establishing that care can be provided in the community for a wide range of people;
— comparing quality and costs of care in the community with care in hospital;
— indicating that there are some groups for whom community care may be problematic;
— identifying needs for health and social care, and highlighting special needs;
— evaluating various types of residential care;
— evaluating models of domiciliary care, and particular service components, that contribute to packages of care;
— evaluating professional interventions and treatments;
— determining the broad order of costs for care in the community, and the cost distribution between agencies;
— testing methods of targeting and developing care-packages;
— developing methods of assessment and case-management;
— documenting conditions and services conducive to enabling people to remain at home.

One of the main methods adopted by the research programme has been to evaluate innovative models of service provision. By doing this, and by clarifying client and patient needs, a significant picture has been pieced together across the programme of what constitutes high-quality community care.

Other Departmental objectives have been concerned with the organizational structures, financing and the processes needed to deliver community care; with supporting carers and enhancing the roles of the private and voluntary sectors. Research contributing to all these objectives will be found in the collection summarized here. The main challenge in the future will be to support research which can indicate how to target care on those most in need, and how to tailor community services which have the greatest beneficial impact on those who use them. It is hoped that this reference document will be a useful starting-point.

Jenny Griffin
Diana Robbins

Chapter 1

Managing and Delivering Services

Managing and Delivering Services

This Chapter incorporates summaries of research concerned with management systems and techniques for delivering services. Much of the work is directly concerned with services for elderly people, although the findings of many of these projects have a more general relevance to community care.

Evaluations of innovations in the delivery of services – studies of experimental case-management projects, assessment and care-packaging, targeting and collaboration – are included here. The implications of the development of a mixed economy of care for management, and 'ground-clearing' studies, which consider the service context in which this development is to take place, are also covered.

The organization and deployment of staff in the new situation is the focus of a number of projects. Specific topics include ways of establishing community nursing establishments; the implications for care staff of caring for people with learning disabilities in the community; the transferability of specialist nursing skills from one context to another; the organization of teams; and the nature of liaison between hospital and the community.

Finally, there are a number of projects dealing with management issues which cut across all user-groups. Summaries cover a major study of ethnic monitoring, evaluations of self-help support and Opportunities for Volunteering, the role of catalyst organizations in promoting collaboration and user participation, and the implications for the personal social services of the development of community schemes.

Case-Management Studies: An Overview of the Kent, Gateshead, Darlington and Lewisham Findings

These studies examined a particular model of case-management, which involved providing case managers, who worked with relatively small caseloads of the most vulnerable elderly, with devolved budgets.

The findings are remarkably consistent. In all settings there was a reduction in the use of institutional care facilities, and all the available data indicate that the quality of life of elderly people and their carers receiving these case-management services improved significantly more than those receiving the usual services. Furthermore, these gains were achieved at no greater cost than costs for existing services over the same time-period, indicating greater efficiency in care provision.

Quality of Life
Costs
Efficiency

The findings throw light on a number of aspects of case-management, including who should receive it; whether budgets can be devolved; the availability and skills of staff; linkages between health and social care, and the managerial implications of this new system of services.

Targeting

The Kent, Gateshead and Darlington studies were carefully targeted on those for whom there was considerable potential for substituting home-based for institutional care. Although improvements in welfare and similar costs were found, indicating greater efficiency, the results did not on the whole indicate significant cost-savings. It is therefore probable that if the same case-management approach were applied to those with a slightly lower level of need, where the opportunity for substitution of community care for institutional care is less, then costs might rise. This is because individuals whose needs fall just below that of present institutional care currently receive relatively low levels of provision, and case-management with more detailed assessments could well lead to expenditure beyond that currently incurred. It follows that careful targeting must be one of the factors associated with the positive effect of these studies upon admissions to institutional care, which supports evidence from other, larger-scale case-management schemes.

Financial Devolution

The evidence indicates that control over resources is an important factor in enabling case managers to respond more effectively to the varied individual needs of elderly people, not only in the UK but also in other countries. Without this control, the case manager may be in a situation in which s/he *asks* for services to be provided but has relatively little power to ensure their adequacy, or coordinate them effectively. Much better outcomes are possible when case managers are able to adapt care plans flexibly, to reflect the individual circumstances of users and carers. It is the capacity to influence both **the type and content** of service available that permits genuine individualization of care.

If more responsive patterns of care depend on the devolution of decisions, and therefore budgets to individual case managers, changes will be needed in public sector organizations to achieve effective decentralization as well as accountability. The challenge of making such changes should not be underestimated.

Style of Case-Management

Within the case-management literature, there is a debate about two differing styles of case-management which may be characterized as 'administrative' and 'clinical' approaches. Some agencies regard the core tasks of case-management as administrative rather than tasks requiring human relations skills. However, in common with some other studies, those undertaken in Kent, Darlington and Gateshead indicate that successful case-management involves combining practical care with the use of human relations skills, including counselling and support, not only to carers and users but also to direct care staff. The 'administrative' model implies that inputs like these are resources which must be purchased separately, where necessary.

This problem is clear from the debate about the separation of assessment and provision – the so-called 'purchaser–provider split'. Given the variety of case-management programmes, any definition which treats the provision of human relations skills and emotional support as only part of the 'provider' role alone is too dogmatic, and quite inappropriate in good practice. The essence of the assessment process involves engaging a person, forming a relationship, giving advice; and therefore, at any early stage, a range of human relations skills. Even the indirect work of case-management – involving coordination and linking formal and informal networks – requires the case manager to support and train key workers in close contact with the service user. The *clinical* model of case-management requires a combination of direct and indirect work, and the integration of casework and service arrangement. It is a useful counter to the risk of bureaucratization and insensitivity in the new care arrangements, which may be particularly great in the absence of appropriately trained staff to act as case managers.

Links with the Health Care System

It is clear that effective health care provision, as well as social care, is vital to the well-being of elderly people receiving case-management services who, by definition, are on the margins of institutional care. The opportunities for locating case-management services with health care services is dependent obviously upon the pattern of development of those health care services.

There are two main contexts in which community care may be linked with health care settings. Firstly, *primary care* provides a setting for case-finding, with the development of screening in general practice for the over-75 population. Secondly, *developments in geriatric medicine and psychogeriatrics* in the United Kingdom also suggest that these environments offer potential for case-management services which are targeted on the very frail. This is particularly true of community-based services.

Matching Case-Management Arrangements to Client and Local Area Circumstances

Within the two models outlined above, case-management arrangements vary in relation to a number of factors including setting, and form of separation of purchaser and provider. Evidence from both UK and overseas studies suggests that the most effective arrangements will be those which vary according to the circumstances of different groups of clients, local area characteristics and the nature of their local health and social care systems.

The Organizational Infrastructure of Case-Management

Discussion of the case-management process often takes place as if it should only be seen as a *client-level activity*, rather than as *part of a system* contributing through assessment and information systems to service planning. Effective client-level work in fact depends upon appropriate organizational infrastructures. The devolution of budgets is one element in this: managers also need to consider factors such as improved information systems and new management approaches to quality assurance, rather than traditional bureaucratic procedures. Without change at all levels in organizations providing care, there is a risk that change will be slight and existing patterns of care will simply acquire new labels without real change in the experience of service users and their families. In the UK context, this could happen if budgets are not devolved, while organizations follow to the letter the principle of separating assessor/purchaser from the provider of care. Bulk purchasing on a large scale may well have no impact for the user, since it may only be substituting an insensitive private/voluntary monopoly provider for an insensitive public sector provider. This is not a recipe for developing client-centred approaches.

In view of the kinds of changes in the pattern of community care which are wanted, and policy-makers' expectations of the role of case-management in the process, it is obviously essential to be clear about target populations, models of case-management which work, degrees of freedom permitted to practitioners within these models, the management of these services and how they relate to health care. In the absence of such clarity, investment in case-management systems could simply become a more expensive response which fails to produce real gains in welfare or changes in the pattern of provision.

Researchers

Dr David Challis and Professor Bleddyn Davies

Personal Social Services Research Unit, University of Kent, Cornwallis Building, Canterbury, Kent CT2 7NF. (0227 764000; FAX 0227 764327)

Publications

Challis, D. (1985) 'Community Care Schemes: An alternative approach to decentralisation', in S. Hatch (ed.), *Decentralisation and Community Care*, London, Policy Studies Institute, 40–54.

Challis, D. (1987) 'Case Management and Consumer Choice', in Clode, D., Parker, C., and Etherington, S. (eds), *Consumers, Welfare and the new Pluralism*, Aldershot, Gower, 91–104.

Challis, D. (1989) 'Elderly Dementia Sufferers in the Community: the Needs, Service and Policy Background', in Morton, J. (ed.), *Enabling Elderly People with Dementia to live in the Community*, London, Age Concern Institute of Gerontology, King's College, 1–9.

Challis, D. (1989) 'Lessons from the Past and Possibilities for the Future', in Social Services Inspectorate (ed.), *Home Care – Facing the Challenge of Change*, Department of Health, 6–13.

Challis, D. (1990) 'Case Management: problems and possibilities', in Allen, I. (ed.), *Care Managers and Care Management*, London, PSI, 9–25.

Challis, D. (1990) 'Practice and Management in the UK Community Care Schemes', in Howe, A., Ozanne, E., and Selby-Smith, C. (eds), *Community Care Policy and Practice: New Directions in Australia*, Melbourne, Public Sector Management Institute, Monash University, Australia, 73–99.

Challis, D. (1991) 'Assessment and Case Management in practice', *Geriatric Medicine*, January, **21**, 1: 14.

Challis, D., Chessum, R., and Luckett, R. (1988) 'Long term care for the elderly: evaluation of the Kent Community Care and related schemes', in Murphy, E. (ed.), *Home or Away*, London, NUPRD/Guy's Hospital, 9–32.

Challis, D., and Chesterman, J. (1985) 'A System for Monitoring Social Work Activity with the Elderly', *British Journal of Social Work*, **15**: 115–132.

Challis, D., and Chesterman, J. (1986) 'Devolution to Fieldworkers', *Social Services Insight*, June 21: 15–18.

Challis, D., and Chesterman, J. (1986) 'Feedback to front line staff from computerised records: some problems and progress', *Computer Applications in Social Work*, **3**, 3: 12–14.

Challis, D., Chesterman, J., Traske, K., and von Abendorff, R. (1990) 'Assessment and Case Management: some cost implications', *Social Work and Social Sciences Review*, **1**: 147–162.

Challis, D., and Davies, B. (1985) 'Towards more coordinated care for the frail elderly', in Jenkins, R., and Mann, A. (eds), *Continuity of Care for the Elderly Mentally Ill*, USA, Royal Free Hospital/Columbia University Centre for Geriatrics and Gerontology, **10**: 1–12.

Challis, D., and Davies, B. (1988) 'The Community Care Approach: an innovation in home care by Social Services Departments', in Wells, N., and Freer, C. (eds), *The Ageing Population: Burden or Challenge?*, London, Macmillan, 191–202.

Challis, D., and Davies, B. (1991) 'Long Term Care: Service-Based and Case Management Focused Models of Care in the United Kingdom', in Wells, L. (ed.), *An Ageing Population*, University of Toronto Press, 43–61.

Davies, B. P. (1986) 'American Experiments to substitute home for institutional-based care: policy, logic and evaluation', in Phillipson, C., Bernard, M., and Strang, P. (eds), *Dependency and Interdependency in Old Age: Theoretical Perspectives and Policy Alternatives*, Beckenham, Croom Helm.

Davies, B. P. (1990) 'Community Care in Australia and elsewhere', in Howe, A., Ozanne, E., and Selby-Smith, S. (eds), *Community Care Policy and Practice: New Directions in Australia*, Melbourne, Australia, Monash University, 260–264.

Davies, B. P. (1990) 'New Priorities in Home Care: Principles from the PSSRU experiments', in Howe, A., Ozanne, E., and Selby-Smith, S. (eds), *Community Care Policy and Practice: New Directions in Australia, ibid.*, 47–72.

Davies, B. P. (1990) 'The Australian situation: A British perspective', in Howe, A., Ozanne, E., and Selby-Smith, S. (eds), *Community Care Policy and Practice: New Directions in Australia, ibid.*, 107–118.

Davies, B. P., and Challis, D. J. (1986) *Matching Resources to Needs in Community Care*, Aldershot, Gower.

'Kent' (Thanet) Community Care Scheme

CASE-MANAGEMENT IN SOCIAL CARE

The model of case-management which was developed in Kent provided the foundations of the subsequent case-management schemes. It was designed to ensure that improved performance of the core tasks of case-management – case-finding and screening, assessment, case-planning, and monitoring and review – could contribute towards more effective and efficient long-term care. Control of resources was devolved to individual social workers, acting as case managers, so that more flexible responses to needs and the integration of fragmented services into a more coherent package, could lead to the development of a realistic alternative to institutional care. The experiment involved locating a small team, consisting of a senior social worker and two basic-grade staff with administrative support, alongside existing services in one area.

Users and Carers

Outcomes

Care Planning

The Case-Management Model

The scheme was targeted on the most frail elderly people, whose needs placed them on the margin of entry to long-term institutional care. Clients were recruited primarily from existing service providers. The case managers had smaller case-loads (about 25–30 cases) and were recruited as being more trained/experienced than is usual in work with elderly people, reflecting the needs and problems of these clients, the responsibility of the work and the cost-consequences of inappropriate decisions. Qualifications and experience in social work were seen as providing a suitable background.

The case managers were responsible for setting up a care plan, and its costs were set against a notional budget for the service. They controlled a budget that could be used to purchase or develop additional services beyond (or instead of) those currently available, to permit a wider range of responses to clients' needs. The overall weekly cost of an individual package of care was limited to two-thirds of the cost of a place in a residential home, reflecting the approximate 'care costs' of that setting: higher expenditure on individual cases was allowed but required management approval. This was designed to permit flexibility within an overall framework of accountability.

The record system had three main elements aimed at improving accountability and supplementing the usual case-notes: assessment information, covering the circumstances and needs of clients; the use of a structured case review at least four times a year covering case manager activities, client problems and the range of resources deployed; and weekly costings of the care-packages for each client. The records made it possible to monitor caseloads, the mix of client problems, case manager activities and costs, and periodically to provide summaries.

The Service in Practice

During the period in which the scheme was monitored, 92 elderly people and their families received the service. The average age was 80 years, and three-quarters were women. All the clients experienced problems with daily, practical activities, such as cleaning, and most needed help taking baths and preparing meals. More than a third were incontinent, a quarter suffered from confusion, and two-thirds were at risk of falling.

Case managers, able to provide more varied services because of their flexible budget, tended to undertake more broad-ranging assessments than before. In addition to using additional services, the budget was used to employ local people as helpers to provide care at times and in ways that existing services did not. The evidence suggested that paid helpers did not displace existing informal care; they were motivated by factors other than money, and payment permitted the involvement of a higher proportion of older and working-class people. Once service packages had been established, case managers continued to assume responsibility for clients, monitoring and adjusting care as required.

It was found that a number of problems often associated with the breakdown of care, such as severe stress on carers, confusion and risk of falling were more effectively managed at home than is usually the case. Apart from practical care, case managers were able to provide for aspects of psychological and emotional well-being which, if neglected, can lead to 'giving up'.

Outcomes

Elderly people involved in the case-management scheme were compared with similar people receiving existing services in an adjacent district, providing 74 matched pairs in all. Elderly people and their carers were interviewed at entry to the services and again one year later, with cost data being collected over the same period.

Table 1.1 indicates that a significantly higher proportion receiving the case-management scheme remained at home – 69 per cent compared with 34 per cent – and fewer entered institutional care than those receiving existing services. Over a four-year period, the reduction in admission to institutional care was still greater for those receiving the case-management scheme – 23 per cent remaining at home compared with 11 per cent of those receiving the standard range of services.

Table 1.1: *Destinational Outcomes for Matched Cases at One Year – Kent*

	Kent Social Care	
	Project	Control
	%	%
Own home	69	34
Local authority home	4	22
Private or voluntary home	8	5
Hospital	4	5
Died	14	33
Moved away	1	1
No. of cases	74	74

Table 1.2 shows that elderly people receiving the case-management service fared significantly better on a range of indicators of subjective well-being, such as morale and mood, and also quality of care, such as need for personal care and household care, than those receiving existing services.

Table 1.2: *Outcomes for Elderly People and their Carers: Mean Change Scores Over One Year – Kent*

	Kent Social Care	
	Project	Control
ELDERLY PEOPLE		
Social and Emotional Needs		
Loneliness	−1.46	0.36
Depressed mood	−0.68	−0.17
Morale	2.99	−1.00
Dissatisfaction with life development	−0.38	0.23
Felt capacity to cope	5.03	0.66
Going out/social visits	5.66	−0.77
Quality of Care		
Need help with		
Rising and retiring	−0.58	0.13
Personal care	−9.47	−1.29
Daily housework	−6.68	−1.71
Weekly housework	−4.77	−1.94
Need for extra services	−2.44	0.69
CARERS		
Stress and Burden Indicators		
Lifestyle effects	−2.5	−1.74
Subjective burden	−1.12	−0.33
Mental health difficulties	−0.82	−0.25
Level of strain	−1.24	−0.5

Although only a relatively small number of people in this study were closely involved with informal carers, due to its location in a retirement area, the evidence suggests that carers also benefited from the case-management scheme. The scheme made little difference to the practical problems experienced by carers, such as restrictions on their social life, but they *did* experience reductions in psychological stress and subjective burdens. The cost to the social services department, NHS and society as a whole was not significantly different from that of providing existing services (table 1.3).

Table 1.3: *Costs for Different Parties Over One Year – Kent*

	Case-Management Scheme	Control Group
	£s	£s
KENT SOCIAL CARE (1977 PRICES)		
Social Services Department	639	702
National Health Service	778	708
Social Opportunity Cost	2670	2498

SUBSEQUENT DEVELOPMENTS IN KENT

Between 1980 and 1987, schemes were developed across a number of areas in Kent alongside the home-help service and social work teams. In 1987–8 the County Council formulated a policy to develop an integrated approach to home support for elderly people, bringing these previously separate elements of services together. This new approach was entitled the Home Care Service, and involved the integration of the roles of social worker, community care case-manager and home-help organizer into one – that of home-care manager. Home-care managers were to act as case managers, hold limited budgets for care services and control allocations of home-help time. The service was targeted upon elderly people who were more dependent than the usual recipients of home-help services. Help at home for people with less severe needs, including predominantly domestic help, was provided through alternative services in the independent sector, supported by the local authority. This development is the subject of a study currently in progress.

Researchers

Dr David Challis and Professor Bleddyn Davies

Personal Social Services Research Unit, University of Kent, Cornwallis Building, Canterbury, Kent CT2 7NF.   (0227 764000; FAX 0227 764327)

Publications

Challis, D. (1982) 'Evaluating Community Care: Some General Principles', in Taylor, R., and Gilmore, A. (eds), *Current Trends in British Gerontology*, Aldershot, Gower, 125–138.

Challis, D. (1982) 'Towards more creative Social Work with the Elderly', in Glendenning, F. (ed.), *Care in the Community: Recent Research and Current Projects*, Beth Johnson Foundation, 43–60.

Challis, D., and Davies, B. (1980) 'A New Approach to Community Care for the Elderly', *British Journal of Social Work*, **10**: 1–18.

Challis, D., and Davies, B. (1981) 'Community Care Projects: Costs and Effectiveness', in Henrad, J. C. (ed.), *Santé Publique et Vieillissement*, Paris, Les Colloques de l'INSERM, 317–326.

Challis, D., and Davies, B. (1984) 'Community Care Schemes: A new approach to domiciliary care for the elderly', in Caird, F. I., and Grimley-Evans, J. (eds), *Advanced Geriatric Medicine*, London, Pitman, **4**: 135–144.

Challis, D., and Davies, B. (1984) 'Home Care of the Frail Elderly: Matching Resources to Needs', *Home Health Care Services Quarterly*, Fall, **V**, 2–3.

Challis, D., and Davies, B. (1985) 'Decentralised Budgeting', *Public Money*, **5**, 3: 21–24.

Challis, D., and Davies, B. (1985) 'Home Care of the frail elderly in the United Kingdom: matching resources to needs', in Trager, B., and Reif, L. (eds), *International Perspectives on Long Term Care*, Haworth Press, 98–108.

Challis, D., and Davies, B. (1985) 'Long Term Care for the Elderly: The Community Care Scheme', *British Journal of Social Work*, **15**: 563–579.

Challis, D., and Davies, B. (1986) *Case Management in Community Care*, Aldershot, Gower.

Challis, D., and Davies, B. (1987) 'Een Nieuwe Weg in de Bejaardenzorg: The Community Care Approach', *Eerstelijnszorg*, 4th May, **1022**: 1–15.

Challis, D., Davies, B., and Holman, J. (1980) 'Bringing Better Community Care to Fragile Elderly People', *Social Work Today*, **11**, 22: 14–16.

Challis, D., Davies, B., and Knapp, M. (1984) 'Cost-effectiveness Evaluation in Social Care', in Lishman, J. (ed.), *Research Highlights 8: Evaluation*, Jessica Kingsley/University of Aberdeen, 104–117.

Challis, D., and Davies, B. (1988) 'Long Term Care for the Elderly: The Community Care Scheme', in Bayens, J. P. (ed.), *Gérontologie et Gériatrie*, Société Belge de Gérontologie et de Gériatrie, Leuven, Belgium, ACCO, 107–126.

Chesterman, J., Challis, D., and Davies, B. (1988) 'Long Term Care for the Elderly: A four year follow-up', *British Journal of Social Work,* (Supplement), **18**: 43–54.

Davies, B., and Challis, D. (1980) 'Experimenting with New Roles in Domiciliary Service', *Gerontologist*, **20**: 288–299.

Davies, B., and Challis, D. (1981) 'A Production Relations Evaluation of the meeting of needs in the Community Care Projects', in Goldberg, E. M., and Connelly, N. (eds), *Evaluative Research in Social Care*, Heinemann, 177–198.

Davies, B., and Challis, D. (1986) *Matching Resources to Needs in Long Term Care*, Aldershot, Gower.

Davies, B., and Missiakoulis, S. (1988) 'Heineken and Matching Processes in the Thanet Community Care Project', *British Journal of Social Work,* (Supplement), **18**: 55–78.

Davies, B. P. (1990) 'New Priorities in Home Care: Principles from the PSSRU experiments', in Howe, A., Ozanne, E., and Selby-Smith S. (eds), *Community Care Policy and Practice: New Directions in Australia*, Melbourne, Monash University, 47–72.

Qureshi, H., Challis, D., and Davies, B. (1979) 'Motivations and Rewards of Informal Care Givers', *Journal of Voluntary Action Research*, **8**: 1–2, 47–55.

Qureshi, H., Challis, D., and Davies, B. (1983) 'Motivations and Rewards of Helpers in the Kent Community Care Scheme', in Hatch, S. (ed.), *Volunteers, Meanings, Motives*, Volunteer Centre, 144–168.

Gateshead Community Care Scheme

The case-management approach, which originated in Kent, was further developed in Gateshead, providing a basis for testing the model in an *urban setting*. A case-management team of two social workers and a senior was established with its own budget, directly responsible to an Assistant Director.

Costs
Outcomes
Use of volunteers

CASE-MANAGEMENT IN SOCIAL CARE

The Service in Practice

During the period of monitoring the scheme, 101 cases were referred and accepted as appropriate. They were a frail group with an average age of 81, who were predominantly female and rather more dependent than those in Kent. One-third suffered from incontinence and confusion, a slightly higher proportion from immobility, and over one-half were at risk of falling. Most required help with key activities of daily living and all needed help with household chores. Over two-thirds had identifiable informal carers, of whom two-thirds were seen as under stress.

Case managers were responsible for undertaking a comprehensive assessment, in line with the scheme's aim of creating individual, flexible packages of care which were responsive to changes in need. It was clear that a devolved budget encouraged assessments which were more detailed and less constrained by existing services. An individual care-plan was based on the detailed assessment, and took into account the choices expressed by the elderly people and their carers. New forms of help were developed using the budget under the case managers' control. As with the Kent scheme, a group of local 'helpers' were employed, who could work flexibly and be paid on a sessional basis, to undertake the wide variety of tasks which often do not fall within the remit of traditional services. They included activities such as ensuring an adequate diet, providing personal care, helping to manage incontinence, giving social support, and assisting people with dementia through reassurance and reality orientation. In some cases, helpers worked to improve mobility following a stroke, under the supervision of a physiotherapist. Case managers regularly monitored the care provided and reviewed their cases using a standard format.

Outcomes

A matched group of elderly people receiving the usual range of services from adjacent areas within Gateshead provided a comparison group for the evaluation: in all, 90 matched pairs of cases were identified. Both groups of elderly people and their carers were interviewed upon identification and followed up a year later. The costs of services were monitored over a one-year period for both groups.

Table 1.4 shows the outcomes in terms of *destination* at one year for the 90 matched pairs of elderly clients. While 63 per cent of those who had been involved in the scheme remained in their own homes, only 36 per cent of the control group clients did so. Roughly similar numbers of each group were in long-stay hospitals, although there was a very marked difference in the rate of admission to residential homes: 1 per cent compared with 39 per cent. There was no significant difference in the death rates or length of survival between the two groups. Over one year, those involved in the scheme remained in their own homes on average for 43 weeks, compared with only 33 weeks for those receiving the usual range of services.

Table 1.4: *Destinational Outcomes for Matched Cases at One Year – Gateshead*

	Gateshead Social Care		Gateshead Health and Social Care	
	Project	Control	Project	Control
	%	%	%	%
Own home	63	36	64	21
Local authority home	1	37	4	50
Private or voluntary home	0	2	4	0
Hospital	7	4	0	4
Died	28	20	28	25
Moved away	1	1	0	0
No. of cases	90	90	28	28

Table 1.5: *Outcomes for Elderly People and their Carers: Mean Change Scores Over One Year – Gateshead*

	Gateshead Social Care	
	Project	Control
ELDERLY PEOPLE		
Social and Emotional Needs		
Loneliness	−1.1	−0.4
Depressed mood	−4.1	−1.9
Morale	2.1	1.66
Dissatisfaction with life development	−0.5	−0.3
Felt capacity to cope	5.3	2.9
Going out/social visits	1.0	−0.9
Quality of Care		
Need help with Rising and retiring	−2.3	−0.5
Personal care	−41.3	−8.6
Daily housework	−16.5	−5.4
Weekly housework	−7.3	−3.8
Need for extra services	−6.4	−2.3
CARERS		
Stress and Burden Indicators		
Lifestyle effects	−2.1	−1.39
Subjective burden	−0.60	−0.33
Mental health difficulties	−0.60	−0.16
Level of strain	−1.18	−0.41

Table 1.5 shows the outcomes, which were observed over one year, on a range of *quality of life* and *quality of care* indicators for the elderly people. For all of the social and emotional need indicators, except the overall morale indicator, there was a significant positive advantage for those involved in the scheme. They were more likely to have improved in terms of depression, loneliness, satisfaction with life, their level of social activity and perception of their capacity to cope. In terms of quality of care and need for help with daily living, reductions of need were consistently significantly greater for those in the scheme than for the comparison group.

Carers' problems of lifestyle – factors such as effects on domestic routine and social activities, as well as strain, expressed burden and mental health problems – were significantly reduced compared with those receiving existing services.

Table 1.6 shows the average annual costs per case incurred by the social services department, the NHS and society as a whole. There was no significant difference between the community care scheme and standard provision. However, irrespective of whether the client received the scheme or standard provision, the health service costs were lower in the inner city, due to the lower utilization of acute hospital beds.

Table 1.6: *Costs for Different Parties Over One Year – Gateshead*

GATESHEAD (1981 PRICES)	Case-Management (Scheme) £s	Control Group £s
SOCIAL CARE		
Social Services Department (Revenue net cost)		
Non inner city	1609	1798
Inner city	2008	1535
National Health Service (Assuming 5% capital allowance)		
Non inner city	1798	1588
Inner city	1505	483
Social Opportunity Cost (capital element discounted at 5%)		
Non inner city	5220	5203
Inner city	5333	3847
HEALTH AND SOCIAL CARE		
Case-Management Team	1570	–
Other Social Services Department (Revenue net cost)	606	1899
Other National Health Service (Assuming 5% capital allowance)	1162	1584
Case-Management Team, SSD and NHS	3338	3483
Social Opportunity Cost (capital elements discounted at 5%)	5159	5070

CASE-MANAGEMENT IN PRIMARY HEALTH CARE

Additional funds were made available to add to the existing team of three social workers, a part-time doctor, a full-time nurse and a part-time physiotherapist with a flexible budget split equally between health and social services. This case-management service was designed to focus upon the most frail of the population, on the margins of institutional care. It was based around a large group practice, and all patients receiving the service were patients of this group of GPs. The pattern of accountability developed for this multi-agency scheme is shown in Figure 1.1.

Figure 1.1: *Accountability in the Health and Social Care Scheme*

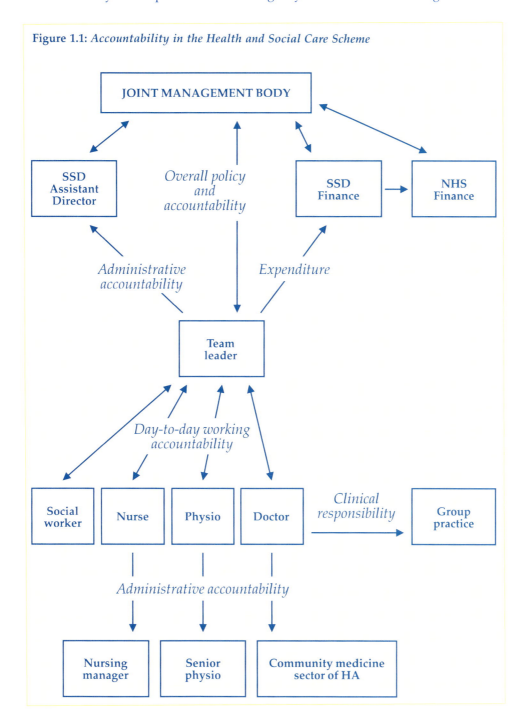

Since this was a pilot scheme with a relatively small number of cases, the only outcome data available relate to destination for a small sample of matched cases (28). After twelve months, 62 per cent of those receiving the case-management service remained at home compared with only 21 per cent receiving the usual services – a similar result to the earlier findings (table 1.4). There was a marked reduction in admissions to institutional care, and those people who died were able to do so within their own homes. As in the social care scheme, there was no significant difference in costs for the case-management approach compared with the existing provision of services to similar cases (table 1.6).

Researcher

Dr David Challis

Personal Social Services Research Unit, University of Kent, Cornwallis Building, Canterbury, Kent CT2 7NF. (0227 764000; FAX 0227 764327)

Publications

Bowns, I., Challis, D., and Tong, M. S. (1991) 'Case Finding in Elderly People: validation of a postal questionnaire', *British Journal of General Practice*, **41**: 100–104.

Challis, D., Chessum, R., Chesterman, J., Luckett, R., and Traske, K. (1990) *Case Management in Social and Health Care*, University of Kent, Personal Social Services Research Unit.

Challis, D., Chessum, R., Chesterman, J., Luckett, R., and Traske, K. (1992) 'Case Management in Health and Social Care', in Lackzo, F., and Victor, C. (eds), *Social Policy and Older People*, Aldershot, Avebury/Gower.

Challis, D., Chessum, R., Chesterman, J., and Woods, R. (1988) 'Community Care for the Frail Elderly: An Urban Experiment', *British Journal of Social Work*, **18**, (Supplement): 13–42.

Challis, D., Chessum, R., Chesterman, J., and Woods, R. (1988) 'Community Care for the Frail Elderly: An Urban Experiment', in Bayens, J. P. (ed.), *Gérontologie et Gériatrie*, Leuven, Belgium, Société Belge de Gérontologie et Gériatrie, ACCO.

Challis, D., Chessum, R., and Luckett, R. (1986) 'Long Term Care for the elderly: Evaluation of the Kent Community Care and related schemes', in Murphy, E. (ed.), *Home or Away*, London, NUPRD/Guy's Hospital, 9–32.

Challis, D., Chessum, R., and Luckett, R. (1983) 'A new life at home', *Community Care*, March, 21–23, 24.

Darlington Community Care Project

CASE-MANAGEMENT IN GERIATRIC CARE

Costs
Outcomes
Carers

The project in Darlington was planned to provide home-care to physically frail elderly people who would otherwise require long-stay hospital care. The project sought to extend the case-management approach used in Kent and Gateshead into a geriatric multi-disciplinary team, using multi-purpose care-workers (home-care assistants) to reduce overlap between personnel. The project team, employed by the social services department, consisted of a project manager, three service managers whose role was to act as case managers, and a team of home-care assistants. The service managers had to cost the service they provided to clients, working to an average budget of two-thirds of the cost of a long-stay hospital bed. The case managers were members of the geriatric multi-disciplinary team, through which all referrals were directed.

The Service in Practice

One hundred and one elderly people with an average age of 80 years, two-thirds of whom were female, were discharged from hospital to the project. Over 90 per cent had been in hospital for two years or less. The most common cause of impairment was stroke, which afflicted over one-third of the clients. Most clients had severe mobility and self-care problems, and about two-thirds experienced problems in maintaining continence. Depression or anxiety appeared to affect the majority of the group and nearly one-third suffered from confusion. On the basis of the Behaviour Rating Scale from the Clifton Assessment Procedures for the Elderly, the project clients were similar to patients in an acute medical ward.

Clients who were to receive the service were assessed by the geriatric multi-disciplinary team, comprising medical staff, hospital and community nursing staff, social workers, paramedical staff and the service managers from the project. The service managers coordinated the assessments of the elderly persons from the different professionals in the multi-disciplinary team, and took responsibility for assessing the family and the potential support network. In about half the cases, a home visit was undertaken so that the suitability of the elderly person's home environment could be assessed.

Each service manager was allocated a budget for their caseload of about 20 clients. A large percentage of this budget was allocated to home-care assistant time, but resources were also spent on paying for additional services from members of the community; and the input of other health and social services resources was also costed. Home-care assistants were instructed and used by a variety of different professionals, in an attempt to integrate much of the work of several different providers into the activities of one single care-worker. In this way, the functions of a home-help, auxiliary nurse or an aide to an occupational group were combined in one person. The service managers' prime function – in consultation with the multi-disciplinary team – was to develop, coordinate and review regularly a package of care, linking together all the necessary resources from a range of different providers. As well as the tasks of monitoring, liaison and coordination, this role also involved the service manager in providing emotional support and advice to elderly people and their families, complementing the activities of informal carers, as well as supporting the home-care assistants and resolving conflicts in the care network.

Outcomes

The study, also funded by the Joseph Rowntree Foundation, compared individuals receiving services from the project with a similar group of patients identified in long-stay wards of an adjacent health district, which was seen as providing a reasonably similar style of geriatric service. Their informal carers were also interviewed, focusing on the experience of care and degree of burden, and compared with a third group of carers of elderly people receiving the usual range of health and social services while living in the community.

About two-thirds of the experimental group were still in their own homes after six months, and only three people were in institutional care; the remainder had died during the period (table 1.7). After 12 months, over 50 per cent were still at home. Although there was a significantly higher death-rate in the project group after six months, this was not the case at 12 months, after allowing for the higher proportion of project clients who were terminally ill. Over the first six months (182 possible days), project clients were at home for an average of 137 days, and the number of days in any form of institutional care was very small.

Table 1.7: *Destinational Outcomes at 6 and 12 Months – Darlington*

Location	Project Group		Control Group	
	6 months	12 months	6 months	12 months
	%	%	%	%
At home	66	56	12	9
Institutional care	3	4	78	60
Dead	31	40	11	31
No. of cases	101	101	113	113

The effects of the project were measured by examining the differences between interview data collected before hospital discharge and six months after discharge, and equivalent measures were derived for the control population. Results in relation to *indicators of subjective well-being* are shown in table 1.8. For the elderly people involved in the project, there was a significant improvement in overall morale and some improvement in satisfaction with their current life situation, as well as a reduction in depression and apathy, compared with the control group. In terms of more *practical indicators of quality of care*, the project clients experienced a significantly reduced need for additional care, and participated in significantly more social activities compared with the long-stay patients.

Carers of project clients were compared with two other groups: carers of elderly people who attended the day hospital in Darlington but otherwise received traditional support at home, and carers of elderly people in long-stay hospital care who were part of the client control group. Project carers carried out significantly fewer care tasks than other carers, experienced less distress about the elderly person's behaviour and about the restrictions upon themselves and their household, and suffered less overall psychological stress.

Table 1.8: *Client Well-Being: Mean Change Scores Over Six Months – Darlington*

	Project Group	Control Group	Significance Level
Subjective Well-Being			
General satisfaction	0.79	0.08	0.056
Satisfaction with life development	0.18	0.10	ns
Morale	1.74	0.21	0.037
Depression	−2.88	−1.05	<0.01
No. of cases (minimum)	41	72	
Behavioural indicators (CAPE BRS)			
Physical disability	0.19	0.17	ns
Apathy	−0.62	0.12	0.014
Communication difficulties	0.07	0.11	ns
Social disturbance	0.60	0.09	ns
BRS total score	0.33	0.56	ns
No. of cases	66	99	
Quality-of-Care Indicators			
Need for improvement in level of care	−4.94	−0.22	<0.001
Social activity level	6.48	2.08	0.011
No. of cases (minimum)	42	76	

Table 1.9 indicates the *costs of care* over a six-month period. Two different figures are given for NHS costs since long-stay beds for elderly people in Darlington were mainly provided in an acute hospital; elsewhere, beds would be in a lower-cost setting, reflected in the second cost estimate which is based on the costs of the control-group hospital. Even using the lower unit cost for hospital care – the most conservative assumption – there was an apparent cost advantage to the main agencies from the project. Social opportunity cost figures, also using the lower unit cost for hospital care, indicated a significant cost advantage to the project.

Table 1.9: *Costs for Different Parties, 1986–87 Prices – Darlington*

	Project Cases		Control Cases	
	Over 6 months £	Per week alive £	Over 6 months £	Per week alive £
Community Care Project	2850	143	–	–
Other SSD (revenue net cost)	30	1	115	4
Other NHS (5% capital allowance)				
1. DMH base	870	51	9838	398
2. Geriatric base	659	39	6205	251
Total Agency Cost				
1. DMH base	3750	195	9953	402
2. Geriatric base	3539	183	6320	255
Total Social Opportunity Cost				
1. DMH base	4977	254	10493	424
2. Geriatric base	4766	242	6859	277

Notes:
1. Long-stay hospital costs at Darlington Memorial Hospital level.
2. Long-stay hospital costs at geriatric hospital level.

Researcher

Dr David Challis

Personal Social Services Research Unit, University of Kent, Cornwallis Building, Canterbury, Kent CT2 7NF. (0227 764000; FAX 0227 764327)

Publications

Challis, D., Darton, R., Johnson, L., and Stone, M. (1988) 'One Face of Care', *Social Work Today*, 4th August, **19**: 12–14.

Challis, D., Darton, R., Johnson, L., and Stone, M. (1988) 'Services, Resource Managment and the Integration of Health and Social Care in the Darlington Project for Elderly People', in Cambridge, P., and Knapp, M. (eds), *Demonstrating Successful Care in the Community*, Personal Social Services Research Unit, University of Kent at Canterbury, 41–46.

Challis, D., Darton, R., Johnson, L., Stone, M., and Traske, K. (1990) 'Supporting Frail Elderly People at Home: The Darlington Community Care Project', *Social Care Research Findings*, Joseph Rowntree Memorial Trust, 7th June.

Challis, D., Darton, R., Johnson, L., Stone, M., and Traske, K. (1991) 'An Evaluation of an Alternative to Long Stay Care for Frail Elderly Patients: Part I: The Model of Care', *Age and Ageing*, **20**: 236–244.

Challis, D., Darton, R., Johnson, M., Stone, M., and Traske, K. (1991) 'An Evaluation of an Alternative to Long Stay Hospital Care for Frail Elderly Patients: Part II: Costs and Effectiveness', *Age and Ageing*, **20**: 245–254.

Challis, D., Darton, R., Johnson, L., Stone, M., Traske, K., and Wall, B. (1989) *Supporting Frail Elderly People at Home*, Personal Social Services Research Unit, University of Kent at Canterbury.

Lewisham Case-Management Scheme – Preliminary Report

CASE-MANAGEMENT IN PSYCHOGERIATRIC CARE

The Lewisham Case-Management Scheme involves the establishment and evaluation of a model of case-management based on the principles of the original Kent Community Care Scheme, which was initiated in Thanet in the late 1970s and developed in Gateshead and Darlington. These schemes have involved the decentralization of control of resources to frontline social workers acting as case managers, so that they can devise more flexible and appropriate packages of care to meet the needs of very vulnerable elderly people. The Lewisham project is unique inasmuch as it focuses on providing care to people with dementia living in their own homes, and their carers; and the service is based in an established multi-disciplinary and multi-agency community mental health team for the elderly.

Dementia
'Key carer'
Multi-disciplinary teams

The Service in Practice

This case-management scheme is designed to provide an effective long-term care component to the work of one of the mental health teams. The teams provide an assessment, treatment, rehabilitation and support service to elderly people with mental health problems living in the catchment area, and have developed a key-worker system to ensure follow up and allow constructive involvement of all members of the team in an overall treatment plan. The team approach is designed to improve case-finding through an open referral policy, and through the range of resources available, the team is able to undertake detailed assessments of need. However, it is often less successful in supporting clients with long-term care needs, since much of the time of team members is taken up with the demands of new referrals and initial assessments, involving acute episodes and short-term interventions. Clients with long-term care needs, in particular those with dementia, are in need of very flexible and individually-focused care services, often requiring extra resources, which take time and financial flexibility to create and sustain.

The objective of the new scheme in Lewisham is to examine whether a sub-group concentrating on long-term care within a multi-disciplinary team can tackle the needs of a long-term care population more effectively, by developing the method of case-management with devolved budgets described above. The case managers are in addition to the existing community care service and are providing extra support and care to a group of clients with whom that service is also often involved, but finds difficult to support.

Two senior social workers, funded by Research and Development in Psychiatry, were appointed as case managers to the scheme in January 1990, employed by Lewisham Social Services Department and based in the Community Team for Mental Health in the Elderly. Administratively, the case managers are part of the hospital social work team, but clinically, they are very much part of the Community Team, with a clearly-defined role which allows them to carry out their long-term case-management function while drawing on the specialist resources in the team.

The case managers are responsible for the long-term support of clients accepted on to the scheme. Because of the frail nature and long-term needs of elderly people with dementia, case managers were expected to deal with a limited caseload of around 20 active cases each, and this has been found to be the limit of other community care projects with frail populations of elderly people. All cases were expected to come to the case managers via the Community Team, after assessment and diagnosis. However, some cases have come directly to the scheme, as its existence has become known.

The scheme is still in progress and early analysis indicates that nearly all cases were women over the age of 75 and suffering from severe cognitive impairment. Nearly all had informal carers, most of whom were experiencing marked stress: less than half of these lived with the elderly person. As in other schemes, case managers in Lewisham have used their budget to recruit paid helpers as a means of providing more individualized care, in addition to deploying existing services. A core group of full-time helpers is currently being recruited to meet the need of people with dementia, particularly those living alone, for a 'key carer'. Experience has shown that these key helpers can act almost as the eyes, ears and mind of a severely impaired person.

Outcomes

The analysis of the effectiveness of the scheme will involve a comparison of the experience of elderly people and their carers supported by the case-management scheme with that of people receiving the usual range of services in the locality.

The study is still in progress, but it is possible to make some preliminary comments. Of the first 20 cases supported by the scheme, half were discharged from hospital or saved from imminent admission as a result of the presence of the scheme. Secondly, there are two organizational findings, which are consistent with the evidence of other case-management schemes:

1. for a case-management scheme involving devolved budgets to work most efficiently, the provision of effective management and administrative support is needed to ensure that individual case managers are able to spend most of their time on activities at the client level; and
2. in supporting elderly people with dementia in the absence of a live-in carer, the role of the 'key carer', organized and supported by the case manager, can be crucial.

Researcher

Dr David Challis

Personal Social Services Research Unit, University of Kent, Cornwallis Building, Canterbury, Kent CT2 7NF. (0227 764000; FAX 0227 764327)

Costs and Welfare Outcomes of Case-Managed Community Care for the Frail Elderly in Two Routine Programmes

- These contrasting schemes mark a stage in the development of community care for the elderly in Kent from a pilot project in a small district (Thanet) to part of mainstream services throughout the county.
- They were the first community care schemes evaluated by the PSSRU not to involve a substantial contribution from the Unit in initiating and maintaining the schemes, and therefore indicate what might be possible when a local authority sets up a scheme with a minimum of outside help.
- Using a quasi-experimental design, elderly people supported by the scheme were assessed by an evaluator just before community care intervention and a year later to obtain information on their disabilities and physical/mental health, social and housing circumstances, quality of life and quality of care received, and how these all changed over the year. Similar interviews were conducted on a matched control group of elderly people receiving standard services. Annual costs were determined for each group.
- Analysis of the information allowed the impact of the scheme on the quality of life of the elderly people to be judged, and its dependence on costs.

Quality of life
Costs
Carers

Some Basic Characteristics of Sheppey and Tonbridge

	Sheppey	Tonbridge
Situation	An island on the North Kent Coast	A town in the heart of West Kent
Population	30,000	40,000
Proportion aged 75 or over	6.3%	5.7%
Employment	Industrialized, with steel works, docklands and chemical laboratories	Some light industry though much of the working population commutes to London
Unemployment	High (13%)	Low (6%)
Proportion in partly skilled/ unskilled occupations	37%	17%
Housing	A high proportion of owner-occupied housing in both areas, much of it Victorian and sometimes lacking modern facilities such as an indoor WC, bathroom, adequate heating or easy-to-manage steps or staircase.	

Table 1.10: *Capacity of the Community Care Schemes to Maintain Frail Elderly People at Home*

Location of matched cases after one year	Sheppey		Tonbridge	
	Community Care	Comparison Group	Community Care	Comparison Group
	%	%	%	%
Own home	62	44	75	60
Local authority residential care	16	13	4	9
Private residential care	–	9	4	9
Hospital care	3	6	4	9
Died	16	28	13	13
Moved away	3	–	–	–
Total number of cases	32	32	23	23

Thus:

(1) Community Care in each area allowed a greater proportion of elderly to remain at home after 12 months than a similar group receiving standard services.

(2) This reduced the numbers being admitted to institutional care.

(3) In Sheppey there was also evidence that the scheme may have played a part in reducing the proportion of elderly dying within the year.

Table 1.11: *Impact of the Schemes on the Quality of Life and Quality of Care of Elderly People and their Informal Carers*

	Significance of improvement in community care group compared with comparison group	
	Sheppey	Tonbridge
A) Social/emotional needs		
Felt capacity to cope	0.001	ns*
Anxiety	0.001	ns
Depressed mood	<0.01	0.06
Dissatisfaction with life development	ns	0.07
B) Care needs		
Need for extra help — rising and retiring	<0.01	<0.01
— daily housework	<0.01	<0.001
— weekly housework	0.08	<0.05
Reliability of help	<0.001	ns
Need for extra services	<0.001	<0.05
No. of severe life events within past year	0.09	ns
Social resource impairment	<0.001	<0.001
C) Health needs		
Activities of daily living impairment rating	0.1	0.07
General health problem index	0.1	ns
Risk of falling	<0.05	ns
Number of cases — community care	30	24
— comparison group	35	27
D) Needs of informal carers		
Backstrain through lifting	Samples	<0.05
Expressed burden	too small	0.08
No. of cases with informal carer — community care	4	9
— comparison group	17	15

*ns=Not significant (>.05)

Table 1.12: *The Costs of the Scheme*

Cost account	Cost £[a]					
	Sheppey			Tonbridge		
	Community Care	Comparison Group	Significance level, p	Community Care	Comparison Group	Significance level, p
A) Annual Costs						
SSD net revenue cost	2059	911	<0.001	1376	958	0.10
NHS opportunity cost[b]	844	1610	0.06	648	1967	0.05
Combined opportunity cost[b] to SSD and NHS	3185	2830	ns	2150	3080	ns
Private residential care	0	254	0.06	179	165	ns
Informal carers	25	47	ns	104	92	ns
B) Weekly Costs						
SSD net revenue cost	41.63	18.56	<0.001	27.33	19.69	ns
NHS opportunity cost	19.20	44.28	<0.05	12.69	41.72	<0.05
Combined opportunity cost to SSD and NHS	66.34	69.07	ns	42.59	64.55	0.08
Private residential care	0.00	4.94	0.06	3.52	3.17	ns
Informal carers	0.63	0.94	ns	2.02	1.77	ns
Number of cases	32	32		23	23	

[a]All costs apply to values in 1982–83.

[b]Includes estimated capital cost discounted at 5%, assuming upgrading of hospital building or purchase of new residential home.

Although the annual combined cost to the social service department and National Health Service shows no significant difference between groups in either area, the social services costs taken alone are very significantly greater for community care cases in Sheppey, the significance level in Tonbridge being 0.1. At the same time, costs to the National Health Service are significantly reduced. This reflects a shift in the bulk of the financial provision from the social services department to the National Health Service as a result of reduced expenditure on acute and long-stay hospital care.

CONCLUSIONS

In the absence of any substantial outside support from the PSSRU, it was still possible for the principal aims of the scheme to be met in the contrasting areas of Sheppey and Tonbridge.

- The frail elderly were enabled to spend longer at home, with fewer admissions to long-term institutional care.
- Many aspects of quality of life, quality of care and health status of the elderly people supported by the scheme and their informal carers improved significantly over the year, when compared with a similar group receiving standard services.
- These improvements were achieved at no significant extra combined cost to the social services department and National Health Service. Moreover, in Tonbridge the average weekly combined cost was reduced to a degree which was almost significant (p=0.08).

Researchers

John Chesterman, Bleddyn Davies and David Challis

Personal Social Services Research Unit, University of Kent, Cornwallis Building, Canterbury, Kent CT2 7NF. (0227 764000; FAX 0227 764327)

Resources, Needs and Outcomes in Community Social Services for the Elderly

The aims of the project were to:

Coordination
Targeting

DESCRIBE *who* gets how much of what service, where, and at what costs, and with what effects, among recipients of community-based social services.

Definitions

'who'
— degree and nature of disability
— degree of informal support, and stress on principal informal carers
— material living conditions

'how much, of what service'
— home-help and home-care
— home-delivered meals
— day-care
— social work support
— community nursing

'where'
— differences between 12 areas in ten authorities in England and Wales

'costs'
— opportunity cost to the social services departments (SSDs) or NHS

'with what effects'
— outcomes for users and carers
— costs to users, carers, SSDs, NHS

EXPLAIN the patterns from evidence based on observation; interviews with field personnel and managers; extensive interviews with users and their principal informal carers at their first receipt of services, and six months later.

EVALUATE the patterns, developing from the evidence arguments about equity and efficiency in the provision of care and the use of public funds.

SUGGEST ways of improving equity and efficiency, and develop arguments about how to improve equity and efficiency in the use of publicly-funded resources.

RESULTS

This summary of results focuses on issues of targeting, and the effects of resource variation on outcomes.

Targeting

Unmet need. The proportion of people with the risk characteristics associated with priority need in the mid-1980s, who were actually receiving services, was lower than the proportion of recipients who did not have these risk factors. In other words, persons with unmet needs appeared to exceed the number of recipients who were *not* in priority need. However, new policies make the targeting criteria of the early 1980s inappropriate. These new policies aim to concentrate resources on the most needy; give 'higher priority to the practical support of carers'; 'develop services to enable people to live in their own homes wherever feasible and sensible'; and ensure payment 'of what they can reasonably afford towards their costs' by users.

Consistency and bias in response to needs. The responsiveness to need of amounts consumed was found to be greater and more consistent than some policy critiques of the period had suggested. Responsiveness seemed in most respects *not* to vary between areas. However, the results suggested bias against the support of informal carers, and more variation between areas in responsiveness to the needs of users *living with others* than to the needs of persons living alone. They also suggested that the consistency of response could be increased.

Interdependence of health and social care needs. The analysis of costs confirmed the importance of a group of heavy users of health and social services, and the lack of coordination of the two sets of services. There is a great and – to some extent – predictable variation in expected lifetime costs for the social services. This should become a more important factor in care planning in the new social services system, with better case-management of potentially more expensive cases, and the consolidation of financial responsibility for them in the SSD.

Effect of charge levels on use. The price of a home-help to the user did not in general affect use. The proportion of expenditure recovered by charges varied according to the proportion of the relevant age-group which was at risk of low income, and the political complexion of the Council.

Analysis has found very different predictors for:

A. *high current need*

> a high benefit–cost ratio, for expensive interventions with only short-term impacts;

and

B. *high reducible risk*

> a high ratio of benefits to costs, with high spending to reduce deterioration and likelihood of admission.

A shift in policy priorities to reducing risk of admission will involve considerable retargeting. B also demands the prediction of lifetime costs and benefits of varying the levels of community-based care. Estimates and predictions of lifetime costs of home-care and the total of home and residential care suggest great variations, and that the predictors depend on factors other than those which create high current dependency.

Costs to principal carers and costs to the social care agencies. The research developed a new method of estimating costs to carers. Applying this method confirms that in the UK, as in some other countries, the greater the level of dependency of the user, the higher the proportion of the overall costs of care borne by the principal carer.

Effects of Increasing Service Inputs on Outcomes

Effects on probability of admission. We failed to find that higher service inputs reduced the probability: there were no effects on the number of days spent in community-based care, and the number of days in residential institutions receiving long-term care.

Effects on user and carer morale were limited to some groups only; there were few effects on felt risks and unmet needs, but larger effects on workers' views about problems tackled. However, there were general effects on clients' perceptions of the risk of continuing to live in the community, clients' perceptions of their capacity to carry out tasks of daily living, field personnel's perception of the impact of the services, and principal carers' perceptions of the difficulties of caring.

These results suggest that avoiding inappropriate and unwanted admissions to institutions for long-term care would require improvements in the *impact of additional services* as well as *changes in the selection of clients*.

Effects on short-term outcomes. Higher service levels are associated with users' perceptions of their value, particularly in the case of the home-help/care service.

The costs of achieving improved outcomes of varying kinds were estimated, as well as the outcomes of a range of case-mixes.

CONCLUSION

It is easier to improve the impact of resources, for more complex cases, by better coordination of inputs than by attempting to make one service have high impacts for every kind of outcome and at all levels of input. The results of the project argue for the development of a logic for fitting local care-management arrangements and policies to dependent and carer circumstances, as well as the characteristics of the area system. The logic is based on the analysis of international evidence about the effectiveness of different arrangements.

Researcher

Professor Bleddyn Davies

Personal Social Services Research Unit, University of Kent, Cornwallis Building, Canterbury, Kent CT2 7NF (0227 764000 x 7587)

Publications

Bebbington, A., and Charnley, H. (1990) 'Community care for the elderly: Rhetoric and reality', *British Journal of Social Work*, **20**: 409–432.

Bebbington, A., Charnley, H., Davies, B., Ferlie, E., Hughes, M., and Twigg, J. (1986) 'The Domiciliary Care Project: Meeting the needs of the elderly. Interim Report', University of Kent, Canterbury, PSSRU Discussion paper 456.

Charnley, H., Baines, B., Bebbington, A., Davies, B., Lawson, R., Netten, A., and Whitley, A. (1989) 'Managing to manage in a post-Griffiths world: Resources, targeting and effectiveness in community care for elderly people', in *Social Services Insight*, 25.10.89 as 'Deciding one's destiny at the drawing board', University of Kent, Canterbury, PSSRU Discussion paper 670.

Davies, B. (1987) 'Allocation of services in England: Facts and myths about the equity and efficiency of social care services', *Revue d'épidémiologie et de santé publique*, June, **35**: 17–26.

Davies, B. (1987) 'Equity and efficiency in community care: supply and financing in an age of fiscal austerity', *Ageing and Society*, **7**, 2: 161–74.

Davies, B. (1987) 'New managerialist argument and the supply and financing of care', in di Gregario, S. (ed.), *Social gerontology: New directions*, Beckenham, Kent, Croom Helm, 75–89.

Davies, B. (1988) 'Making a reality of community care: a critique of the Audit Commission Report', *British Journal of Social Work Supplement*, **18**: 173–188.

Davies, B. (1989) 'Les Besoins en Soins: leur couverture et leur coût en établissement ou à domicile', *Gérontologie et Société*, **47**: 54–70.

Davies, B. (1990) 'Community care of the elderly: On the evaluation of strategic innovations and change', in Kraan, R., *et al.*, *Significant innovations in the community care of elderly people: An analysis of policy and schemes in England and Wales, the Netherlands, and Sweden*, Frankfurt, Campus/Westview, 203–227.

Davies, B. (1992) 'On resources, needs and outcomes: The nature of the challenge', in Morgan, K. (ed.), *Gerontology: Responding to an ageing society*, London, Jessica Kingsley.

Davies, B., Darton, R., and Goddard, M. (1987) 'The effects of alternative targeting criteria and demand levels for the opportunity costs to the SSD of care in local authority homes', University of Kent, Canterbury, PSSRU Discussion paper 484.

Lawson, R., and Davies, B. (1991) 'The home help service in England and Wales', in Jamieson, A. (ed.), *Home care for older people in Europe: A comparison of policies and practices*, Oxford, Oxford University Press, 63–98.

Netten, A., and Davies, B. (1991) 'The social production of welfare and the consumption of social services', *Journal of Public Policy*, **10**: 331–347.

Quine, L., and Charnley, H. (1987) 'Evaluating the malaise inventory as a measure of stress in carers of mentally handicapped children and elderly people', in Twigg, J. (ed.), *Evaluating support to informal carers*, Social Policy Research Unit, University of York. University of Kent, Canterbury, PSSRU Discussion paper 551.

Twigg, J. (1986) 'Carers: Models of carers: How do social care agencies conceptualise their relationship with informal carers', *Journal of Social Policy*, **18**: 53–67.

The Care in the Community Demonstration Programme

The Care in the Community demonstration programme was funded by the DHSS between 1984 and 1989 to explore different ways of moving long-stay residents and resources from hospital to the community. Grants totalling £25 million (at today's prices) were made over three years to 28 pilot projects supporting people with mental health problems (8 projects), learning disabilities (11), adolescents with multiple disabilities (1), physically disabled adults (1), elderly people with mental health problems (4), and elderly physically frail people (3). The PSSRU monitored and evaluated the programme.

Organizing services

PRINCIPLES AND PRACTICES

Service philosophies were based in care practices developed locally or imported from outside. Care-management, normalization, and a commitment to user involvement were among the widely-adopted principles. Implementing normalization sometimes proved difficult, particularly if the implementation was badly conceived, inflexibly applied, or run contrary to the expressed preferences of clients. Allowing clients to take risks and make the 'wrong choices' had to be balanced against public expectations of professional accountability. If some of the underlying principles of care proved unworkable or at least disappointing in implementation, they nevertheless encouraged staff to strive to achieve the best for clients, and challenged the narrow preconceptions of others.

If projects were to put their various care principles into practice, they needed adequate funding, some influence over the resources of provider agencies, and willingness at user and management levels to link service responses to needs. In these respects, they resembled all community care services. But they were cushioned against some difficulties by the relatively generous DHSS grants, and the high degree of financial and operational independence which protected funding offered. The funds provided help with capital outlays – in effect, double funding for the period when hospital cost savings were negligible – and usually meant that resources could be established in the community before clients left hospital. The conditions of central funding ensured that joint liaison and planning were at least attempted, and they generally succeeded. Another recommendation – the use of some form of care-management – helped to raise the 'target efficiency' of community care.

Finances. The crucial significance of social security payments in the successful operation of projects was clear from the evaluation, and was consistent with other evidence. There was, for example, a thin dividing line between flexibility and instability; social security funds reduce the constraints often imposed by agency budgets, but are themselves subject to unexpected changes of value and eligibility.

A second difficulty was that the income from benefits was not always adequate to provide desired standards of care, let alone compensate for the lack of social contacts, employment opportunities and personal belongings which often accompany former hospital residents. However, by introducing care-managment, most projects were able to help clients claim their benefit entitlements. Thirdly, although the programme reduced the disincentives to providing appropriate care by subsidizing costs from central grants, the benefits system still made it financially more attractive to offer residential rather than domiciliary care.

Similar questions arose in relation to dowries, double-running costs and the protection of funding. Can *future arrangements* allow for the sort of practice which took place within the programme with such success? Pilot projects enjoyed protected funding for three years, with mainstream health or social services funding promised thereafter.

Staffing. Through lack of experience, poor information, or simply over-optimistic assumptions, many projects underestimated community support needs. As a result, some of them were left with inadequate numbers or types of staff, and inadequate funds to meet the costs of overtime, promotions and pay settlements. These difficulties were in addition to the considerable and continuing demands which community care makes on staff. If these demands are to be met, training and support must be taken seriously.

Some community care arrangements need skills different from those conventionally expected of hospital staff. They also need flexibility in their deployment. The challenge, therefore, is to ensure that training strategies produce the right mix of abilities, the right blend between 'therapeutic' and 'basic' skills, and the right balance between professional abilities and simple caring attitudes. In the multi-agency community care systems envisaged by the 1990 Act, conventional professional needs and boundaries may not survive.

Some of the staffing difficulties in the programme were undoubtedly the result of the initiative being seen by some people as short-term. Similar difficulties of recruitment and retention may reappear in the new mixed economy, if the links between purchasers and providers are dominated by comparatively short contracts.

Accommodation and services. Between them, the projects offered many different accommodation and day-support arrangements, although most encountered local constraints. For example, while the range of accommodation included residential homes, sheltered housing facilities, hostels, staffed group homes, core and cluster networks, supported lodgings, home-care (foster) placements and independent living, only a handful of projects were able to offer clients this wide a choice. Most people were offered more choice than they had come to expect in hospital; but this does not mean that one of the core aims of the 1989 White Paper – enhanced user choice – had been achieved. The availability of the right kind of housing proved to be a major constraint.

Accommodation plans and practices were often strongly influenced by a desire to emphasize the contrast with hospital. Even if normalization was not an overt objective, community living arrangements were often designed to provide a domestic, integrated and 'ordinary' setting. There were, as a result, large differences between the physical and social environments of the hospital wards that clients had left and the community placements to which they moved. By every criterion we used, accommodation in the community was more 'normal' and less institutional than hospital.

There were also better standards of day-care, support and leisure provision. Difficulties arose in achieving the degree of community integration and participation that many projects sought, especially in relation to education services and employment. Integration in the community is often a matter of chance – the availability of the right kind of housing in the right area, vacancies in adult education classes, a buoyant labour market – so that community care agencies can often have only limited influence. But this should not divert attention from the difficulties experienced by many projects in overcoming inertia and obstructive attitudes. Projects with independent workers acting as *welfare entrepreneurs* probably had greater success in overcoming these problems.

SERVICE ORGANIZATION

The service systems set in place within the programme share many features with the likely future organization of community care. Some kind of care-management was used, occasionally with devolved budgets. There was widespread improvement of joint-working relations, and occasionally joint purchasing. When projects employed what might now be called community care brokers, they were beginning to behave like enabling agents within a quasi-market.

Care-management. There had been care-management experiments in Britain before the launch of the programme, but these were confined to services for elderly people. The programme offered a chance to examine this kind of organization in new fields. Because the programme was not prescriptive, a variety of styles emerged, each giving different emphasis to the five core tasks of case-finding and referral, assessment and selection, care-planning, monitoring, and case-closure. Devolution of responsibility for decision-making is central to the community care changes introduced by the 1990 Act. The majority view from the projects was that benefits flow from greater autonomy in decision-making, policy formulation and budgetary control.

Joint working. The programme contained five models of joint working between health and social services authorities: the unitary agency, semi-independent agency, lead agency, joint agency, and multi-agency models. Joint working was welcomed by most projects as an opportunity to improve local inter-agency cooperation. Even within the lead agency model, it was essential to coordinate planning and service monitoring. The voluntary sector was involved rather less in community care planning than many would have wished, and the private sector was only really involved as a provider of residential care.

Some familiar organizational issues arose. Clarity of roles and responsibilities – for example, through joint documents, strategies, transfer agreements and personnel policies – helped avoid inter-agency and purchaser-provider conflicts. Existing joint-planning machinery often proved useful for arbitration, advice and steering. Reorganization – where it occurred in social services departments or the health service – proved demoralizing and distracting. Geographical isolation required special liaison to prevent services becoming managerially remote. Devolved responsibilities and budgets helped to promote accountability and flexibility, and made services more responsive to individual needs and local circumstances. Case review was better conducted outside residential or day-care settings, and on an integrated basis. Access to policy-making processes and to information on finance and budgeting helped generate positive working attitudes and staff commitment.

A mixed economy. The successful establishment of a mixed economy of provision and management owed more to chance and tradition than to the intentions and structures of the demonstration programme. Success often seemed to depend mainly on the voluntary sector's access to information, its energies and its contacts. A number of obstacles block the path to a more mixed-care economy, even when the political and professional wills exist. Establishing care-management and devolving budgets takes an authority some way towards the enabling role foreseen for authorities in the White Paper; and more than half of the pilot projects illustrated some of the benefits of contracting with voluntary agencies for the provision of certain services.

Service users and outcomes. The people who moved from hospital were likely to need less care support in the community than the 'typical' long-stay hospital resident. Predictably, given a well-targeted community-care system, we found evidence that greater needs as assessed in hospital prior to discharge, and also as assessed in the community some nine months later, were associated with the receipt of more care support and higher costs. Although the clients were on average less 'dependent' than those who remained in hospital, they posed many challenges for agencies and staff. Most suffered from the well-known effects of institutionalization. A majority of the elderly, physically frail clients had lost contact with their families and friends. Almost all clients had under-developed life-skills, and most clients with learning disabilities required special management or support. Most had few personal possessions.

Outcomes. Hospital closure gives rise to obvious fears about the consequences for people discharged into an unfamiliar, potentially hostile community. One of the most important achievements of the programme was, simply, the successful resettlement of a large number of people. The projects established support systems to counter the widely-feared failings of removal from hospital: no one was homeless; no one spent any time in prison or a police cell. Mortality and hospital readmission rates were no higher than would be expected of a general population with these characteristics. *It was the distinctive approach of the programme which provided safeguards and contributed to success.* The common failings of community care are often due to poor resourcing and poor management. The future success of community care will be conditional upon the availability of adequate and pro-tected funding, and upon effective use of those funds through rigorous care-management.

Improvements in quality of life after leaving hospital were very marked for most of the people with **learning disabilities** included in the evaluation. Statistically significant improvements were found along a number of dimensions. The cost of community care was higher than the cost of hospital for more than half the sample; but higher costs bought better quality care and better quality of life. Smaller and more domestic community settings were associated with better client outcomes: in other words, normalization appeared to work. The fundamental policy question suggested by these results is whether local agencies are able or prepared to incur the higher costs of community care in order to reap these obvious benefits.

Clients with **mental health problems** enjoyed many improvements in lifestyle after leaving hospital: some moved to ordinary housing; integration into the community was by no means complete, but was an improvement over hospital. They expressed more positive attitudes, and were exercising more choice than had previously been possible. Low incomes and low levels of staffing nevertheless often severely limited projects' and clients' options. Although there were few noticeable changes in quality of life or clients' characteristics, there were on average no deteriorations, and costs were lower. For this group of people with mental health problems, community care was therefore no lower in quality but significantly lower in cost than hospital. When community care costs rose above the average this tended to reflect greater needs and better client outcomes.

Quality of life in the community for **elderly people** was certainly no worse, and in some respects better, than life in hospital. There was no deterioration in skills and behaviour, nor in satisfaction with activities and social contacts, while client self-reported morale had improved. Clients moved to better physical surroundings, and were given more choice and greater opportunities; community care costs were lower than in hospital. The programme therefore demonstrated the scope for resettling elderly people within the community after long-term residence in hospital.

CONCLUSION

The evidence accumulated from the Care in the Community programme shows that it is possible to organize community care so as to make better use of resources – either spending less than before (elderly people, and those with mental health problems), or spending more but reaping better client outcomes (people with learning disabilities) – and to target services effectively at needs. The ways in which these successes have been achieved resemble some aspects of the new organization of community care envisaged by the 1990 NHS and Community Care Act.

Researcher

Professor Martin Knapp

Personal and Social Services Research Unit, University of Kent, Cornwallis Building, Canterbury, Kent CT2 7NF. (0227 764000)

Unit Costs of Personal Social Services in Inner London – Progress Report

The purpose of the research is to investigate the unit costs of personal social services expenditure in inner London in order to determine why they are higher than elsewhere in England. The research seeks to distinguish cost-raising factors which are beyond the control of local authorities from those which are potentially avoidable, and will provide background information about inner London costs. It will also provide cost evidence relevant to decisions about the provision of residential and domiciliary care.

Costs
Level of Provision
Staffing

Background

Inner London authorities spend much more on social services than do other local authorities – in 1988/9, total gross expenditure *per capita* was three times the average elsewhere in England. There has been concern not only about the equity of this situation but also about the ability of inner London to sustain such a high financial burden.

Ten years ago, the main explanation offered for this differential was the high levels of provision made by inner London authorities. The reasons for these high levels have been heavily researched. Some investigators have focused on the high levels of need and the shortage of low-cost substitutes. Others considered that it was in part the product of local discretion, fuelled by anomalies in the system of local government finance, which caused London authorities to be favoured by the old method of assessing rate support grant used before 1981. This was combined with a relatively low proportion of inner London authorities' income falling to the domestic ratepayer, so that political accountabitility provided little check to increased expenditure. A third type of explanation has focused on differences in efficiency.

Over the last decade, volume growth of social services has been restrained, significantly more so in inner London than elsewhere. At the same time, the unit costs of all services have shown very large increases – the real cost of the main services for children has more than doubled, while over all main services, the average increase is estimated at about 60 per cent[2]. The result is that unit cost differentials have become increasingly significant in explaining variations in expenditure between local authorities; and inner London authorities have always maintained much higher average unit costs.

Table 1.13 shows the differential in 1988/9. The trend appears to have been spreading in that over the last decade, these much-higher-than-average costs have also been appearing among many outer London boroughs.

---

[2] Unit costs throughout this report are based on Department of Environment Revenue Out-turns and Department of Health Activity Statistics.

Table 1.13: *Differential Between Inner London Authorities and the National Average for the Gross Unit Cost of Main Personal Social Services in 1988/9*

Homes for the elderly	28%
Homes for people with learning disabilities	28%
Day-centres for the elderly	28%
Administration (per £ spent)	40%
Social Work (per child in care)	48%
Home-help (per hour)	53%
Day-nurseries	68%
Community homes for children	69%
Boarding-out children	72%
Meals on wheels (per meal)	76%
Adult training/social care centres	77%

Source: Bebbington & Kelly (1991) 'Unit Costs of PSS in Inner London', PSSRU Discussion Paper 757; also 'Trends in Unit Costs', PSSRU Discussion Paper 799.

Methods and Findings

The first stage of the London Unit Costs project has been looking at explanations for the higher unit costs in London based on available statistical evidence. The results so far offer some useful pointers—

- Neither the high volume of provision, nor special local factors affecting needs, are likely to be important cost-raisers in London for adult client-groups, although they are for children.
- The high unit costs do not result from missed opportunities for using low cost substitutes, such as community rather than residential services or private and voluntary sector provision. London authorities have generally been progressive in this respect.
- Although political control affects volume of provision, it does not appear to produce high unit costs.
- Capital costs are not sufficiently great to make much difference.

The most frequently-voiced explanation for the high unit costs in inner London is the high cost of staff, which averages around 35 per cent more per employee, more than double the London-weighting allowance. This is attributed partly to grade drift and partly to the higher turnover and absenteeism in London, and the apparently much higher cost of providing cover. In addition, employee productivity – the ratio of output to staff – is lower in inner London for many services. In its 1987 report, the Audit Commission pointed out low occupancy and capital productivity among residential and day-services in London, although our initial investigations do not confirm this. Whether this low productivity is due to an attempt to provide a higher quality service, to special problems in providing services in London, or to inefficiency, we do not yet know.

Stage two of this project is currently under way. It is investigating unit costs in much greater detail through case studies in 5–6 local authorities, which include both inner London authorities and local authorities in other inner cities, and will be exploring further the issues raised above. Part of the task is to ensure the comparability of the statistical and accounting data which underpin these conclusions – and indeed many of the assumptions that are used in preparing grant assessments.

Researcher

Andrew Bebbington

Personal and Social Services Research Unit, University of Kent, Cornwallis Building, Canterbury, Kent CT2 7NF. (0227 764000; FAX 0227 764327)

Collaboration and Cost-Effectiveness

The Study

Planning
Joint finance
Barriers to
collaboration

This study (undertaken between 1985 and 1989) was designed to investigate one of the most important means of implementing community care – **inter-agency collaboration and joint planning** – and one of the principal policy instruments to facilitate joint planning – **joint finance. Its broad aim was to acquire a detailed understanding of the role, productiveness and inter-relationship of joint planning and joint finance in the changed context following NHS restructuring in 1982 and the Care in the Community initiative**.

The research itself was a collaborative exercise between the Centre for Research in Social Policy (University of Loughborough) and the Centre for Health Economics (CHE, University of York)[3].

This work consisted of four detailed 'core'-site studies and two issue-based studies: (i) of high DHA finance take-up; and (ii) of innovations in joint-management arrangements.

FINDINGS

Joint Finance

Joint finance *had* acted, as intended, as an incentive to collaboration: it was instrumental in the launch of most of the schemes in the joint-management study, and it had produced some significant net additions to local community services and facilities.

There had been generally slow progress in changes in procedures, following on from DHSS guidance on joint finance[4]. Some, such as agreeing funding criteria and establishing timetables for bids, had been improved; but option-appraisal, cost-effectiveness analyses and monitoring procedures remained unsystematic or non-existent.

Joint finance was always dependent for success upon continuing growth in social services budgets: a pre-condition for the successful implementation of community care policies is the alignment of service and resource policies.

Joint Planning

Formal joint-planning machinery remained officer-dominated while Joint Consultative Committees typically were only token bodies. Joint planning also remained an essentially bilateral exercise between health and social services. The

---

[3] For an account of the CHE's part of the project, see page 47.
[4] DHSS (1983) Health Service Development: Care in the Community and Joint Finance, Circular HC(83)6/LAC(83)5, London, DHSS.

involvement of education, housing and voluntary bodies was minimal; partly because the machinery was designed as a bilateral forum and partly because, for voluntary organizations in particular, involvement was restricted by a lack of planning resources.

The most coherent and well-developed joint-planning arrangements were found in areas which had *complex* rather than stable and simple relationships between organizations. In the latter areas, there was greater reliance on informal networks and processes and less on elaborate joint machinery.

Concrete evidence of the benefits of joint planning was limited: there was no evidence of the comprehensive, joint-client-group strategies envisaged when joint planning was first introduced. However, our findings were: first, that such comprehensiveness is unrealistic because planning resources are scarce and need to be deployed selectively; second, that joint planning itself needs to be carefully planned, monitored and adjusted to take account of changing local needs; and third, that planning should be seen as evolutionary and dynamic, with the emphasis on the process itself rather than intermittent, tangible outputs. The beneficial outputs of this process are essentially *intangible*: mutual organizational learning; a clarification of agency and professional differences; an upward spiral of trust; and growing consensus about aims, principles and priorities.

Although there was considerable evidence of partial joint planning at the level of individual services and facilities, the research confirmed that – if judged by the standards of the initial Circulars – there was little or no genuinely joint planning.

Barriers to Inter-Agency Coordination

Structural	• fragmentation of service responsibilities across agency boundaries, within and between sectors; • inter-organizational complexity and non-coterminosity of boundaries.
Procedural	• differences in planning horizons and cycles; • differences in budgetary cycles and procedures.
Financial	• differences in funding mechanisms and bases; • differences in the stocks and flows of financial resources.
Professional	• differences in ideologies and values; • professional self-interest and concern for threats to autonomy and domain; • threats to job security; • conflicting views about clients'/consumers' interests and roles.
Status and Legitimacy	• organizational self-interest and concern for threats to autonomy and domain; • differences in legitimacy between elected and appointed agencies.

The barriers we identified indicate the scale and complexity of the challenge which coordination posed for health and local authorities.

One important caveat to criticisms about the record of collaboration is that performance has not been uniformly poor. Both the Audit Commission and Griffiths observed that examples of successful coordination, although generally on a small scale, could increasingly be found. In our study of innovations in management arrangements, we examined in detail a number of such examples, including projects which appeared to have overcome the barriers and moved beyond the mere rhetoric of joint working.

Our overall finding was that these jointly-managed schemes are inherently fragile, and vulnerable to the organizational pressures that threatened their sustained development. They operate on the periphery of parent bodies and may be viewed as either an administrative inconvenience or a threat to the professional or organizational *status quo*; they may rely too much on mutual trust and altruism; and they may similarly be over-reliant on the personal networks of their original champions.

We identified four key factors which would contribute to the survival and success of these schemes: clarity of purpose; commitment and shared ownership; robust and coherent management arrangements; and organizational learning. Successful collaboration remains a key to implementing the Government's current community care policies. Our research suggests that to succeed there must be both an understanding of the nature of the barriers to coordination and a belief in the possibility of overcoming them.

Researchers

Brian Hardy (Research Fellow); Gerald Wistow (Senior Lecturer in Health and Social Care Management)

Nuffield Institute for Health Services Studies, University of Leeds, Fairbairn House, 71–75 Clarendon Road, Leeds LS2 9PL.

A. Turrell

Business Manager, Queen's University Hospital, Nottingham.

A. L. Webb

Professor of Social Policy, Department of Social Sciences, Loughborough University.

Publications

Reports to DHSS (DH):

Pilot Survey Report (1986)

Hardy, B., Turrell, A., and Wistow, G. (1988) *Innovations in Management Arrangements: Interim Report.*

Hardy, B., Turrell, A., and Wistow, G. (1989) *Innovations in Management Arrangements: Final Report.*

Hardy, B., Turrell, A., and Wistow, G. (1989) *Collaboration and Cost-Effectiveness: Final Report.*

Wistow, G., Hardy, B., and Turrell, A. (1987) *Joint Planning and Joint Finance in Bedfordshire.*

Wistow, G., Hardy, B., and Turrell, A. (1987) *Joint Planning and Joint Finance in Cambridgeshire.*

Wistow, G., Hardy, B., and Turrell, A. (1987) *Cross Financing or a Joint Budget?: DHAs' Use of Joint Finance.*

Wistow, G., Hardy, B., and Turrell, A. (1988) *Joint Planning and Joint Finance in Sunderland*.

Wistow, G., Hardy, B., and Turrell, A. (1988) *Joint Planning and Joint Finance in Calderdale*.

Books:

Hardy, B., Wistow, G., and Turrell, A. (1992) *Innovations in Community Care Management*, Aldershot, Gower.

Wistow, G., and Brooks, T., (1988) *Joint Planning and Joint Management*, RIPA.

Wistow, G., Hardy, B., and Turrell, A. (1990) *Collaboration under Financial Constraint*, Aldershot, Gower.

Chapters:

Wistow, G. (1988) 'Beyond Joint Planning: Managing Community Care', in G. Wistow and T. Brooks (eds), *Joint Planning and Joint Management*, RIPA.

Wistow, G. (1988) 'Health and Local Authority Collaboration: Lessons and Prospects', in G. Wistow and T. Brooks (eds), *Joint Planning and Joint Management*, RIPA.

Wistow, G. (1988) 'Off-loading Responsibilities for Care', in R. Maxwell (ed.), *Reshaping the National Health Service*, Policy Journals and Transaction Books.

Wistow, G. (1989) 'Planning and Collaboration in a Mixed Economy', in *Community Care in a Mixed Economy: Meeting the Challenge*, Nuffield Institute Seminar Series.

Wistow, G., and Hardy, B. (1986) 'Transferring Care: Can Financial Incentives Work?', in A. Harrison and J. Gretton (eds), *Health Care UK 1986*, Policy Journals (an extended version of a paper first published in *Public Money*).

Wistow, G., Hardy, B., and Turrell, A. (1988) 'Community Care and NHS Spending of Joint Finance', in A. Harrison and J. Gretton (eds), *Health Care UK 1988*, Policy Journals.

Articles:

Hardy, B., and Wistow, G. (1989) 'Avoiding the Pitfalls', *Social Services Insight*, **4**, 19: 25–27.

Wistow, G. (1986) 'Keeping it in the Health Service', *Social Services Insight*, **1**, 15: 16–18.

Wistow, G. (1986) 'Caring in the Community', *Finance and Accountancy*, 31 October, 8–10.

Wistow, G. (1987) 'Joint Finance: Promoting a New Balance of Care in England?', *International Journal of Social Psychiatry*, **33**, 2: 83–91.

Wistow, G. (1988) 'Joint Working', *Community Care*, 30 June.

Wistow, G. (1989) 'Joint Planning, Joint Finance and Joint Management', in I. Mocroft (ed.), *Collaboration in Planning and Working*, ARVAC Occasional Paper No 10.

Wistow, G., and Hardy, B. (1991) 'Joint Management in Community Care', *Journal of Management in Medicine*, **5**, 4: 40–48.

Other:

Wistow, G. (1989) 'Joint Planning in Practice', *Involving Voluntary Agencies in Joint Planning*, West Midlands Regional Health Authority.

Wistow, G. (1990) *Community Care Planning: A Review of Past Experience and Future Imperatives*, Community Care Implementation Document 3, DH.

Wistow, G. (1990) Address to 'Making it Happen', Conference (Queen Elizabeth Conference Centre, London). 1. Department of Health and Social Security (1983): *Health Service Development: Care in the Community and Joint Finance*, Circular HC(83)6/LAC(83)5, London, DHSS.

Managing the Mixed Economy of Care

Introduction

This two-year study had two main aims:

- To map actual and intended reductions in the direct provider role of social services departments (SSDs), together with the scale and nature of non-statutory provision and its potential for further development.
- To identify the key elements and principal management tasks of a managing agency role for SSDs.

There were two main research tasks. First, an analysis of available statistics on the balance of provision and funding of social care. Second, a detailed examination of the plans and intentions of a sample of English social services authorities. The latter involved interviews (conducted between December 1990 and April 1991) with Directors and Chairs of Social Services in 24 authorities and with representatives of voluntary organizations, private sector agencies and health authorities.

Study Findings

Enabling and the Mixed Economy

The term 'managing' a mixed economy implies diversity of supply, and a purchasing function capable of specifying requirements in terms of identified need, together with systematic procedures through which an appropriate volume, mix and quality of supply can be purchased and monitored. The evidence from our study is that although some of these components were being developed by the majority of local authorities, very few were developing comprehensive arrangements and seeking to create a market in social care. A common argument was that 'social care is different' and that market mechanisms are inappropriate. However – although concepts like competition, purchasing and market creation had limited appeal – most authorities gave equally little support to maintaining the *status quo*.

Developing the Supply Mix

Although there was virtually universal support for the service principles embodied in the legislation and guidance, there were widespread reservations about this enabling role. These reservations were expressed as a slow, or cautious, development on the one hand and a selective development on the other hand.

Five main reasons were given for the relatively slow development of the mixed economy: the general policy context; reservations about social-care markets; pride in public sector provision; scant potential outside the public sector, and a range of other perceived disincentives and obstacles.

(1) Authorities had other priorities for April 1991 – the deadline for establishing inspection units and complaints procedures – and faced considerable uncertainty: for example, whether the funding changes would be implemented in 1993 and local authorities would continue to have the lead role. There was also a widespread view that a mixed economy of care had existed for many years anyway.

(2) Whilst some authorities thought it premature to prepare market development plans before they had mapped needs and agreed broad service strategies, others simply questioned the idea that they should be 'market making'. The main objection to markets and the primary source of scepticism about the benefits of competition was again that 'social care is different'. This view transcended political boundaries.

(3) Authorities generally acknowledged a tendency towards inflexible and unresponsive public services. However, the majority felt that the public sector had provided good quality public services and should continue to do so.

(4) Authorities generally reported significant supplier-related constraints to the development of a mixed economy: a lack of alternative suppliers; the unwillingness of alternative suppliers; the under-development of alternative suppliers; and the increasing shortage of volunteers.

(5) Among the other disincentives and obstacles contributing to authorities' slow and cautious development were: socio-economic factors (such as labour market changes, and land and property prices); deficiencies in information technologies; certain VAT anomalies; skill shortages within SSDs; and a disjunction between the agendas and timetables of health and local authorities.

Most local authorities expressed a clear preference for working with voluntary agencies rather than the private sector. Three main reasons were given. First, voluntary bodies engender greater trust because their directors or trustees gain no financial benefit if the organization prospers. Second, many voluntary organizations have long track records and good reputations, with management boards often sharing the service philosophies and principles of local authorities. Third, the transaction costs of contracting with voluntary agencies were perceived to be lower than with private agencies.

Most of the interest in diversifying supply concerned the establishment of not-for-profit 'trusts' for residential care of those adult client-groups attracting welfare benefits: with no immediate financial pay-off, day and domiciliary care were rarely mentioned. It was, however, generally agreed that some homes should be retained in local authority control both to provide a benchmark for standards and to ensure that statutory obligations can be fulfilled.

Developing the Purchasing Function

Only a third of authorities in the study had yet to decide how to map need, mainly because they saw this as a priority for 1991/92.

As regards service specifications and contracts, we identified five broad types of authority. Two 'conscientious objectors', which had considered and rejected the arguments for tighter specifications and contracts. Four 'floating voters' had yet explicitly to consider this issue. Five 'new beginners' had decided to use service specifications and contracts but had yet to introduce new arrangements. The largest group of authorities – nine 'incrementalists' – had decided to expand their use of contracts, though carefully and relatively slowly. Finally, three 'proven enthusiasts' had already drawn up service specifications or contractual links for many of their services.

These gradual developments in contracting procedures were largely confined to the voluntary sector: generally, however, examples of tendering are rare.

CONCLUSIONS

A significant shift in attitudes was discernible, at least amongst senior officers and leading members. There is a growing acceptance of an enabling role for local authorities: an acceptance of a reduction in the near-monopoly of public sector provision, and an increasing diversification of supply.

However, local authorities have different views of what the enabling role entails; and this accounts for the wide variations in the ways in which implementation was being approached. There was a widely-held belief that local authorities should remain significant service providers – but of a set of much more tightly-defined services. Many authorities were also reluctant to reduce public sector provision rapidly, because alternative suppliers either do not exist, are not willing, not competent, or are unsuitable by virtue of being profit-motivated.

Our findings suggest both the beginning of cultural change within the personal social services and also that some of the components of the White Paper's enabling model are beginning to be developed. In what is a rapidly changing field, the pace and direction of change can be expected to accelerate.

Researchers

Gerald Wistow and Brian Hardy

Nuffield Institute of Health Services, University of Leeds, Fairbairn House, 71–75 Clarendon Road, Leeds LS2 9PL. (0532 459034; FAX 0532 460899)

Martin Knapp, Julien Forder and Caroline Allen

PSSRU, University of Kent, Cornwallis Building, Canterbury, Kent. (0227 764000; FAX 0227 764327)

Publications

Wistow, G., Knapp, M., Hardy, B., and Allen, C. (1992) 'From providing to enabling: local authorities and the mixed economy of social care', *Public Administration*, **70**, 1 (Spring): 25–45.

Cost-Effectiveness and Collaboration: An Analysis of Joint Finance in Seven non-London Health Authorities

This analysis formed part of a three-year project carried out in collaboration with the Centre for Research in Social Policy at the University of Loughborough[5]. The aim of the project was to assess cost-effectiveness and collaboration in English NHS and local authorities, with particular reference to the expenditure on joint finance. The research was prompted partly by Parliamentary worries that joint finance was not being spent in a way which befitted NHS authorities, or which reflected good accountancy practice or cost-effectiveness analysis.

Joint Finance Packages of care

This summary is based on data from joint-finance programmes in seven non-London health authorities. The data are analysed in terms of the beneficiaries of the programmes, the agencies involved, the nature of community services provided and the financial arrangements used in funding projects.

FINDINGS

1. Client User Groups

Table 1.14: *Client Users of Joint Finance (Number of Projects)*

Health Authority	Mentally-ill people	People with learning disabilities	Elderly people	Elderly mentally-ill people	Physically-handicapped people	Miscellaneous	**Total**
A	3	8	7	–	2	3	23 (8%)
B	6	4	10	–	2	3	25 (8%)
C	7	11	12	1	–	21	52 (17%)
D	3	23	8	2	1	19	56 (18%)
E	2	8	6	1	1	9	27 (9%)
F	6	18	19	2	3	22	70 (23%)
G	11	15	3	1	2	20	52 (17%)
Total No. of Projects(%)	38 (12%)	87 (29%)	65 (21%)	7 (2%)	11 (4%)	97 (32%)	305 (100%)

Table 1.14 indicates the range of client-groups benefiting from individual schemes across each health authority's joint-finance programme over a fixed period. A large number of schemes have been devoted to services for people with learning disabilities (87—29 per cent) and for elderly people (65—21 per cent). This is not surprising since, in both cases, progress in the development of community care has

[5] For an account, see page 39.

been more prolific than for groups such as mentally-ill people, elderly mentally-ill people and physically-handicapped people.

Thirty-two per cent of schemes did not fall into the five main priority-groups identified. This miscellaneous category includes schemes aimed at other priority groups (e.g. alcoholics, under-fives), schemes which either cannot be attributed to any one group or may serve a particular mix of clients, and schemes involved with administratively-related problems. The presence of this miscellaneous group reflects the diversity covered by the concept of community care – much of which remains to be evaluated in terms of cost and outcome.

Expenditure analysis also indicated that people with learning disabilities and elderly people in this sample tended to be major beneficiaries of joint finance programmes. The average expenditure on services for people with learning disabilities and elderly people was 19 per cent and 28 per cent of the total respectively. The variation between districts, however, was large.

2. Provider Agencies

At the time of the analysis – two years after the introduction of the new arrangements for joint finance – collaboration remained dominated by local authority social services and health authorities: progress towards more comprehensive collaboration in these seven study localities had been slow. Only seven local authority housing schemes, two voluntary schemes and one local authority education department scheme had been successful participants, representing small proportions of the local joint-finance budgets. Health authorities themselves had secured 78 schemes (an average of 17 per cent of total expenditure) and a further 12 held jointly with social services. This relative health sector dominance may reflect some of the local authorities' concerns about using joint finance.

This apparent lack of progress in extending the range of agency participants was predictable. The 'rolling' nature of the joint-finance revenue programme makes for the slow introduction of new agencies. Any local system currently heavily committed to funding existing revenue schemes has relatively less of an annual joint-finance allocation available for supporting new schemes.

3. Service Provision

If community care is to offer the flexibility and diversity necessary to meet the individual needs of people, a range of community-based services is needed. These fall into five basic categories: residential, domiciliary, day-care, respite and primary health services. By selecting different combinations of particular services within each broad category, packages of individual care can be provided.

The analysis showed that joint finance had contributed to the enhancement of all five aspects of community living. In particular, the areas of day-care, domiciliary care and primary health services appeared to have important places in the programme.

The data clearly indicated that service improvements and developments are the key areas on which joint finance has focused, although one authority did spend joint finance on staff training schemes. There are few research schemes, which suggests a lack of evaluation of innovative ideas, despite their being tested out in a pilot situation.

Further analysis of schemes supporting improvements and developments to service models shows the extent to which joint finance is supporting populations *already in the community*. The resource consequences of running down large institutions in parallel with the building of new community-based services, in most instances, exceed the capabilities of joint finance, and regional health authorities formulate their own funding arrangements for this purpose. **Joint finance in reality is focusing on reducing demand from the community for long-stay hospital care**.

4. Financial Arrangements

An analysis of the financial arrangements used in joint finance is important from a funding point of view: joint finance was first envisaged as providing an appropriate balance between capital and revenue in order to contribute to both the transfer of resources *to* the community and a build-up of resources in the community. In particular, the programme was expected to consist of approximately two-thirds of capital projects and one-third revenue. With increasing financial stringency imposed upon local government budgets, many have found it difficult to support the revenue consequences of capital projects and so the composition of the joint-finance programme is different from initial expectations.

This research showed that there are five main divisions to be made in relation to future revenue commitment. The first group consists of capital projects with no revenue consequences. The second group includes capital projects with associated revenue consequences – these may include revenue consequences of limited duration or indeed requiring a total commitment after the completion of the tapering process. The third group are revenue projects of limited duration lasting less than the standard seven-year period. The fourth group consists of revenue projects with seven-year periods during which the health authority contribution is phased out. The new arrangements in the 1983 DHSS circular[6] allowed the introduction of extended periods of time, up to a maximum of 13 years, in which sponsoring agencies could respond to the financial consequences of joint finance. This is the fifth and final category.

In the seven health authority localities included in the study, a disproportionately-high number of projects were funded on limited-duration revenue arrangements. This suggested that the initial expectation that joint finance could act as a pump-priming fund to stimulate the transfer and build-up of resources is not always realisitic in the current financial climate.

The lack of response to the new, extended financial arrangements, again, is partly due to the nature of the rolling programme. It is also due partly to the implications such an arrangement has on the remainder of the fixed joint-finance programme. A commitment by a health authority to fund fully the revenue consequences of a project over 13 years can impede the rate of new projects in forthcoming years.

CONCLUSION

Although it is not possible to generalize from this analysis, it seems that although joint finance programmes lack the means and focus to provide an adequate and appropriate bridging fund, they can make important but limited contributions to the community care of particular client-groups.

The results of the small survey show joint finance has been instrumental in pump-priming the development and improvement of day services, respite services and primary health services for elderly people and mentally handicapped people.

---

[6] DHSS (1983) *Joint Finance and Community Care*, HC(83)/LAC(83)6, DHSS.

These service developments and improvements tend to predominate in areas of service provision for groups already living in the community, requiring long-term care or for those considered at risk of future hospitalization. Joint finance does not play a significant role in the direct transfers of people and resources out of long-stay hospitals. There is no reason to believe that the role for joint finance described above will not or could not be extended in the future into similar areas for mentally-ill and physically-handicapped people.

Researchers

Karen Gerard and Ken Wright

Centre for Health Economics, University of York, Heslington, York YO1 5DD. (0904 433646; FAX 0904 433644)

Publications

Gerard, K. (1988) 'An Analysis of Joint Finance in Seven North-London Health Authorities', CHE Discussion Paper 35.

Gerard, K. (1990) 'Economic evaluation of respite care for children with mental handicap: A preliminary analysis of problems', *Mental Handicap*, **18**: 150–155.

Gerard, K. (1988) 'An Appraisal of the Cost-effectiveness of Alternative Day Care Settings for Frail Elderly People', *Age and Ageing*, **17**: 1–7.

Gerard, K., and Wright, K. (1990) 'The Practical Problems of Applying Cost-Effectiveness Analysis to Joint Finance Programmes', CHE Discussion Paper 66.

The Ethnic Monitoring of Social Services Project

In 1990, the Ethnic Monitoring of Social Services Project conducted a survey of all social services departments in England, Scotland, Wales and Northern Ireland. The survey was part of a three-year DH-funded project looking at these departments' development, implementation and monitoring of services for the black and minority ethnic community. Of the 133 departments contacted, 92 responded, achieving a response rate of 69 per cent. Some of the results have been published in the report *Equally Fair*?[7] and this summary is based on that publication.

Record-keeping

Service delivery

Employment policy

FINDINGS

Of the 92 departments which responded to our survey, a number have developed interventions concerning adoption and fostering, translation and interpretation, black and minority ethnic community groups, and services to the elderly, as well as equal opportunities policies and ethnic record-keeping and monitoring systems. In terms of service delivery initiatives, only 8 out of the 92 departments had not taken any of the 11 initiatives which we enquired about. Although a 'larger' New Commonwealth and Pakistan (NCWP) population was associated with a greater number of service delivery initiatives, the association was complex. There appeared to be gaps in provision in areas with larger NCWP populations, while small numbers of people of NCWP origin did not mean that initiatives were not being taken by the social services department.

The variability identified in service delivery initiatives was also reflected in relation to equal opportunities policies and ethnic record-keeping and monitoring systems (see table 1.15). Our analysis further showed that equal opportunities policies for service delivery were often 'younger' than those for employment. The results suggest a variable approach to the *formalization* of the commitment to ensure equality of opportunity for the black and minority ethnic community, and that departments often relied on employing black and minority ethnic people as a vehicle of change.

Our results also illustrated that having an equal opportunities policy for service delivery was not associated with departments having taken any of the 11 service-delivery initiatives. Nor did it suggest that departments had taken, on average, more of these service-delivery initiatives. Factors that were associated with an increase in the average number of initiatives are summarized in table 1.16. The associations were complex, but significant. For example, the average number of service delivery initiatives taken by departments was greater if the department had given priority to services to the black community in the planning process. The likelihood of this priority being given was increased if the department had an equal opportunities policy for service delivery.

---

[7] For details, see *Publications*, page 54.

Table 1.15: *Equal opportunities policies, and ethnic record-keeping and monitoring systems for employment and service delivery*

Employment:
- 78 local authorities and 82 social services departments have an equal opportunities policy for employment;
- fewer local authorities (48) and social services departments (39) have an ethnic record-keeping and monitoring system for employment.

Service delivery:
- 51 local authorities and 59 social services departments have equal opportunities policies for service delivery;
- 40 social services departments have ethnic record-keeping and monitoring systems for service delivery.

In comparison to employment:
- a greater number of service delivery ethnic record-keeping and monitoring systems exist outside an equal opportunities policy for service delivery;
- fewer social services departments, 30 or 34 per cent, have both service-delivery equal opportunities policies *and* ethnic record-keeping and monitoring systems;
- more social services departments, 21 or 24 per cent, have *neither* equal opportunities policies *nor* any ethnic record-keeping and monitoring system for service delivery.

Table 1.16: *Factors influencing the average number of service delivery initiatives taken*

- the size of the NCWP population;
- whether services to the black and minority ethnic community were a priority in the planning process;
- whether policy statements for major services stated the role of equal opportunities.

It was clear that the crucial factor was *not* the existence of a policy for service delivery, but how developed their equal opportunites *policy framework* for service delivery was. Our survey identified four components of this policy framework and these are summarized in Table 1.17.

Table 1.17: *Factors in the equal opportunities policy framework and links with the monitoring of services to the black and minority ethnic community*

Factors in the policy framework:

- the social services department has an equal opportunities service-delivery policy;
- the policy states the aims and objectives in relation to race equality;
- the policy includes a strategy for implementation;
- the policy states who is responsible.

If social services departments had all four of these components it was more likely that they:

- had a commitment to monitor services to the black and minority ethnic community;
- had an ethnic record-keeping and monitoring system for service delivery;
- had a system which did not only record ethnic origin but included other factors such as religion, language or diet.

It is clear that those departments which have made more progress in developing their equal opportunities service-delivery policy and monitoring framework have on average taken more initiatives to progress equality for the black and minority ethnic community, regardless of whether they have 'small', 'medium' or 'large' NCWP populations.

Turning to those 40 departments that do have ethnic record-keeping and monitoring systems for service delivery, it is clear that the computerization of client information has been a critical factor in their ability and commitment to implement them. However, it also appears to be the case, in at least seven departments, that implementation was as much related to the technology now being available as to any formalized commitment to making progress on equality. More significantly, only 14 of the 40 departments that have ethnic record-keeping and monitoring systems for service delivery have actually analysed the information produced by them. Although many of these systems are 'young' compared with equal opportunities policies, it does appear that once implemented – often after long periods of development – they may be very little used.

CONCLUSIONS

From the evidence of our survey, it is clear that there are some departments which are in a position to respond positively to the challenges posed by the new community care regime, and to ensure that their services account for the needs of their black and minority ethnic community. These departments have recognized the importance of equal opportunities policies for service delivery as well as employment. They have ensured that these policies state the aims and objectives in relation to race equality. By combining this with a strategy for implementation, and an indication of who is responsible for implementation, they have gone some way to ensure that these policies are not a paper exercise. In terms of monitoring, these departments have acknowledged the importance of assessing the progress of equality, even though many have not actually analysed the information contained in their ethnic record-keeping and monitoring systems.

The findings suggest that if departments are committed to providing community care services that meet the needs of the black and minority ethnic community, then at the very least they need to consider how coherent and comprehensive their policy and monitoring framework is. While most departments have made some commitment, and a few appear to have made real progress, many have adopted a piecemeal or haphazard approach, which makes it difficult to answer the question of whether they will meet the challenges of community care in the 1990s and beyond.

Researchers

Jabeer Butt and Peter Gorbach

National Insitute for Social Work, Mary Ward House, 5–7 Tavistock Place, London WC1H 9SS. (071 387 9681; FAX 071 387 7968)

Publications

Butt, J. (ed.) (1990) *Ethnic record keeping and monitoring workshop report*, National Institute for Social Work Research Unit, Race Equality Unit, Social Services Research Group.

Butt, J. (1992) 'Monitoring equality: the social services experience', *Assignation*, **9**, 2.

Butt, J. (1992) 'Challenging research: community care research and the black community', in R. Smith, and L. Harrison (eds), *Community Care Research and Community Care Policy*, School of Advanced Urban Studies, University of Bristol, 60–72.

Butt, J. (forthcoming) 'Meeting the challenge of services to the black community', *Social Work Today*.

Butt, J., Gorbach, P., and Ahmad, B. (1991) *Equally Fair? A report on social services departments' development, implementation and monitoring of services for the black and minority ethnic community*, Race Equality Unit, National Institute for Social Work.

Research on Community Nursing Services – Progress Report

Introduction

The growing emphasis on care in the community, and its links with preventive health care, highlights the importance of the role played by district nurses and health visitors. However, little is known on any systematic basis of how establishments – numbers of staff and hours worked – for district nurses and health visitors are set and reviewed. This two-year research project will identify the ways in which community nursing establishments are currently set and reviewed, and will use them as a basis for future guidance.

A review of the literature and contacts with practitioners and managers have already suggested some key factors:

Potential Models for Community Care Organizations

Following the National Health Service and Community Care Act 1990, many models are being explored for purchasing and providing health and social care in the community. Community nursing services, (currently provided by health authority community units,) could continue to be purchased by the District Health Authority, or perhaps by incorporating the DHA, Family Health Services Authority, and possibly the local authority. Alternatively, primary and secondary care purchasing could be separated, and community nursing purchased by the FHSA alone. Another possible purchasing model would be the direct employment of district nurses and/or health visitors by fund-holding GPs.

Changes can now take place on the providing side – for example, by mergers between health-care provider units, between these units and GP practitioners' services, and/or with local authority social care providers. Developments at the interface of primary and secondary care are also increasing in scale and type.

Community Nursing Education and Training

Some community nurse managers are considering the impact on establishments of the likely role of nurses who are now training for registration under 'Project 2000'. These nurses will be qualified to work in both hospital and (supervised) community settings. The United Kingdom Central Council for Nurses, Midwives and Health Visitors is also proposing changes to the education of registered nurses wishing to work in the community. Such changes would introduce a new discipline of 'community health nursing', with a potential reduction of emphasis on the current professional boundaries between district nursing and health visiting.

Skill Mix

The search for optimum value for money from finite resources for health care has prompted many nurse managers to review the activities and skills of their nursing staff. Opinions vary about the best mix of skills and acceptable standards of care, but if purchasers are to identify the best ways to spend their limited resources,

Establish-ments
Training
Purchaser–provider split

providers will need to be explicit about the nature, cost and standard of services they provide.

Role Overlap

Problems of overlapping roles are most obvious between district nurses/health visitors and practice nurses, and social workers. More collaboration (both formal and informal) between health authorities, local authorities and family health services authorities will help to clarify service boundaries and professional responsibilities.

Information Systems

Effective planning and review of services need good information systems. In the context of community nursing, such systems should be able to provide information on service need, activities and outcomes. Currently, a range of data-collection systems are in use, contributing different levels and quality of information as a basis for managers' deployment of staffing resources.

The Project

The project is being carried out in two stages and will focus the issues outlined above. First, there is a survey of current practice in a representative sample of health authorities. This will be followed by a more detailed study of a smaller number of authorities, chosen to represent different approaches to tackling the issues involved. A report on Stage I was prepared in 1992.

Researchers

Jane Lightfoot and Nicola Walsh

Social Policy Research Unit, University of York, Heslington, York YO1 5DD. (0904 433608)

Transferability of Mental Handicap Nursing Skills from Hospital to Community

PRELIMINARY FINDINGS

Learning disabilities

Staffing

The two-year project was assigned to collect information on

(a) the employment of Registered Nurse Mental Handicap (RNMH) nurses across both the statutory sector (health and social services) and independent sector (voluntary and private);

(b) the role and functions of RNMH qualified staff in various settings and with clients of different levels of learning disability, when compared with staff with other or no professional qualifications.

Phase 1 of the project consisted of a survey of all health and social services departments in England along with voluntary and private agencies which could be identified from various sources. The survey was conducted by means of a postal questionnaire, with a response from agencies representing about 5,461 RNMH nursing staff.

Information collected in Phase 1 covered a wide range of areas. The most distinctive finding was that while many in different sectors recognized the comprehensive nature of the RNMH background, reservations were expressed about 'institutional approaches' from RNMH nurses. This even applied to District Health Authorities who were, not surprisingly, the major employers of such staff. In Phase 2, it was possible indirectly to gauge the extent to which this 'image' was based upon RNMH practice, through analysis of data from case-study areas. One area was chosen for each of health, social services and the independent sector.

Phase 2 involved a number of methods of data collection, including the construction of an observational checklist – the Staff Activity Checklist (SAC) – covering 22 activities. Those activities involving interactions with service users and informal carers were evaluated on the basis of a value statement, and against explicit criteria. The SAC complemented interview data and material from a self-completion questionnaire which asked staff for background information about their employment, training and qualifications, and career plans. Data were collected on staff in three qualification groups – those with RNMH, with other professional qualifications and those with no professional qualifications. Senior and middle managers without direct care responsibilities were interviewed, but not observed.

Initial analysis of the observational data suggests that there may be no statistically significant difference between the activities and performance of the three groups of staff. Further work on these analyses is in progress. RNMH staff, however, contributed a particular combination of activities and what are called 'skills plus' factors.

In addition, the findings of the project as a whole will highlight issues such as:

▶ equity

▶ motivation

- ► organizational constraints
- ► comparability

All of these will be discussed in the final report, currently in preparation.

Researcher

Mr John Brown

Department of Social Policy and Social Work, University of York, Heslington, York YO1 5DD. (0904 433494)

Assessment and Care-Packaging after the White Paper

Introduction

The object of this research is to define good practice in assessment and care-packaging, with a view to identifying ways of delivering a more efficient, appropriate and good quality service. The project examines ways in which current challenges to established professional perspectives may provide the starting-point for generating changes that will allow assessments to be made more effectively.

Interviews with community care practitioners and their managers across two counties in North Wales have been completed, and an observation phase – involving accompanying professionals on assessment and review visits to elderly people – is nearing completion. Findings reported in this abstract relate only to the first two phases of this study.

The two follow-up phases were planned for 1992.

Training
Targeting
Attitudes

Summary of Early Findings

The findings from the first two phases indicate that:

- Information and training designed to motivate front-line staff is needed to maintain the momentum of implementation.
- Although much discussion and planning of reforms is happening at managerial levels, assumptions cannot be made about levels of knowledge amongst more junior staff. Insufficient copies of policy documents and/or failure to circulate them were reported.
- The training needs identified by the respondents in this study suggest that there may be benefit in canvassing opinion about training more widely. Joint or multi-disciplinary training may provide an opportunity to narrow professional divisions.
- Training should emphasize the therapeutic aspects of the assessment process even when no service results. Over-emphasis on 'those in greatest need' as being the only legitimate beneficiaries of full assessment, and service provision, may be counter-productive.
- Negative perceptions about the White Paper proposals should be taken into account when planning training, implementation and how best to motivate staff. More can be done to highlight the ways in which the intended reforms could result in more satisfactory outcomes for both client and worker.
- Rumours about budget-holding and role-change (case/care-management) resulting in insecurity and anxiety could be minimized by better communication and interpretation of policy at all levels.
- Referral procedures may need to be re-examined. The information on referral forms leads to decisions about what sort of assessment an individual will eventually receive. Inaccurate or inadequate information can lead to poor targeting of assessments and subsequent services.
- Recent experience of working with practitioners suggests that agreed definitions and directions have not always filtered down to those at the level of client

contact. It is important that this is rectified so that development and debate take place at all levels, and between all levels of seniority. The comments and observations made by some practitioners suggest that they do not see themselves as being able to effect change through the present mechanisms of the management structure.

- The persistence of professional divisions and the lack of communication between agencies suggests an urgent need for action: joint debate, training and planning is likely to be necessary if care-management policies requiring multi-disciplinary cooperation are to work well.

- Community care workers say that they need and want better to understand the roles of other professionals working in the community, so that cross-referrals may be made more appropriately. This might be done through local liaison groups, where members of each agency or profession could in turn make a presentation or answer questions about their professional role to others.

- There was considerable anxiety amongst practitioners about targeting services on those most in need. The long-term consequences of targeting should be monitored in order to identify its impact on *preventive* work. Many practitioners said that the importance of cleaning services should not be forgotten in moves towards more personal care. Further research into the consequences of withdrawing basic services to elderly people with lower levels of needs is required, as well as more information about what the *consumers of services actually want*.

- It was recognized that home carers would be asked to care for increasingly vulnerable elderly people. In order to meet this challenge, a more structured and broader training was seen as necessary. Much remains to be done in clarifying roles and responsibilities and/or agreeing cooperative practices between district nursing and home-care services.

- Policy makers must consider the potential for development of the private and voluntary sectors in context: the service infrastructure of rural areas must be taken into account in setting objectives.

- The anxieties of community care workers about the private and voluntary sectors must be understood, and where possible accommodated. In order to gain their support and create enthusiasm during a time of change and uncertainty it is vital that a participatory approach to the planning and implementation of changes is taken.

The question of resources is fundamental to many of the findings outlined here. Major reforms to the nature and style of community care are in prospect; but consistent and sustained planning for the future will be difficult to achieve in an uncertain financial climate.

Researcher

Ms Kerry Caldock

Centre for Social Policy Research and Development, University of Wales, Bangor, Gwynedd LL57 2DG. (0248 351151)

Publications

Caldock, K. (1992) *The Management of Community Care for Elderly People After the White Paper: Practitioner perspectives*, University of Wales, Bangor, Centre for Social Policy Research and Development.

Caldock, K. (1991) *Assessment After the White Paper: practitioner perspectives*, University of Wales, Bangor, Centre for Social Policy Research and Development.

Service Packaging and Learning Disabilities: Interim Report

Research into service packaging is one of several studies linked to the evaluation of the All-Wales Mental Handicap Strategy. The aims of the service packaging project are to:

Consumer views
Carers
Individual planning

- explore the level of satisfaction with services of both persons with a learning disability and their family carers;
- describe the nature and functions of services which are valued by these user groups;
- evaluate how such service packages contribute to the opportunity of users to lead normal, independent and high-quality lives;
- evaluate how service packages for family carers contribute to stress reduction and satisfaction with their caring role;
- account for the variations in personal and social circumstances which affect these outcomes;
- assess the relative merits of different methods of packaging services; and
- inform policy-makers on the basis of these findings.

The research was in two parts; the first phase involved sending a postal questionnaire to all family carers living in seven local authority districts in Wales. Altogether, 752 families participated in the survey, a response rate of 76 per cent. Besides the usual demographic data, the questionnaire sought to discover the extent of service use and professional contact with family carers and users, and carers' appraisals of service quality. Further questions on the nature of user and family carer participation in service planning, their hopes for the future, and some basic indicators of the impact of services on their lives were also included. The second stage will be concerned with tracing the impact of services on the lives and lifestyles of a sub-sample of individuals and their families.

Findings – first phase

The findings have so far underlined the importance of particular service *process* factors to an understanding of how individuals appraise services (intermediate outcomes). The next step is to evaluate how those processes are related to an understanding of the lives and lifestyles of individuals and their families (personal outcomes).

The results suggest that services appear to be targeted primarily at families with children or adults with poor physical capacities. As has been found in other studies, families reporting challenging behaviour do not seem to be receiving the attention that might be expected. The data indicate a continued need for more adequate service response to families reporting challenging behaviour of the service user.

Only about a fifth of carers noted that there was an agreed service plan for themselves and their relative, although nearly half reported having been involved in some form of individual planning meeting in the previous 12 months, and 64 per cent claimed to have a key worker. Surprisingly, there appeared to be little targeting in terms of age, physical capacity or the level of reported challenging behaviour in the allocation of key workers. The discrepancy between the proportion reporting a key worker and a service planning meeting suggests that workers have difficulties maintaining a consistent programme of reviews.

More important is the large number of carers with key workers who do not acknowledge the existence of any service plan. As earlier studies have shown, key workers and individual plan systems have not developed at the speed anticipated by policy. The importance of extending and providing more opportunities for families to participate in individual planning is clearly demonstrated. Only 11 per cent of families reported having an individual plan as opposed to other types of case-planning meetings, and these families were significantly more likely to see the meeting as useful and to be satisfied with the progress of the decisions made than those involved in other types of meetings.

Although over half the families were very or quite satisfied with service packages received, just under a fifth (18 per cent) expressed definite dissatisfaction, and on all indices of service sufficiency used, such as the need for help to enable the family to lead a more normal life, between a third and two-fifths indicated service shortfalls. High proportions of carers expressed feelings of isolation (45 per cent), deleterious effects of the caring role on their health (40 per cent) or restrictions in their social life (62 per cent). These indicators suggest that there is a long way to go before services could be said to be tailored to the needs and wishes of individuals.

The presence of a key worker, involvement in an individual planning meeting and the existence of a service plan were associated with general overall service satisfaction and an increased likelihood of carers believing the professionals were able to empathize with themselves and their relative – an aspect of service delivery which emerged as highly significant in carers' appraisals of services. The existence of mechanisms for involving carers at the case level can therefore be seen as being linked to some key indices of service quality.

On the one hand, key worker systems and a more recent history of family involvement in meetings about the service user both appear to impinge on the prospects of people having access to something resembling a service package. *Participation in the mechanisms for involvement at the individual case level* appears to offer the best guarantee for those who want to gain access to the services concerned: it is also likely to lead to satisfaction with services in general and with the professional support provided. These service arrangements do not, however, impinge so strongly on views of service deficiencies, needs expressed, or on indicators of stress such as effects on the carer's health or their social isolation. Other service processes emerge as more important here: especially, *the perceived ability of professionals to empathize* with the needs and views of persons with learning disabilities and with family carers; and the *reluctance carers feel about contacting professionals* for help. These three factors, reflecting aspects of rapport between professionals, service users and carers, affect all the nine intermediate outcome measures so far analysed. The findings are relevant to an understanding of effective care-management arrangements, strategies for involvement of users and carers, and their relationship to service quality.

Researcher

Dr Gordon Grant

Centre for Social Policy Research and Development, University of Wales, Bangor, Gwynedd LL57 2DG. (0248 351151)

Publications

Grant, G., Ramcharan, P., and McGrath, M. (1991) *Appraising service packages: initial findings of a phase one questionnaire survey of 376 families*, University of Wales, Bangor, Centre for Social Policy Research and Development.

McGrath, M., Grant, G., and Ramcharan, P. (1991) *Service packages: factors affecting carers' appraisals of intermediate outcomes*, University of Wales, Bangor, Centre for Social Policy Research and Development.

McGrath, M., Ramcharan, P., and Grant, G. (1991) *Points of view: carers' perceptions of service packages*, University of Wales, Bangor, Centre for Social Policy Research and Development.

Ramcharan, P., Grant, G., and McGrath, M., (1990) *Reconciling Value-directed and Value-relative Approaches to Evaluation Research: the case of the service packaging project*, University of Wales, Bangor, Centre for Social Policy Research and Development.

Service Developments under the All-Wales Mental Handicap Strategy

The All-Wales Mental Handicap Strategy was initiated by the Welsh Office in 1983 and was aimed at the development of locally-available community-based residential, day, family, support, respite and professional services for people with learning disabilities. It sought also to promote equal access for such people to generic services and the general resources of the community. It promised additional investment of £26 million over a ten-year period, paid outside the Revenue Support Grant, to build local service infrastructure and support change. The Strategy stressed the development of structures for multi-agency planning, and consumer representation in planning, at local and county levels.

Service planning
Consumer involvement
Collaboration

Service Development in Wales: 1983–1988

A. Residential Provision

The number of people living in hospitals decreased from 2,087 in 1983 to 1,735 in 1987. Between 1983 and 1988, local authorities and private and voluntary bodies opened 45, 30 and 26 new settings respectively, with the median size of residence in operation falling to between 5 and 7 places. However, 59 per cent, 57 per cent and 44 per cent of residents in staffed local authority, private or voluntary accommodation still lived in settings with 16 or more places. It is generally believed that there has been an acceleration in the growth of community provision and in the rundown of the large hospitals since 1988. Yet the Welsh Office Annual Report for 1989/90 showed an estimated total need for ordinary housing accommodation for adults of 3,702 places, of which only 986 (26.6 per cent) had been provided. The pace of change has been slower than was hoped for, despite the concerted central government policy and financial lead. A more detailed survey of provision in 4 districts suggests the same conclusion. Between 1986 and 1990 there was an increase of 26 places in group home or staffed house provision: 32 people out of a total residential population of 168 lived in such facilities, implying a further 21-year period of redevelopment at the rate achieved over the study period.

B. Day Services

The number of places in adult training centres, including special needs provision, rose from 2,997 in 1983 to 3,192 in 1988, with average unit size decreasing from 81 to 76 places. There has been an increase in sessional attendance with a complementary expansion in alternative forms of day occupation, particularly opportunities for work experience and access to colleges of further education. There has also been a modest expansion of small businesses and rural/horticultural projects; and a number of schemes have been set up which focus on local community activities on an individual basis.

C. Family Support

Family support has been a major focus for service delivery in the early years of the Strategy. Domiciliary support services have become widespread, growing rapidly from 41 individuals/families served in 1983 to 1,840 by 1988. Family-based respite-care and respite in locally-available staffed housing both increased over ten-fold in the same period. Twenty-eight per cent of the additional allocations available under the Strategy to that date had been used to provide such services. However, 59 per cent of one-parent families in the survey of four districts in 1990 (and 48 per cent of two-parent families) received neither domiciliary support nor respite care and only 11 per cent (and 15 per cent) received both. The Welsh Office Annual Report for 1989/90 indicates that only 18 per cent of the need for short-term care in domestic settings, and 55 per cent of the need for domiciliary support in the home is being met.

D. Professional Input and Service Coordination

The establishment of community mental handicap teams as a means of coordinating professional and service contact with individuals and their families was an early priority of the Strategy. The professional infrastructure has continued to grow, accounting for 25 per cent of the Strategy allocations to 1988, although recruitment difficulties – particularly in psychology and speech therapy – can mean that vacancies exist. Team staff are often central to the process of individual planning, but evidence from a variety of studies suggests that this is still only being done for about a third of potential clients. Information on professional involvement from a survey of four districts shows 69 per cent of the sample in touch with GPs in a six-month period in 1990, but only 37 per cent in contact with social workers, 20 per cent with community nurses and between 5 per cent and 11 per cent with psychologists, physiotherapists or speech therapists.

E. Service Planning and Management

The Strategy has given local authorities the role of lead agency in the context of pluralistic provision – by statutory, as well as private and voluntary bodies. The development of a single plan for each county, to which all parties can contribute, has been introduced; and most counties have strengthened their central resources by appointing service development officers. Training has been provided to develop attitudes and working practices in keeping with the principles of the Strategy, and concerted efforts have been made to foster advocacy, and encourage integration in schooling. It has also become clear that people with challenging behaviour received fewer benefits in the early years of the Strategy, and were identified as a priority group for attention in the mid-term review of the Strategy in 1988.

Scope of a Comprehensive Community Service

The definition of a comprehensive community service has become more sophisticated, as initiatives under the Strategy have begun to replace inadequate institutional provision with a range of local alternatives. Table 1.18 illustrates components of a modern local service. Given a largely institutional starting position, with wide territorial inequalities in services and service expenditures, and the need to switch a large proportion of existing resources between managing agencies, the current situation is inevitably patchy. This is true even in areas which have made considerable progress in recent years. No locality has adequate provision across all components of a comprehensive service.

CONCLUSION

The All-Wales Mental Handicap Strategy has provided the impetus for organizational reform, but progress has been modest and experience has varied in different localities. It is clear that the determination to see through the planned change has to be sustained over decades, rather than years.

Table 1.18: *Components of a Comprehensive Service Infrastructure*

Family Support	Specialist Professional Input	Generic Professional Input
* Early counselling	* Community nursing	* General practitioners
* Domiciliary support	* Social work	* Dentistry
* Home teaching	* Psychology	* Chiropody
* Family-based respite	* Psychiatry	* Audiology
* Short-term care	* Physiotherapy	* Ophthalmology
* Sitting-in services	* Speech therapy	* Paediatrics
* Genetic counselling	* Specialist teams, eg	* Psychiatry
* Housing adaptations	Challenging behaviour,	* Other consultants
	Sensory Handicap	

Education	Day Services	Residential Services
* Home teaching	* Community leisure	* Support in own home
* Support in mainstream	* Community-skills training	* Group homes
schools	* Employment placement	* Staffed housing
* Special schools	* Supported employment	* Fostering
* Further Education	* Work experience	* Adult family placement
* Adult Education	* Small businesses	* Shared tenancies
	* Vocational training	
	* Special needs provision	
	* Social centres	
	* Retirement services	

Advocacy	Coordination and planning	Other Service Components
* Self-advocacy	* Individual planning systems	* Volunteer coordination
* Citizen advocacy	* Keyworker systems	* Resource and activity
	* CMHT structures	library
	* Care-management	
	* Service brokerage	

The experience of the early years of the Strategy bears witness to the challenge it set to the existing service culture. The clear provision targets set by the Strategy, and the system of monitoring plans developed by the Welsh Office both proved to be essential. Service authorities had to learn how to collaborate with each other and consumer groups in order to produce joint county plans. New mechanisms, such as individual planning or care-management, have to be resourced and implemented on a wide scale if strategic service development is to be based on an understanding of individual needs and requirements. Counties have invested in development workers and in training in an attempt to adjust to the new circumstances.

The implementation of the new arrangements for community care will produce similar demands on service authorities in England. The community care policy aims to promote individual opportunity, choice and independence, and to encourage a range of service providers to operate a variety of tailor-made services locally. Purchaser authorities will contract services through systems of care-management focused on the assessment of individual need. Experience in Wales suggests that the sustained effort required to change the planning and provision culture should not be underestimated.

Researchers

Dr Stephen Beyer, Mr Stuart Todd, Mr Gerry Evans and Dr David Felce

Mental Handicap in Wales: Applied Research Unit, 55 Park Place, Cardiff CF1 3AT. (0222 226188; FAX 0222 641871)

Publications

Beyer, S., Evans, G., Todd, S., and Blunden, R. (1986) *Planning for the All-Wales Strategy: A Review of Issues arising in Welsh Counties*, Cardiff, Mental Handicap in Wales: Applied Research Unit.

Beyer, S., Todd, S., and Felce, D. (1991) 'The implementation of the All-Wales Mental Handicap Strategy, 1983–1988', *Mental Handicap Research*, **4**, 2: 115–140.

Evans, G., Todd, S., Beyer, S., Felce, D., and Perry, J. (in press) 'Assessing the Impact of the All-Wales Mental Handicap Strategy: A Survey of Four Districts', *Journal of Intellectual Disability Research*.

Evans, G., Todd, S., and Beyer, S. (1992) *A Four Year Longitudinal Study of the Impact of the All-Wales Strategy on the Lives of People with Learning Difficulties*, Cardiff, Mental Handicap in Wales: Applied Research Unit.

Policy Implementation Studies – the All-Wales Mental Handicap Strategy

Following the launch of the All-Wales Mental Handicap Strategy in 1983, the Centre was commissioned to study the early stages of strategy implementation and impact. The research covered three areas of direct concern to community care policy:

Multi-disciplinary working

Consumer views

the **development of community mental handicap teams** as a means of integrating the delivery of services to individuals and their families;

the design of **inter-agency planning mechanisms intended to promote the participation of users and their families in decision-making;** and

the **impact of these arrangements from the perspective of families.**

Community mental handicap teams were the subject of a survey in 1987, which produced the following results.

The teams studied varied in membership from three to over 20 members. Social workers and community mental handicap nurses constituted over 50 per cent of the membership of the 37 teams in Wales, but a range of other health professions was also represented. Although most of the teams had been in existence for less than three years, many had appointed service organizers with responsibility for promoting and maintaining specialist services – including respite care, community living, family aide, voluntary and welfare rights services. Their existence helped teams to develop new services while enabling other team members to concentrate on casework or individual planning.

The survey suggested the existence of four categories of teams, based on an analysis of professional membership: all categories showed high levels of mutual trust and support between team members, and mutually accepted patterns of working had largely been established – often across professional boundaries. Their achievements included significant new service developments, including flexible use of domiciliary support services and respite care, a shift away from dependency on residential services, and the institution of individual planning systems.

Multi-disciplinary teamwork, aimed at developing needs-led services in consultation with service users and their families, appeared to work best when three conditions were present:

1. the existence of a team coordinator, accepted by all the professions involved;

2. team control over the deployment of existing services and resources; and

3. a community care contingency budget which could be used to tailor service packages to individual requirements.

Some problems remained however. Progressive thinking about values, philosophy and joint work was often in advance of that of higher management, so that management accountability and control, and unclear agency policy could inhibit teams from developing needs-led services. Workload problems meant that individual plans could not be drawn up for all users, and information was patchy. The links between teams and the rest of the service system also needed to be strengthened.

The research also explored the effectiveness of *arrangements for involving service users and their families in local and strategic inter-agency planning and management of services*.

The findings suggest that progress had been made in empowering family carers – mostly parents – by providing for their involvement in most of the key planning and decision-making forums within each county in Wales, but this is not true of people with learning disabilities themselves. There is still therefore a strong tendency, supported by the structures for planning, for parents to speak on behalf of, or as representatives of, their sons and daughters. Parental interests may not always match those of their relatives, and separate means of representation for both services users and parents in planning systems are desirable if the ultimate goal is to be services tailored to individuals.

The research confirmed that there are no easy solutions to involving users and their family supporters – even parents – in these processes: by far the majority did not want to be involved in local or strategic planning at all. They simply wanted someone like a key worker to visit them in their own home in order to ensure that they were informed about developing services, and about how their own and their relative's needs and wants could be met. Although uneven, progress towards involvement of users and families in planning and management became an important force for redistributing power. But the experience of the Welsh mental handicap strategy suggests that involvement that falls short of helping users to take calculated and informed risks about their own life choices will not be widely welcomed by users, nor by many of their families. Involvement of users and families worked best when there was a clear framework for inter-agency collaboration at all levels from individual to strategic planning and management of services.

The *new arrangements and the way they impacted upon families* were broadly welcomed. The opportunity to be consulted, the right to access to an individual plan meeting, the knowledge that assessment of individual needs was not to be the result of professional assessment alone, and the chance to help shape strategic thinking and operational planning were principles receiving widespread support. However, the consultative arrangements were seen as a key link in ensuring that new resources would be available. Without the link, it is doubtful whether this major experiment would have succeeded to the extent that it has.

There were inevitable frustrations about the time and effort required to establish new structures for planning, and this led to delays in formulating local plans: new services did not come on stream as quickly as many people would have liked. Even so, families welcomed the increased contact with the service system and the improved flow of information about service aims and intentions. It is only now, with the steady growth of new services, that the true gains to services, users and families can be gauged. This is the subject of continuing research in the Centre.

Researcher

Dr Morag McGrath

Centre for Social Policy Research and Development, University of Wales, Bangor, Gwynedd LL57 2DG. (0248 351151)

Publications

Grant, G. (1986) 'Joint teams with joint budgets? The case of the All Wales Strategy', in S. Hatch, and I. Allen (eds), *Health and Social Services Collaboration in Community Care*, London, Policy Studies Institute Report.

Grant, G. (1990) *Consumer Involvement and the All Wales Strategy: a research note for the All Wales Advisory Panel sub-group on Consumer Involvement*, University of Wales, Bangor, Centre for Social Policy Research and Development.

Grant, G. (1990) 'Hidden pearls: a personal view of the All Wales Strategy', *LLais*, **18**: 3–4.

Grant, G. (1990) 'Researching user and carer involvement in mental handicap services', in G. Wistow, and M. Barnes (eds), *Researching User Involvement*, Nuffield Institute for Health Service Studies, University of Leeds.

Grant, G., Humphreys, S., and McGrath, M. (eds) (1986) 'Community Mental Handicap Teams: Problems and Possibilities', in *Community Mental Handicap Teams: Theory and Practice*, Kidderminster, British Institute of Mental Handicap Conference Series.

Grant, G., Humphreys, S., and McGrath, M. (eds) (1986) *CMHTs: Theory and Practice*, Kidderminster, British Institute of Mental Handicap.

Grant, G., and Jenkins, S. (1990) 'Community Mental Handicap Teams: Involving Voluntary Organisations and the Community', in S. Brown, and G. Wistow (eds), *The Roles and Tasks of Community Mental Handicap Teams*, Aldershot, Avebury.

Grant, M., and McGrath, M. (1990) 'Need for respite care services for caregivers of persons with mental retardation', *American Journal on Mental Retardation*, **94**, 6: 638–648.

Grant, G., McGrath, M., and Humphreys, S. (1987) *Some initial findings of a survey of 190 families supporting people with a mental handicap in the Gwynedd vanguard area*, University of Wales, Bangor, Centre for Social Policy Research and Development.

Humphreys, S. (1987) 'Participation in Practice', *Social Policy and Administration*, **21**, 1: 28–39.

Humphreys, S., McGrath, M., and Grant, G. (1986) 'Reflections on an All Wales Strategy vanguard area', *Mental Handicap*, **14**: 143–147.

McGrath, M. (1988) 'CMHTs in Wales', *Mental Handicap*, **3**: 101–104.

McGrath, M. (1988) 'Inter-agency collaboration in the All-Wales Strategy', *Social Policy and Administration*, **22**, 1: 53–67.

McGrath, M. (1989) 'Consumer participation in service planning – the AWS experience', *Social Policy and Administration*, **1**: 67–89.

McGrath, M. (1989) 'Domiciliary support services', *Llais*, Sept/Oct.

McGrath, M. (1989) 'Models of domiciliary support – Providing support to individuals at home and their locality', in G. Evans (ed.), *Report of a conference*, Gregynog, Powys, jointly organized by CSPRD, Bangor and Mental Health in Wales, Applied Research Unit, Cardiff.

McGrath, M. (1991) *Multi-disciplinary Teamwork*, Aldershot, Avebury.

McGrath, M. (in press) 'Whatever happened to teamwork: reflections on CMHTs', *British Journal of Social Work*.

McGrath, M., and Grant, G. (1992) 'Supporting needs-led services: implications for planning and management systems', *Journal of Social Policy*, **21**, 1: 71–97.

McGrath, M., and Humphreys, S. (1990) 'CMHTs at work: the Welsh experience', in S. Brown, and G. Wistow (eds), *The Roles and Tasks of Community Mental Handicap Teams*, Aldershot, Avebury.

Ramcharan, P. (1991) 'Avoiding the fate of Sisyphus', *Llais*, Winter 1991, Issue 9.

Ramcharan, P. (1991) 'Individual Planning, the All Wales Strategy and the Community Care White Paper', *Llais*, Winter 1991, Issue 9.

Ramcharan, P., McGrath, M., and Grant, G. (eds) (1990) *Individual Planning and the All Wales Strategy in the light of the Community Care White Paper*, Report of a One-Day Conference held at Gregynog, Powys, 6 December.

Community Mental Handicap Teams: Organization and Operation

Community Mental Handicap Teams (CMHTs) evolved in the mid-1970s as a response to the fragmentation of services for people with learning disabilities, and awareness that services were at best partial. During the 1980s they became one of the central means for developing services for people with learning disabilities and testing ways of working in a multi-disciplinary context.

Multi-disciplinary teams

Individual planning

Collaboration

This research project investigated the organization of CMHTs, the working procedures which teams have developed and the impact which teams have made on the patterns of responsibilities which care agencies undertake. It included a major survey of CMHTs in England; the examination of the policies of social services departments and health authorities; and detailed case-studies of selected teams.

FINDINGS

The teams

In the late 1980s about 350 CMHTs were in existence and only 12 health authorities did not have one operating in their area. Almost all included a nurse and social worker and the majority involved either a clinical psychologist, a psychiatrist or both.

Table 1.19: *Professions Represented on CMHTs*

	% of teams
Nurse (CMHN)	94
Social Worker	92
Psychologist	69
Psychiatrist/MH consultant	52
Occupational therapist	43
Speech therapist	40
Physiotherapist	39
Other specialist therapist	4
Teacher	4
No. of Teams	303

There were a range of related models: small core-teams comprising one to four staff, extended teams of up to about ten workers and still larger collections of staff operating more as a service network than a team. The different types of CMHT did not appear to vary with respect to caseload.

Table 1.20 lists the issues which prompted the formation of CMHTs.

Table 1.20: *An Agenda of Issues*

- the remoteness of services from individuals and their families

- the difficulties faced by families and clients in accessing services

- the organizational and professional fragmentation of services, so that families and clients are unclear about who is doing what

- the discontinuity of services, so that families and clients fall into gaps between services

- the lack of extensive liaison between statutory agencies and voluntary or informal care networks

---

CMHTs have contributed substantially to the development of policies and services for people with learning disabilities. They have worked towards the *development of a service infrastructure*, the implementation of *individualized programme plans* and *the coordination of care systems*.

They have been active in the difficult but necessary task of appraising need – not only at the individual level, as part of casework, but by mapping out the structure of need within local populations through undertaking need surveys and compiling registers.

Table 1.21 shows some of the common characteristics of the teams which were studied.

Table 1.21: *Common Characteristics*

- referral routes of clients to teams are different for social-worker members compared with community-nurse members;

- there is little case reallocation amongst members of the team;

- social workers and nurses develop different patterns for visiting clients and families

- nurses and social workers keep separate case record systems and use different methods for recording case details

---

For many CMHTs the team framework does little to alter the traditional and separate approaches to professional practice which have existed between health and social service staff. Their experience points to three general conclusions about multi-disciplinary teams:

1. Without clearly-defined roles, team members will drift towards the common ground between them.

2. Where team members have no actual or perceived authority to coordinate services, they will create their own service niche to fill.

3. Where a team has little direct control over service resources, its own role will be limited to using its personnel as resources.

Management and Support

Management provides a key to fostering effective multi-disciplinary working. Many CMHTs suffered from the differences in the style and culture of management between different professions. It proved difficult to establish common patterns of accountability, both between line-managers and fieldworkers and between middle and higher management.

Some solutions lie in the clarification of roles, responsibilities and objectives within teams. More comprehensive and shared information systems, and the establishment of performance indicators and standards are helpful, and can lead to improved communication.

Resources and Access to Them

Lack of resources – both in terms of services or money – caused some teams to focus on service delivery at the expense of service provision, and others to revert to familiar individual case work. A vicious circle may be created. Team members believe (sometimes rightly) that they cannot create the resources they need, and stop trying: the momentum for service change and improvement may be lost. Problems are made worse if team members from different professions and agencies do not have access to all available resources.

CONCLUSIONS

CMHTs have managed to protect resources and services for people with learning disabilities during a period of severe resource constraint. They have focused attention on important policy goals: the need for inter-professional cooperation and more responsive and comprehensive community services.

Most of the work done by most of the teams is not highly skilled or specialist, which may reflect the constraints mentioned above. It is also a response to a real need for routine surveillance, combined with help and advice to clients or families as everyday problems arise.

In the increasingly sophisticated world of community care management, simple services should not be overlooked. Resource allocation decisions must, therefore, be based on reliable information concerning need. Effective service delivery also requires clarity and mutual understanding about the contributions that can be made by different professions, understanding of the professional cultures that shape formal procedures, and careful scrutiny of patterns of work. CMHTs provide an example of one possible model.

Researchers

Stephen Brown and Terri Griffiths
Contact: Dr Jill Vincent and Professor Robert Walker

Centre for Research in Social Policy, Department of Social Sciences, Loughborough University of Technology, Loughborough, Leicestershire LE11 3TU. (0509 223372; FAX 0509 238277)

Publications

Brown, S. (1987) *Case Management Practice: An Examination of Casework in CMHTs*, CRSP Working Paper.

Brown, S. (1988) *Professional Orientations to the Casework Task*, CRSP Working Paper.

Brown, S. (1990) Community Mental Handicap Teams: CRSP Practice Papers Series:
  Number One: *Variations on a Theme*
  Number Two: *Professions in Teams*
  Number Three: *The Developmental Role*
  Number Four: *Managing Care*

Brown, S. (1990) *Community Mental Handicap Teams in England: A Register of Information*, CRSP Working Paper.

Brown, S., and Wistow, G. (1990) 'Horses for Courses', in S. Brown, and G. Wistow (eds), *The Roles and Tasks of CMHTs*, Aldershot, Gower.

Brown, S., and Wistow, G. (1990) *The Roles and Tasks of CMHTs*, Aldershot, Gower.

Care in the Community for People with Learning Disabilities: the Implications for Direct-Care Staff

The study was concerned with two groups of staff. The first group worked in an NHS long-stay hospital, which was subject to a closure programme; the second group worked in a new, local authority, staffed housing scheme, providing care in the community to people discharged from the hospital.

The project covered a wide range of issues relating to staff and their recruitment, management, training and morale. An intensive study was carried out which included unstructured observation, a postal survey with a standardized question-naire, and extended interviews with a random sample of hospital and community staff and with management of the two organizations. A full report was prepared and the results were published as the book *Care Staff in Transition*.[8]

Recruitment and Organization

We found that the recruitment of age- and gender-appropriate staff was difficult in the community; young women were the most likely employees. High rates of mobility helped produce a very unstable organization, which had high turnover. Organizational stability in the hospital was largely due to factors which could be duplicated to some extent in community services. These factors were:

- the employment of part-time staff, usually women with young dependent children; and
- the organization of the work around a variety of shift-working arrangements.

The flexibility of the shifts suited part-time women who subsequently remained in service for much longer periods than full-time staff. We noted that part-time staff were often marginalized within the service, and that this was a short-sighted view.

A fixed shift system – such as the traditional social services model involving 'sleep-in shifts' – lost this advantage. The scale of community operation also implied a lack of flexibility in staffing. A pool of available staff would provide back-up in the community, and more variety in shift patterns would permit the employment of less mobile staff.

The small units typical of the community service were much more sensitive to client behaviours. Even quite mild behavioural oddities could cause big disruptions and increases in staff stress. The shift system involving residential sleep-in exacerbated this problem, since staff could find themselves isolated for long periods. This highlights the importance of having back-up staff and expert assistance.

Hospital closure

Staff stress

Training and support

---

[8] For details, see *Publications*, page 77.

Ex-hospital staff were appropriate employees in the community setting, but all staff in the community needed an adequate induction programme. This was because the service was new and the job itself was evolving. Consequently, there was considerable ambiguity in the role assigned to basic-care staff who have to perform as independent practitioners.

We found that the stress experienced by community staff was best predicted by levels of ambiguity. We further found that those who reported the highest levels of ambiguity and isolation were subsequently more likely to leave the service. We also found that those who had been given a one-week induction training felt less ambiguity in their role and were less likely to leave the community service. Thus the stress and dissatisfaction in the job, and the consequent high turnover, could be reduced by an induction programme.

Hospital Closure

Within hospitals that are evolving new methods, or closing down, the villa/ward managers were clearly identified as the critical staff grade. They should be the prime targets for managerial support and training resources, especially with regard to the managerial aspects of their role.

There is a very real need for management to emphasize that services are in transition rather than in decline, since the latter is not only incorrect, but leads to a narrow focus among staff and low morale. Staff need to know, in advance, what the precise strategy is; and they need to be allocated to new roles well in advance.

Because new community services must work closely with traditional hospitals, there are many opportunities for professional conflicts. Disagreements tend to centre on the practicalities of providing the 'right service'. Early clarification at all levels of the proposals, to deal with the *most challenging clients* is likely to be the most effective intervention that planners can make in ensuring cooperation between service providers.

A key theme of the study was *uncertainty*: this was the major feature underlying the problems we discovered. Policy and strategic uncertainty was mirrored in tactical uncertainty within the declining hospital service. Detailed advance planning was lacking. Uncertainty over the role expectations in the community also led to lower staff morale and heightened turnover. Basic grade staff cannot be expected to 'make the job up' on their own and supervisors cannot be expected to manage them without appropriate training and support.

Researchers

Peter Allen, Jan Pahl and Lyn Quine

Centre for Health Services Studies, University of Kent, Cornwallis Building, Canterbury CT2 7NZ. (0227 764000)

Publications

Allen, P., Pahl, J., and Quine, L. (1988) *Staff in the Mental Handicap Services: a Study of Change*, University of Kent, Centre for Health Services Studies.

Allen, P., Pahl, J., and Quine, L. (1990) *Care Staff in Transition*, London, HMSO.

Allen, P., Pahl, J., and Quine, L. (1990) 'Long stay hospital closure: managing the staff', *Health Services Management*, **86**, 2: 84–86.

Liaison and Continuity of Nursing Care

INTRODUCTION

Continuity of care between hospital and home is important to patients and clients as consumers of the service, to nurses in the development of their professional role and to managers of the service in making the best use of resources. The purpose of this study was to explore where the problems lay in ensuring continuity, and to identify the practical factors which would contribute to improved continuing care for patients moving between hospital and home.

Hospital discharge

Coordination

Health and social care

The research was carried out in two phases of two years each, between 1985 and 1989.

Phase 1: Hospital Community Liaison Links in Nursing

In the first two-year phase, the research covered:

- The concept and status of liaison nursing between hospital and community;
- current, existing patterns of liaison;
- the meaning of continuity of care to nurses working both in hospital and community.

Findings

The process of liaison consists of two key elements:

- communication between nurses in hospital and community;
- discharge planning for patients.

They are affected by three major concepts:

- community awareness of hospital staff, including—
  - knowledge of community services,
  - perceptions of the roles of community-based staff,
  - recognition of the effects of patients' home background on their subsequent health and well-being;

- attitudes and beliefs of hospital staff regarding the concept of continuity of care and its importance relative to the remainder of patient care;

- organizational factors – that is, the structure and setting in which liaison takes place.

Three models of liaison were identified, relating to the organizational structure within which liaison takes place.

Model 1

Liaison between nurses working in rural community hospitals, and those in the community was direct, with face-to-face interaction in a shared base.

There were no liaison nurses, nor was there seen to be any need for them, since communication of information and discharge planning was regarded as satisfactory.

Senior nurses had a liaison responsibility within an overall managerial framework.

Patients and staff were often a fairly static population and a high proportion of non-specialist nursing and medical care was provided.

Model 2

Nurses in district general hospitals communicated directly with those in the community for any continuing care arrangements.

There was no liaison nurse.

Communication on discharge was generally regarded as unsatisfactory by community nurses, who felt that the information they received was often inappropriate and lacking in both quality and quantity.

Model 3

Indirect liaison took place via liaison nurses between nurses in district general hospitals and the community.

The role of liaison nurses varied in content.

The amount of time spent on liaison ranged from full-time, to a half-day-a-week activity which comprised little more than a clerical function for passing on referrals to community nurses.

Liaison nurses were found to be most effective when functioning in a **support** role, helping hospital nurses to develop their community awareness and providing advice about community services. In this way, an element of responsibility for discharge planning remained with the hospital nurse.

These findings were fed into the second two-year phase of the study.

Phase 2: Liaison and Continuity of Nursing Care

This phase took the form of an action-research study. Hospital and community nurses and their managers were involved in identifying practice problems and issues in discharge planning and liaison, and in systematically evaluating change.

A small sample of patients was also interviewed to introduce a consumer perspective.

Findings

Many of the subjects identified as problems were common to all three groups. They are summarized below, together with the action taken by the group members.

Problem	Action
1. Verbal Communication	
The quality of personal communication was a recurrent problem, and the absence of it seen as a block to the transfer of the kind of information which promoted good discharge planning and continuity of care.	Ways of overcoming inadequacies included giving hospital-wards lists of community nurses with names, telephone numbers and best contact-times. Hospital staff were also asked to sign and date discharge forms so that community nurses would be able to contact a nurse who knew the details of a patient's care for any query.
2. Written Communication	
Discharge forms were the subject of lengthy discussion in all three areas. There was already a plethora of discharge forms being sent to unknown destinations for uncertain purposes.	Two groups felt that a nurse-to-nurse referral form with full nursing information was essential, and devised a document to be sent home with the patient. This would be retained at home, and be available at the time of a district nurse's first visit.
The internal postal system contributed to lengthy delays over short distances in another group.	Agreement was negotiated for discharge forms to health visitors to be sent by first-class mail.
3. Wasted Visits	
The absence of information given to district nurses by GPs when patients were admitted to hospital or died, resulted in unnecessary visits and often caused distress to nurses, relatives and neighbours.	A number of solutions were discussed and developed between district nurses and GPs: — coloured stickers on notes of patients visited by community nurses; — whiteboard for GPs to write names of patients admitted to hospital; — weekly computer-lists of patients visited by district nurses.
4. Duplicated Visits	
On a number of occasions, visits by district nurses and health visitors were duplicated.	Regular meetings were arranged in one group to examine patients' records for the appropriate visit. Where district nurses and health visitors were in separate bases, meetings proved more difficult.

Problem	**Action**

5. Role of the Health Visitor

Hospital nurses in all groups expressed concern about incomplete knowledge of the role of the health visitor and – especially in relation to the elderly – their consequent inability to assess whether it was appropriate to refer patients to her.	The three groups proposed different solutions: — all new staff members and those already in post should be offered a short period of time with a health visitor; — sisters/charge nurses should be invited to accompany a health visitor for a day; — student nurses should be informed during training in order to create awareness in future qualified staff.

Clarification of the health visitor's role also highlighted the lack of differentiation between health visiting and social work, and generated discussion about appropriate referral.

As provision of health care becomes increasingly varied, it will be even more important for one individual to be responsible for liaison. The liaison nurse could become a key figure in monitoring specified standards of care in contracts which cover hospital and community care. The difficulty of defining role boundaries between health and social services in community care was highlighted in the action-research study. Health and social needs are interlinked, and with changing community care and the development of case-management, it will become increasingly important for health and social services staff to communicate effectively. Agreement will be needed on joint assessment, monitoring and evaluation procedures.

Researcher

Dr Sue Armitage

Temple of Peace and Health, Cathays Park, Cardiff CF1 3NW. (0222 231021; FAX 0222 238608)

Publications

Chapters:

Armitage, S. K. (1991) 'Conclusion: Liaison in Context', in S. K. Armitage (ed.), *Continuity of Nursing Care*, London, Scutari Press.

Jowett, S. A., and Armitage, S. K. (1991) 'The Liaison Complex', in S. K. Armitage (ed.), *Continuity of Nursing Care*, London, Scutari Press.

Articles:

Armitage, S. K. (1989) 'Liaison Nurse: The Key to Continuity of Care', *Good Practices in Community Nursing*, Community Nursing Monograph Number Two, Department of Nursing, University of Manchester.

Armitage, S. K., and Jowett, S. A. (1987) 'Liaison Links between Hospital and Community', (short report), *Nursing Times*, **83**, 41: 66–67.

Armitage, S. K., and Jowett, S. A. (1988) 'Hospital/Community Liaison links in Nursing', Unpublished research report.

Armitage, S. K., and Jowett, S. A. (1988) 'Hospital/Community Liaison links in Nursing: the role of the liaison nurse', *Journal of Advanced Nursing*, **13**, 5: 579–587.

Armitage, S. K. and Jowett, S. A. (1989) 'Liaison Links in Nursing', *Primary Health Care*, **7**, 1: 6.

Armitage, S. K., and Williams, L. (1989) 'Action Research', (short report), *Nursing Times*, **85**, 22: 54.

Armitage, S. K., and Williams, L. (1990) 'Communication in primary health care', *Nursing Times*, **5**, 1: 34–35.

Armitage, S. K., and Williams, L. (1990) 'Liaison and Continuity of Nursing Care', Unpublished research report.

Development of Community Schemes

This project examined the feasibility of using community-based schemes as a means for achieving flexibility, variety, and choice in service provision. It considered the management, organization, staffing and practice implications for social services if this approach is to become a commonplace and important feature in the work of area offices.

SSD area offices

Elderly people

The project found that there were more schemes in area offices that had high overall staffing levels; a high proportion of specialist staff; were located in the more rural areas; had given a 'lot of effort' to formal inter-agency liaison; and had a forum open to the public.

The project also found that social workers were more likely to be involved in schemes in areas:—

- which were organized on a geographical basis;

- where the team leader was perceived as encouraging such work;

- where social work attitudes favoured a community approach;

- where there was a formal workload measurement system; time off *in lieu* or overtime were recognized; and there had been a formal assessment of the needs of the area.

The qualitative material suggested that the success of strategies for promoting schemes for elderly people was likely to depend on the commitment of the area manager, the knowledge of community groups and key personnel in outside organizations, the protection of staff from competing demands, funding for the rent of suitable premises, and the general social context – for example, the availability of volunteers.

Researchers

David Crosbie and Anne Vickery

National Institute for Social Work, Mary Ward House, 5–7 Tavistock Place, London WC1H 9SS. (071 387 9681; FAX 071 387 7968)

Publications

Crosbie, D., and Vickery, A. (1988) 'Schemes in area offices: time and partnerships required to undertake schemes', in P. Wedge (ed.), *Social Work – A Third Look at Research into Practice*, Proceedings of the Third Annual Joint Universities Council – British Association of Social Workers Conference. Birmingham, BASW.

Crosbie, D., and Vickery, A. (1989) 'Community Based Schemes in Area Offices', (report to DH), London, National Institute for Social Work Research Unit.

Crosbie, D., Vickery, A. V., and Sinclair, I. A. C. (1988) 'Schemes and social workers: issues of time, pressure and training', *Social Work Education*, **7**, 3: 30–34.

Miller, C., Crosbie, D., and Vickery, A. (1991) *Everyday Community Care: A Manual for Mangers*, London, NISW.

Sinclair, I., Crosbie, D., and Vickery, A. (1990) 'Organisational influences on professional behaviour: factors affecting social work involvement in schemes', *Journal of Social Policy*, **19**, 361–374.

The Development and Implementation of a Consumer-Orientated Inter-Agency Strategy on Community care

Progress Report

The Birmingham Community Care Special Action Project (CCSAP) was a time-limited project established to develop an inter-agency, user-orientated strategy for community care. The establishment of CCSAP was prompted by an awareness of an actual and increasing shortfall in resources available to provide community care services.

Consumer views
Evaluation
Agency change

A small project team was established which saw its underlying purpose as changing the culture of service provision, and challenging the bureaucracy. The evaluation was established in order to learn from Birmingham's experience, and to facilitate the further implementation of such a strategy in Birmingham and elsewhere.

The Evaluation

From our initial analysis of CCSAP, we identified four dimensions of the project which we are using to structure the evaluation.

◆ *Community care* – what are the principles on which the policy should be based and how have these been applied in practical service developments.

◆ *User involvement* – who has been involved, what has been the process of involvement, and what have been the outcomes of this for the users and carers themselves, as well as for service development and for the service organizations involved.

◆ *The inter-agency approach* – what agencies/departments have been involved and what has this meant for inter-agency working as well as for the development of community care policy and practice.

◆ *CCSAP's role as a time-limited catalyst* aiming to have an impact on the development of mainstream services.

These dimensions are being studied through an analysis of four key streams of activity initiated by CCSAP.

1. *A series of consultations with carers.* These consultations led the definition of '11 Action Points' on which the city committed itself to take action. The evaluation is looking at the mechanisms set up to promote action, and what progress has been made in response to the key problem areas defined by carers. In addition, questionnaires have been sent to all carers attending the consultations, and interviews have been conducted with a random sample of those responding to the questionnaires.

2. *Developments in day-services for people with learning disabilities* arising from a review undertaken by CCSAP. Developments have focused on two day-centres and on a team of community placement officers in one part of the city. The evaluation has been looking at, for example, changes in the type and range of activities available to people attending the centres; the extent to which resources outside the centres are being accessed to increase the range of options available;

users' perceptions of any changes that have taken place and their ability to participate in decision-making in the centres; and users' perceptions of the extent to which they have broadened their activities and increased control over aspects of their lives through the assistance of the community placement officers.

3. *Employment and training initiatives for people with disabilities*. These initiatives also result in part from comments made by service users during the review of day-services. The major focus of the evaluation is on the inter-agency dimension of these initiatives.

4. *Initiatives designed to give users of mental health services a voice* in service development and provision. The evaluation will focus primarily on the different models of user involvement explored in these initiatives.

The development of monitoring systems to enable both providers and users to review the development of services in terms of CCSAP principles was intended to be a significant part of the evaluation. The definition of evaluation criteria and performance indicators and the design of monitoring instruments are therefore in themselves outcomes of the research.

Researchers

Dr Marian Barnes and Mr Gerald Wistow

Nuffield Institute of Health Services, University of Leeds, Fairbairn House, 71–75 Clarendon Road, Leeds LS2 9PL. (0532 459034; FAX 0532 460899)

Publications

Barnes, M., and Wistow, G. (1991) *Changing Relationships in Community Care. An interim account of the Community Care Special Action Project*, Working Paper No 3, Nuffield Institute for Health Services Studies, University of Leeds.

Barnes, M., and Wistow, G., (forthcoming) 'Sustaining Innovation in Community Care, *Local Government Policy Making*.

Barnes, M., and Wistow, G. (forthcoming) 'Consulting with Carers. What do they think?', *Social Services Research*.

Barnes, M., and Wistow, G. (eds) (forthcoming) *Researching User Involvement*, a collection of papers from a conference at the Nuffield Institute, October 1990.

Jowell, T., and Wistow, G. (1989) 'Give them a voice', *Insight*, **4**, 7: 22–24.

Jowell, T., and Wistow, G. (1990) 'The Total Service', *Insight*, **5**, 4: 22–23.

Wistow, G., and Barnes, M. (1991) *Consumers, Citizens or Survivors. User Involvement and Cultural Change in Community Care*, Paper presented at a conference of the European Group for Public Administration, The Hague, August 1991.

Support for Self-Help: Evaluation of 18 Local Self-Help Support Projects (SHA)

Local networks

Voluntary sector

This programme was one element in the DHSS Helping the Community to Care Initiative, which was announced in July 1984. There were 18 self-help support projects set up across England, evaluated by the Tavistock Institute. The Institute adopted a developmental approach to the evaluation, and encouraged self-evaluation by local projects, while retaining a more conventional research role involving surveys, reports and so on. The research team contributed to the task of the development workers and they – in turn – contributed to the research task. Many of them were partners in a series of research groups formed to explore specific themes and issues.

The main purpose of the programme was to test the effectiveness of a general local support function for self-help in the context of community care. Specific questions to be considered included the influence of the characteristics of the locality; what methods were effective in different conditions; the match between group needs and support; and how to mobilize local professionals and statutory bodies. Support needs of development workers were also considered as well as more general questions about the *limits* of self-help. The extent to which self-help groups were relevant to the health needs of some populations where they were relatively undeveloped – ethnic minorities, for example – was another focus.

FINDINGS

Local projects achieved their overall aims in five broad areas: in setting up *new* groups; in providing support to *existing* groups; in providing support to a *very wide range* of groups; in *networking* – linking groups to each other and to professionals; and in *raising the profile* of self-help locally.

The wide-ranging support services provided included: **information, advice, practical help, office assistance, acting as a go-between, skills development, emotional support, leadership**.

The characteristics of the worker were crucial to the effectiveness of a local self-help initiative. These included: preferred modes of working, conception of self-help, ideology, ethnicity, gender, local knowledge. The first three at least are interconnected: a worker who enjoys taking a development role within groups will tend to adopt or adapt a conception of self-help consistent with that role.

The characteristics of the group interacting with the worker were also relevant: some focused on empowerment, others on therapy, adjustment to a disabling condition, or respite. These interests were not mutually exclusive, and – in the first three cases – were often combined with an interest in education. Ethnicity was another important variable.

The nature of the support provided is primarily a product of the interaction between the characteristics of the worker and the group. But both of course are part of larger systems or networks which affect the transactions between them.

The characteristics of the host agency, within which the project is located, included size, extent of involvement with local voluntary and statutory sectors, the priority given to the project, structure and management, supervision/support, policies and objectives, ethnicity, ideology.

A *laissez-faire* style of management funded gives the worker ample discretion but s/he will probably go elsewhere for support and supervision. A traditional welfare ideology may conflict with the community development ethos of some practitioners. While a participative mode of management may fit in well with the egalitarian focus of self-help among some ethnic minority communities, it is not a feasible approach for an agency which sets objectives for numbers of new groups formed. A black worker will find it difficult to relate to black groups if s/he is operating from a predominantly white agency which does not have credibility with local black communities.

Group affiliations may also be part of the transaction: e.g. membership of a national self-help organization, relations with other local support services, and so on.

Demographic variables are of course relevant – urban/rural distinction, ethnicity, social class. As is the case with many ethnic minorities, effective self-help in dispersed rural populations is achieved not by imposing conventional models, but by building on existing social forms. Segregated working-class communities are more likely to produce generalist groups, orientated towards mutual aid and campaigning. Single-issue groups affiliated to national organizations tend to have a middle-class bias; non-affiliated groups can attract a broader membership provided that they meet in a socially 'neutral' location.

The local pattern of institutions is a second element in the common environment: strength of the local voluntary sector, statutory-voluntary relations, local tradition of self-help.

The factors summarized here form the basis of a contingency theory which makes it possible to recognize connections among a range of variables which impinge directly or indirectly on effective support, and to make predictions.

The qualitative and quantitative data suggest that local support projects can have a distinctive and significant role in self-help support in at least three respects:

— Support strategies can be specific to characteristics of the local population and conditions and can target special needs. For example, a local project can introduce self-help as part of a package of mental health services in planned discharge of psychiatric patients.

— Through independent assessment of local needs, they can promote or support groups for conditions not covered by national organizations, and they can provide specific local support for groups that do have national affiliation.

— Participation in and development of local networks of voluntary and statutory workers enables them to link groups to agencies, services and individual workers relevant to the group's needs. They can also promote networks between groups. Even if a fixed-life support project is not refunded, such networks and connections will often persist.

Research Team

F. Abraham, D. Hills, E. Miller, E. Sommerlad, E. Stern and B. Webb

Tavistock Institute of Human Relations, The Tavistock Centre, 120 Belsize Lane, London NW3 5BS. (071 435 7111; FAX 071 794 4661)

Publications

Abraham, F. (1989) *Delivering Self Help Support: The First Year in the Life of the Self Help Alliance*, Tavistock Occasional Papers.

Abraham, F., and Sommerlad, E. (1989) *Self Help Support and Black People: Start-up strategies in four SHA projects*, Tavistock Occasional Papers.

Abraham, F., and Webb, B. (1989) *Self Help and Mental Health*, Tavistock Occasional Papers.

Hills, D., and Stern, E. (1988) *Self Help in Rural Areas*, Tavistock Occasional Papers.

Miller, E. (1987) *Support for Self-Help: The Origins and Develpment of the Self Help Alliance*, Tavistock Occasional Papers.

Miller, E., and Webb, B. (1988) *Effective Self Help Support in Different Contexts*, Tavistock Occasional Papers.

Sommerlad, E., and Hills, D. (1990) *Managing an innovative Project: issues in the relationship between host organizations and projects*, Tavistock Occasional Papers.

Opportunities for Volunteering: Monitoring and Evaluation

Origins of the Scheme

The Department of Health's Opportunities for Volunteering scheme started in 1982 as a short-term, experimental programme costing £3.3m for one year in England. (Scotland, Northern Ireland and Wales had their own separate arrangements). Today it has a budget of £6.7m per annum and contributes to the funding of over 400 projects. The scheme has three main aims: to develop opportunities for unemployed people to do voluntary work; to expand voluntary work in the health and personal social services; and to 'pump-prime' new schemes. Grants are restricted to voluntary sector participants.

The scheme's administrative arrangements are a pragmatic response to the wide variation in institutional arrangements in the voluntary sector. An original feature of the scheme is the delegation of decisions on funding local voluntary projects to national voluntary bodies (table 1.22).

Voluntary sector

Costs

Efficiency/ effectiveness

Table 1.22: *The Agents for Opportunities for Volunteering*

Age Concern
Barnardo's
British Association of Settlements and Social Action Centres (BASSAC)
Church of England Children's Society
Community Service Volunteers (CSV)
Consortium (General Fund) – representing intermediary bodies
Council of Churches in Britain and Ireland (CCBI) – for schemes sponsored by churches
MENCAP
MIND
National Association for the Care and Resettlement of Offenders (NACRO)
National Association of Leagues of Hospital Friends (NALHF)
Panel of Four – representing people with impaired hearing
Pre-school Playgroups' Association (PPA)
RADAR
Royal National Institute for the Blind (RNIB)
Spastics Society

Monitoring the Scheme

The research brief has evolved over the life of the project, in light of developments in the nature of the scheme and the changing requirements of policy customers in the Department of Health:

1. Answers were required to a set of open questions, including
    'Does this method of funding work?'
    'Do local projects receive suitable grants?'
    'Do they do what they said they would?'

'Are the conditions of the scheme being met?'

'What do the voluntary projects do – can you describe the range and content of the work?'

2. The Department wanted 'management information' rather than research results, including a continuous flow of information on how the money was being spent each year; the size of projects in £s, numbers of volunteers, client-groups served, type of service, and so on.

3. The Department of Health asked for advice based on research activity as a contribution to the consideration of specific policy questions – for example: should the annual programme be changed to a three-year, rolling one; can the scheme be aimed more specifically at the inner cities, or young unemployed people; and (most difficult) is it 'efficient', and how can efficiency be increased?

4. Finally, the research team has been working with agents to promote self-evaluation of projects and to disseminate good practice.

Insights and Lessons

*   The method of delegated funding has been shown to work: the voluntary sector can be relied upon to set up and manage community projects subject to departmental conditions. The scheme has probably added several per cent to the total number of paid organizers of volunteers, and supports about half to one-quarter per cent of the total number of people volunteering in a month. This constitutes value for money. According to the Charities Aid Foundation, a total of about £1b is directed to service-providing and volunteer-deploying bodies, yet the current budget for Opportunities for Volunteering is only £6.7m. Such arguments have provided the basis for the continuation of the scheme, and there is abundant evidence that it is popular with the participating voluntary bodies.

*   The projects funded through Opportunities for Volunteering not only reflect the Department of Health's interests, but also the pattern of voluntary activity in England, which in turn reflects a pattern of constraints. In 1989/90, about 32 per cent of projects served old people as their main client-group, 22 per cent children and families, 14 per cent physically-handicapped people and smaller percentages for people with learning disabilities or mental illnesses, women and minority ethnic groups. Projects primarily provide day-care or activities based in centres (58 per cent) while only a quarter offer domiciliary (home-visiting) services. Recruiting volunteers to visit and support clients in their own homes, while not impossible, has been shown by the research to be inherently more difficult than centre-based activity. This is especially true if a significant proportion of the volunteers are unemployed people looking for something to do and not initially committed to the client-group.

*   It has been found that, to be practicable, a voluntary project usually requires funding for at least one member of paid staff, plus associated running costs. It therefore needs a budget of £10,000–£15,000 per annum. One member of paid staff can usually recruit, deploy and support between 10 and 30 volunteers depending on the difficulty of the task in hand; on the whole it is easier to deploy more volunteers in a club for reasonably healthy old people, for example, than in a scheme to befriend ex-psychiatric patients. The more demanding the volunteer-client relationship, the fewer the volunteers in the scheme.

*   Many voluntary organizations are keen to take on community care duties and purchase-of-service arrangements, and serve the needs of their clients as efficiently as possible. But, as community-based organizations, they do not always respond to bureaucratic demands as easily as community care policy-makers might wish.

- Most voluntary organizations remain quite small, with only small numbers of paid staff. They find it more difficult to respond to changes in policy at short notice and are organizationally 'fragile': a small cut in income or a change in suggested working methods might spell disaster. They depend heavily on support and advice on matters such as management, accountancy, training, contracts, health and safety, from either a national body like Age Concern England, or specialist agencies such as the Volunteer Centre UK. It is also true that the provision of these functions attracts less funding than the agencies would wish.

The Opportunities for Volunteering scheme has been shown to be an effective, efficient and popular mechanism for funding the development of voluntary work; and the close link between research and policy has helped the scheme to adapt to changing circumstances. The evaluation has *not* supported the notion that thousands of volunteers can be summoned to the assistance of community care at little cost, but suggests that the intrinsic characteristics of voluntary organizations necessarily impose constraints on what can be achieved and the method of achieving it. A well-resourced infrastructure to support individual projects and organizations is also of vital importance.

Researchers

Katherine Gaskin, Ian Mocroft and Andrew Shaw

Centre for Research in Social Policy, Department of Social Sciences, Loughborough University of Technology, Loughborough, Leicestershire LE11 3TU. (0509 223372; FAX 0509 238277)

Publications

Doyle, M. (1988) *Some Pointers for Evaluation*, CRSP, OFV42.

Doyle, M., and Mocroft, I. (1987) *A Directory of Projects Funded in 1987–88*, CRSP, OFV21.

Doyle, M., and Mocroft, I. (1987) *Opportunities for Volunteering 1987–88*, CRSP, OFV4.

Doyle, M., and Mocroft, I. (1988) *A Directory of Projects Funded in 1988–89*, CRSP, OFV22.

Doyle, M., and Mocroft, I. (1988) *Opportunities for Volunteering 1988–89*, CRSP, OFV29.

Doyle, M., and Mocroft, I. (1988) *OFV: A Model for Funding the Voluntary Sector*, CRSP, OFV34.

Doyle, M., and Mocroft, I. (1988) *Towards Performance Indicators and Assessable Competencies*, Paper 1, CRSP, OFV32.

Doyle, M., and Mocroft, I. (1989) *Future Funding of Time Expired Projects*, CRSP, OFV35.

Doyle, M., Mocroft, I., and Shaw, A. (1990) *A Directory of Projects Funded in 1988–90*, CRSP, OFV33.

Griffiths, C.T.A (1988) *OFV Preliminary Evaluation of the Project Progress Reports*, CRSP, OFV43.

Mocroft, I., and Doyle, M. (1988) *National Agents Administration of the Opportunities for Volunteering Scheme 1987–88*, CRSP, OFV41.

Mocroft, I., and Doyle, M. (1988) 'Opportunities for Volunteering: A Case Study of the Voluntary Sector', *Health Care UK*, CRSP, OFV31.

Chapter 2

Elderly People

Elderly People

Research summarized in this Chapter covers a whole range of issues relating to the health and social care of elderly people, and reflects the importance of this group in the development of policy on community care. The needs of 'young' elderly as well as frail elderly people are covered by some projects; and the special situation of elderly people from ethnic minorities is the focus of one review, and an element in several others. An extensive review of literature about community care provision for older people in England and Wales, undertaken as part of an EC-wide project, opens the Chapter.

A number of studies have been undertaken which 'map' or evaluate existing services: nursing homes and hospices, private and voluntary residential care, continuing-care accommodation, and multi-purpose homes. Innovations in domiciliary care, projects included in the Welsh Office Elderly Initiative, services relevant to discharge from hospital, or which promote rehabilitation back to the community – all of these have been the subject of research included here.

Other summaries report work which has focused in detail on the elderly people themselves – their health status, their services histories, their views of services and their opportunities to exercise real choice. The problem of the possible abuse of elderly people is raised by one review.

Literature Review of Community Care for Old People in England and Wales (EC Project)

SUMMARY

Quality of life
Informal care
Mixed economy

Background

More than 59 million people over the age of 60 live in the European Community. Problems encountered in implementing effective community care for the minority of these people who are frail provided the impetus for an EC-sponsored programme of research (Age Care Research Europe [ACRE]) into care-delivery systems for them. Nine countries participated in this programme. A major review of the research literature, undertaken by the NISW Research Unit represents part of the English–Welsh contribution. The review covered provision of services by the statutory, voluntary and private sectors and the demographic, historical and socio-economic policy context in which these services are delivered.

The findings are documented in four reports to the Department of Health* which, together with overviews of the historical and social and economic policy context, were published as *The Kaleidoscope of Care* (Sinclair, *et al.*, 1990). This book also includes additional material on housing provision and reviews of the finances available to elderly people for their care, and of services to black and minority ethnic elders.

Issues

Key issues examined included the demographic distribution of elderly people, their disabilities, their housing, and their financial situation; the steps that old people and their carers take to overcome their problems; the quality of life of old people and what determines this quality.

Analysis shows that certain groups of elderly people experience cumulative disadvantage. Serious difficulties such as malnutrition or hypothermia often occur as a result of a combination of disadvantages, including physical frailty and low income. Their difficulties are at least partly structured by features of society – for example, the housing market – whose influence is not restricted to old age. Whereas most old people are capable of looking after themselves, others would find it easier given adequate housing and better incomes.

The case-study of services for black and minority ethnic elders illustrates these processes. The literature is patchy, but it confirms the cultural heterogeneity of ageing and shows that elders experience the 'triple jeopardy' of suffering racism, disadvantages in housing, health, employment and pensions, and services that are not tailored to their general and specific needs. Equality and ethnic record-keeping and monitoring programmes are not as developed as they might be, although there has been progress in this area. *Ad hoc* 'schemes' may compensate, in the short term, for the disadvantages elders face in getting the services appropriate to their needs.

---

* For details, see *Publications*, pages 98, 99.

They do little to counteract the negative processes at earlier points in life – for instance, in relation to housing and employment – which lead to such disadvantages.

However, not all dependency is structured in this sense. Physical and mental frailty does increase with age; and those suffering severe dementia, for example, cannot look after themselves however rich and well-housed they may be.

Solutions proposed for these problems have included greater reliance on informal care, the promotion of independence, improved targeting by the statutory sector and the development of the voluntary and independent sectors. In order to cope with the increasing number of severely handicapped old people, statutory services, in alliance with carers, may need to be targeted on the 5 or so in every 100 who require concentrated short-term help. The longer-term needs of others might be met through the voluntary sector and through the purchase of services, adaptations to accommodation and labour-saving equipment, which would be made possible by the increasing prosperity of old people. By these means, structured dependency might be reduced, carers assisted and services targeted to those who need them most. The book (Sinclair, *et al.* 1990) considers these 'solutions'.

Informal Care and the Promotion of Independence

Care for frail, elderly people by informal carers is, above all, local – a matter of personal contact, co-residence and proximity of support. Care at a distance is manifestly insufficient if the old people need concentrated short-term help, and exhausting if they have regular needs. Heavy care is predominantly a matter for spouses and local daughters. These carers, however, drift into caring and do not generally take old people into their homes specifically in order to care for them. Neighbourly help, while important, is limited in scope and quantity – a situation which fits the wishes of both neighbours and old people. The scope for *increasing* the amount of informal care given to old people who are not living with their spouses and do not have a child nearby is very limited.

However, the scope for *enhancing* informal care seems greater; services can support, supplement and complement carers. More generally, taxation, pensions or social security policy can aim to reward, or at least not penalize carers.

Similar considerations apply to the promotion of independence. Old people's determination to cope is formidable and there is much room for assisting this and relieving the burden it imposes. This, however, is likely to impose additional costs on social services rather than reducing them.

Care and the Statutory Sector

Statutory domiciliary services are reviewed, both as a set of discrete services and as a system of related services which together aim to enable very frail, old people to remain outside residential care. Individual services are generally relevant to the needs of old people, appreciated by them, and effective at reducing particular problems. Considered as a system, services are inadequate in quantity, ill-coordinated at the level of planning, procedures and individual cases, and have paid little attention to enabling old people to do things for themselves. Overall, statutory services do not make systematic provision for: the nagging anxieties of old people (for instance about their gardens); help with bereavement – a major source of unhappiness; certain needs of carers; intensive services over a range of need, or emergency alternatives to residential care which would enable decisions about residential care to be taken other than under the pressure to clear a hospital bed.

Experiments which provide integrated 'packages' of services tailored to particular circumstances have proved more effective, especially where packages are broadened rather than simply increased in quantity. Similarly, services such as day-care, relief care, and sheltered housing are a genuine alternative to residential care only if they form part of a package. A strategy of providing very frail people with such packages will increase costs unless either some less frail people are left without services they appear to need, or the services are directed with very great precision at those who would otherwise enter residential care.

Care and the Voluntary Sector

Despite its central place in recent policy, there is little specific information about the role and scale of the voluntary sector – seen here as including semi-formal organized groups and schemes, volunteers and voluntary organizations – and its contribution can only be assessed by distinguishing clearly between funding, service provision and regulation. Information sources and trends in charitable income illustrate its inherent uncertainty and the dramatic variation in local-authority spending on this sector. There are also wide variations in the provision of voluntary services which bear, if anything, an inverse relationship to need. There may, however, be considerable potential for the encouragement, and thus the redistribution, of voluntary activity when positive policies are adopted by local authorities.

At the level of services there is a need for more detailed research on the significance of assessment and matching, on volunteer training and support, and on the role of paid organizers. Reliable funding and securing referrals from professionals are probably the most significant problems for many voluntary organizations. There may also be difficulties in balancing the supply of appropriate clients with that of helpers. The lack of transport and adequate and acceptable carer cover seem likely to restrict the use of voluntary services and activities which involve leaving home. The distinction between 'in-home' and 'out-of-home' services is important. Greater reliance on the voluntary sector would, in many areas, require considerable investment in development.

The review suggests that the voluntary sector will not be able to ensure equity and wide coverage. A key dilemma is to achieve regulation and accountability without losing the flexibility so highly valued in voluntary activity. Purchase-of-service contracting may overcome weaknesses in the voluntary sector such as insufficient funding and regulation. However, research highlights the importance of improved procedures for ensuring accountability and for monitoring, to avoid the unintended and unfortunate consequences of this kind of contracting which have occurred in the USA.

Care and the Private Sector

The review of present and future levels of disposable income available to elderly people suggests that most have limited funds to spend on services. Those among them who have most need of services are particularly likely to be badly off. Those who have somewhat more money generally place services low on their list of priorities for spending. It is, further, suggested that any development of private services as an alternative to the statutory sector will either shift care away from its traditional recipients or require the private sector to become, effectively, a subsidized agent of the state.

There is a serious lack of information about private-for-profit care-services for elderly people. Developments in the private residential care sector in the 1980s were dramatically affected by changes in the social security system, particularly board-and-lodging allowances; while the private sector responded by rapid expansion, the voluntary sector of residential care did not. The difference in character between private and voluntary residential provision is important to policy-makers and, therefore, also to the way statistics are collected.

In contrast to the situation with residential care, the supply of *organized* private domiciliary help and care remains undeveloped. Unlike private residential care, it seems that the availability of a subsidy has not and would not stimulate its growth or its transformation into formally-organized enterprises. This makes it more difficult for local authorities to consider providing all or part of their domiciliary services by purchase from the private sector.

In general, the private sector is diverse, fragmented, prone to change and often unorganized, with many activities unrecorded. It is small scale, local and relies upon part-time female labour. There are gaps in knowledge about 'market conditions' relevant to planning domiciliary help comprehensively across the boundaries of a mixed economy of welfare. The sector has concentrated on residential rather than domiciliary care and there are massive variations in the extent of its provision between different local authorities or even within the same local authority. Since the private sector operates to make profit and to satisfy demand rather than need, it follows that it is difficult to incorporate it in any integrated plan that is concerned with the distribution of total welfare resources, whether nationally or locally.

CONCLUSION

The researchers concluded that all the proposed solutions had a contribution to make, but that none was of itself sufficient and none would reduce costs. Nor would the changes about to be introduced by the NHS and Community Care Act in themselves ensure an efficient, mixed economy of welfare. In their view, the focus of community care needs to be widened. Community care has failed to specify and achieve the standards of welfare which old people and their carers should expect. Services have not been considered in relation to wider aspects of welfare policy, notably pensions. A range of solutions based on a strong statutory sector will be needed to secure an adequate standard of care.

Researchers

Ian Sinclair – NISW (now at the University of York)
  Roy Parker – University of Bristol (commissioned)
  Diana Leat – Freelance and City University
  Jenny Williams – NISW

National Institute for Social Work, Mary Ward House, 5–7 Tavistock Place, London WC1H 9SS. (071 387 9681; FAX 071 87 7968)

Publications

Leat, D. (1989) *EEC Project, Report 3: Welfare Provision for the Elderly: The Contribution of the Voluntary Sector*, National Institute for Social Work Research Unit.

Parker, R. (1989) *EEC Project, Report 4: Welfare Provision for the Elderly: the Contribution of the Private Sector*, National Institute for Social Work Research Unit.

Sinclair, I., Parker, R., Leat, D., and Williams, J. (1990) *The Kaleidoscope of Care: A Review of Research on Welfare Provision for Elderly People*, London, HMSO.

Sinclair, I., and Williams, J. (1989) *EEC Project, Report 1: Welfare Provision for the Elderly: Social and Demographic Background*, National Institute for Social Work Research Unit.

Sinclair, I., and Williams, J. (1989) *EEC Project, Report 2: Welfare Provision for the Elderly: the Contribution of the Statutory Sector*, National Institute for Social Work Research Unit.

Elderly People – Choice, Participation and Satisfaction

Aim of the research

The purpose of the study was to examine the ways in which elderly people exercise choice in the care services they receive, both in the community and in residential care; the extent to which they participate in decisions about their care; and the extent to which they are satisfied with the care services they receive from all sources. The study was designed to contribute to the much wider debate about the issues of choice, participation and how to hear the voice of the consumer.

Design of the study

The main focus was on elderly people living at the margin of community and residential care. The study took place in three local authorities – an outer London borough, a southern county and a northern county.

We interviewed 100 elderly people in the community and 103 elderly people in residential care, half in local authority homes and half in private homes. We also interviewed 72 carers of elderly people in the community and 74 carers of elderly people in residential care. Finally, we interviewed 40 social workers, 11 domiciliary care organizers, 11 team managers, 19 heads of local authority homes and 24 heads of private homes.

Findings

- There was very little evidence that the elderly people we interviewed were able to operate as 'informed customers' in their use of care services, either in the community or in residential care. Elderly people and carers reported great difficulties in gaining **access to information** about community and residential services. There was a clear need for reliable written and oral information about community and residential care services.

Rationing of information was related to rationing of services and some professionals acknowledged that they did not want to raise expectations that could not be fulfilled. Social workers and domiciliary care organizers often only had a partial and selective knowledge of the community and residential services in their area. They were often reluctant to offer information about the private sector and knew little about the voluntary sector.

- Very few elderly people had extensive **packages of care** services: most elderly people had only one or two services, and some did not have anything in their package at all. There was a need for packages of care to be regularly monitored and reviewed. Some elderly people were entering residential care when they had had little or no support from community services.

- **Targeting of services** on those most in need was already taking place, but the implications of this had not always been assessed. Targeting of community care might well mean that other elderly people lack preventive services and enter residential care before they need to, particularly those being supported by relatives in the community who are less likely to receive services than elderly people living alone.

Packages of care
Targeting
Collaboration

- **'Enabling'** the independent sector in community care will not be easy. There was little evidence of use by elderly people of private or voluntary domiciliary or community services. Most elderly people, their carers and social workers thought that private services were in short supply and very expensive, particularly if personal care was involved. The provision of voluntary services was patchy and thought by social services staff to be contracting.

- Many elderly people had very small informal networks and some had no **informal care** available to them at all. The majority of elderly people interviewed were widowed and a substantial minority had never had children or had no living children. Most informal care devolved on one close female relative or on very elderly spouses.

- Many of the carers were very elderly themselves, with one quarter of the carers interviewed in the community being over 70 and one in ten over 80. Some elderly couples supporting each other were living in very precarious circumstances. More **support for carers** of all ages is needed, particularly respite care, an increase in services directed at the elderly people themselves, and more information on services and benefits.

- **Front-line professional workers need support** in their role of encouraging elderly people to participate in decisions about care services. They were often worried that their implicit practice of prioritizing and rationing would become explicit under the new community care arrangements.

- Many **social workers** were concerned that their skills might become devalued and submerged in the demands of administration, budgeting, management and 'enabling' others to provide services. The dangers of this were pointed out by many social workers, who said that elderly people had emotional as well as practical needs and that it was not always possible to disentangle them.

- There is an urgent need to develop structures and practices which facilitate close **collaboration** between social services staff and colleagues in other professions, particularly in community nursing and general practice. Relationships and links between social workers and GPs were found to be poor, and liaison and communication with other professionals, although more productive, depended largely on proximity and personal acquaintance.

- Few elderly people had much **choice** in what services they received or any say in the time at which the service was delivered, the person who delivered it, or how much they received. Services were generally acknowledged to be in very short supply, access to them was usually controlled by professional gatekeepers, and, in the absence of considerable financial resources on the part of the consumer, they were not readily available in the form or at the time they were needed.

Choice and participation by the elderly people in the community usually took a negative form, with elderly people refusing services or discontinuing them if they found them unsuitable to their needs. There was evidence of unmet demand for services among elderly people and their carers, and concern about a lack of discussion of their needs.

- A substantial minority of elderly people in **residential care** felt they had not had enough discussion or control over the decision to enter. Most elderly people had no choice over which home they entered. Although many were happy to leave the decisions on their entry to residential care to others, some were clearly under pressure, while most felt there were no alternatives. Most of them had entered residential care after a fall, fracture or illness requiring hospital treatment and a quarter had entered straight from hospital. The only group to have behaved like active consumers had mainly entered private residential care at a time when they were reasonably fit.

There was evidence, however, that entry to residential care could be a positive choice. Some elderly people had made a choice to enter residential care because they were very elderly, tired and lonely; others were pleasantly surprised by the relief and security offered by residential homes.

• Many elderly people and their carers were reluctant to **complain** about services, particularly women and those living alone. Local authorities and other service providers should issue clear statements about their policy on complaints, ranging from the apparently trivial to the most serious.

Levels of **satisfaction** with the domiciliary and residential care services received were usually fairly high among the elderly people and their carers, although there was a significant minority of dissatisfied customers. But reported levels of satisfaction with these services are almost always misleadingly high. One of the overwhelming impressions gained in this research, particularly from the elderly people themselves, was that expectations were low. The comment by one elderly woman on her limited package of care – 'I'm satisfied. I don't expect a lot in life . . .' was echoed time and time again by elderly people, both in the community and in residential care.

Researchers

Isobel Allen, Debra Hogg and Sheila Peace

Policy Studies Institute, 100 Park Village East, London, NW1 3SR. (071 387 2171; FAX 071 388 0914)

Publications

Allen, I., Hogg, D., and Peace, S. (1992) *Elderly People: Choice, Participation and Satisfaction*, London, Policy Studies Institute.

Service Histories of Elderly People

Introduction

This project was designed as an integral part of the longitudinal study of ageing which began in 1979. Using a sub-sample of elderly people (n=61), the study focused on:

Consumer views
Assessment
Care-packaging

- consumer perspectives of domiciliary services (user and non-user views);

- the processes involved in becoming a services user and the patterns of use and 'careers' of users thereafter;

- the appropriateness, efficacy and outcomes of services offered, and the ways in which they are (or are not) coordinated, 'packaged' and managed.

The study also examined factors involved in service refusal and service use at both high and low levels of dependency. These data were compared with the views of service providers and managers and the carers of elderly people.

The main findings from the study have implications for the implementation of the 1990 NHS and Community Care Act and are summarized below:

Processes and Patterns in Service Use

Investigation of the processes and patterns of service use indicated that for the most part the process of receipt of services remains predominantly **reactive** to crises of health or social distress. There was little participation in referral processes by those professional groups that could be expected to have a more **preventive** than **reactive** function (e.g. health visitors and social workers).

The Packaging and Appropriateness of Services

Traditional styles of working and expectations of services will need to change if services are to be targeted according to practical need as well as social or psychological factors. Offering inappropriate or unwanted services for social rather than practical need led to wastage, especially of meals services, and ran the risk of producing dependency.

The scope of services remains too narrow and biased towards traditionally 'female' tasks. There was a failure to supply help with traditionally 'male' tasks, such as household maintenance, repairs and gardening, with potentially dangerous consequences.

The concentration of domiciliary services into the normal working week was inappropriate to the needs of elderly people who lacked support in the evenings and at weekends.

There was a specific list of services on offer and elderly people could either 'take it or leave it' within this range. Some people with critical needs received no help because no appropriate service existed.

Support and recognition for the resources, ingenuity and experience that some elderly people and/or their families can bring to bear on the management and organization of their own packages of help was lacking.

Geographical Factors in Service Provision

Generally, the levels of available services were found to be broadly comparable with those in urban areas. However, widespread transport difficulties inhibited access to services, day-care or visiting friends and relatives in hospital. Failure to plan and organize services on a small-area basis led to problems in setting up coordinated, joint-working approaches.

Higher costs may be incurred in providing services in sparsely-populated rural areas where travel times and distances are high; and some services (e.g. meals-on-wheels) do not currently exist.

The Relationship of Dependency to Service Use

It was found that providers need to be encouraged to tailor services to match elderly persons' and their carers' real needs, rather than assess the extent to which their situation warrants the services already available. This finding was supported by the fact that no elderly person (regardless of their level of dependency), living with a younger generation carer, received any practical assistance other than from the community nurse.

Summary

The results of the research suggested the following conclusions:-

- 'Problem-orientated' approaches to community care are common, but do not fully meet the needs of elderly people and their informal carers for support services.
- The use of stereotypes and routinized responses may lead to inappropriate provision which may fail to support or may actually undermine independence.
- A better understanding of informal support networks could enable service providers to make more sensitive and complete assessments of the needs of elderly people. New elements to services will be needed if tailoring and packaging are to become a reality in efforts to sustain the independence of elderly people for as long as possible.
- Against the background of the current emphasis on assessment, the research suggested that account needs to be taken of the ways in which individual professionals and professionals as groups perceive their clients, define their problems and needs and make choices and decisions on their behalf. The way in which professionals conceive of their role, the role of other professional groups and their clients' needs cannot be separated from the practical aspects of policy implementation – especially those that require closer inter-professional planning and joint working.

These points have formed the basis of new research currently in progress, concerning assessment, care-packaging and inter/intra-professional practice.

Researcher

Ms Kerry Caldock

Centre for Social Policy Research and Development, University of Wales, Bangor, Gwynedd LL57 2DG. (0248 351151)

Publications

Caldock, K. (1989) *Consumer Perspectives on Community Care: appropriateness, coordination, packaging and case management*, Centre for Social Policy Research and Development, University of Wales, Bangor.

Caldock, K. (1989) *Processes and Patterns in Service use: User careers of elderly people in rural North Wales*, Centre for Social Policy Research and Development, University of Wales, Bangor.

Caldock, K. (1990) *Responsive Community Services for the Elderly: breaking the mould*, Centre for Social Policy Research and Development, University of Wales, Bangor.

Caldock, K. (1992) 'Domiciliary Services and Dependency: a meaningful relationship?' in F. Laczko and C. Victor (eds), *Social Policy and older people*, Aldershot, Avebury.

Caldock, K., and Wenger, G. C. (1988) *Elderly People and the Health and Social Services (Rural North Wales)*, Report to DH/WO, Centre for Social Policy Research and Development, University of Wales, Bangor.

Caldock, K., and Wenger, G. C. (1990) *Geographical Factors in Rural Health and Social Service Provision*, Centre for Social Policy Research and Development, University of Wales, Bangor.

Caldock, K., and Wenger, G. C. (1992) 'Health and Social Service Provision for Elderly People: the need for a rural model', in A. Gilg (ed.), *Progress in Rural Policy and Planning*, Vol. 2, London, Belhaven Press.

Health Survey of a Random Sample of Elderly People

The aims of the survey are:

— to obtain information regarding morbidity, health status and quality of life among elderly people;

— to obtain information regarding the consumption of prescribed and over-the-counter medication by elderly people;

— to investigate the social networks, lifestyles, cigarette and alcohol consumption of elderly people.

Physical disability
Mental health
Loneliness

A random sample of people aged 65 years and over was drawn from the Family Health Service Authority computer records in Newport, Gwent, (a town identified as 'average' among urban areas in England and Wales). Subjects were approached to be interviewed independently in their own homes by trained, experienced interviewers. The interview schedule included measures of morbidity, health status, quality of life and lifestyles. Specific topics covered were functional disability, dependency, self-perceived health status, anxiety, depression, cognitive impairment, sleep patterns, common symptoms, medication (prescribed and over-the-counter), GP consultations, frequency of falls and fractures, social life, social contact, social support, life satisfaction, and alcohol and cigarette consumption. Where possible, questionnaires included in the interview schedule were those previously validated on community samples.

Preliminary analysis of the data collected has produced the following results:-

— Twenty-eight per cent of the respondents suffered from either moderate or severe physical disabilities and 38 per cent from mild disabilities. *The severity of disability tended to increase with age*; only 12 per cent of those under 70 years and 56 per cent of those 80 years and over were considered moderately/severely disabled. *Women tended to be more physically disabled than men*; 75 per cent women and 52 per cent men had some degree of disability. *Physical disability was associated with marital status*: widowed respondents reported more physical disability than married; 37 per cent widowed and only 19 per cent married suffered either moderate or severe disability.

— Six per cent of the respondents were housebound and 14 per cent went out only with assistance. *Physical disability and mobility were closely associated*: 72 per cent of housebound respondents were severely physically disabled; 84 per cent of respondents who went out without assistance had either no or only mild disability. *Mobility was also associated with marital status*: 9 per cent widowed and 3 per cent married respondents were housebound, 74 per cent widowed and 85 per cent married respondents went out without assistance.

— *Physical and mental health were closely associated*; 76 per cent of those significantly depressed also suffered from physical disability; 15 per cent of those without anxiety and 30 per cent of those with, suffered from a degree of physical immobility. *Memory impairment, unlike anxiety and depression, increased with age*: 6 per cent of those under 75 years and 26 per cent of those 75 years and over suffered from some degree of memory impairment. *Women scored higher than men in all aspects of mental impairment*: 35 per cent women and 18 per cent men were significantly anxious; 11 per cent women and 5 per cent men were significantly depressed, and 23 per cent women and 10 per cent men suffered some degree of memory impairment.

— *Perceived health status was strongly associated with standard assessment of physical and mental health status*: 63 per cent of those who were able to go out without assistance reported good health status and 100 per cent of bedfast respondents reported poor health status; 80 per cent of respondents with no physical disability and only 16 per cent with severe disability reported good health status; 69 per cent without anxiety and only 29 per cent with significant anxiety had good health status; 66 per cent without depression and only 18 per cent with significant depression reported good health status. *Health status, both actual and perceived, deteriorates with age*. But this was true only up to the age of 84 years, where there was a marked improvement: 56 per cent under 85 years and 68 per cent of 85 years and over reported good health status. This would seem to indicate that people over 84 years old, living at home, are often the healthy survivors.

— *Self-reported loneliness increased with age*: 34 per cent under 80 years and 49 per cent of those aged 80 years and over had experienced loneliness. *More women than men experienced loneliness* – 48 per cent women and only 22 per cent men – *and loneliness was associated with both physical and mental disability*.

— Twenty-seven per cent of respondents smoked – 32 per cent under 75 years and only 21 per cent of those 75 years and over. *Smoking was associated with gender*: 32 per cent men and 19 per cent women smoked; 10 per cent men and 3 per cent women smoked 20 or more cigarettes per day. *Smoking and alcohol consumption were closely associated*: 77 per cent of non-smokers did not drink alcohol; of the respondents who smoked 20 or more cigarettes per day, 14 per cent were considered moderate or heavy drinkers and only 5 per cent as non or occasional drinkers.

— *Alcohol consumption was also associated with age and gender*: 87 per cent men and 73 per cent women drank alcohol; 14 per cent men and only 1 per cent women were considered moderately heavy drinkers; 84 per cent under 75 years and 72 per cent of 75 years and over drank alcohol; 8 per cent under 75 years and only 2 per cent 75 years and over were considered moderately heavy-drinkers. *Alcohol was also related to physical and mental health*; as mental and physical health deteriorated so did the alcohol consumption of respondents. Eighty-six per cent of respondents without physical disability and 75 per cent with some physical disability drank alcohol; 83 per cent without significant anxiety and 71 per cent with significant anxiety drank alcohol.

— The results support the view that *a high proportion of elderly people take prescribed medication* and that many are taking several at a time: 68 per cent were taking at least one prescribed medication and 30 per cent were taking more than three different ones. The most commonly used group of drugs were those for the cardiovascular system (38 per cent) and the central nervous system (25 per cent).

— *Forty-six per cent of respondents had trouble sleeping*; 85 per cent woke during the night and 36 per cent woke more than once. Of these, 61 per cent woke to pass urine and 19 per cent woke spontaneously. Ten per cent reported either poor or very poor quality of sleep, 35 per cent felt tired on waking and 29 per cent felt sleepy and lacklustre on waking. Twenty-two per cent took sleeping tablets, the most common were Nitrazepam (27 per cent), Euhypnos (18 per cent) and Dalmane (12 per cent). Of those taking sleeping tablets, 27 per cent reported that they had no or little effect on their quality of sleep. *Physically disabled people were likely to take longer to go to sleep*: 12 per cent without disability and 29 per cent with disability took longer than 30 minutes. *Women were also likely to take longer than men to go to sleep*: 56 per cent women, 31 per cent men took longer than 30 minutes.

— Twenty-four per cent of respondents stated that they had fallen within the previous six months, 43 per cent being indoor falls and 57 per cent outdoor falls. *Falls were associated with poor subjective health status, symptoms of faintness, weakness or muzziness, functional disability, impaired mobility, anxiety and depression. There was a relationship between falls and the taking of prescribed medication;* 79 per cent of fallers and 64 per cent non-fallers were taking prescribed medication; 37 per cent of fallers and 27 per cent non-fallers were taking more than three different types of drugs.

Researchers

Dr Dee Jones, Mrs Sandra Cranton

Research Team for the Care of Elderly People, Department of Geriatric Medicine, University of Wales College of Medicine, Cardiff Royal Infirmary, Cardiff CF2 1SZ. (0222 491000)

Presentations

Chairman and presenter – Sleep patterns and insomnia. Sleep patterns and medication among a random sample of older people, *XIV International Congress of Gerontology*, Acapulco, 18–23 June 1989.

The Discharge from Hospital of Frail Elderly People

Aims of the Research

Home-helps

Users and carers

Effectiveness

This was planned as an exploratory phase for a larger study which aimed to identify effective approaches to the provision of home-help/home-care to elderly patients discharged from hospital.

It aimed to:

1. **Describe** the approaches in terms of

   — organizational models of the home-help service

   — assessment by home-help organizers

   — the roles and tasks of the home-help.

2. **Evaluate** the effectiveness of the approaches in terms of their

   — perceived relevance to elderly people

   — impact on particular problems of daily living

   — impact on the elderly person's morale and experience of well-being

   — effects on carers.

Methods

The exploratory study was conducted in three parts:

1. Discussions by telephone with a relevant principal officer and two social workers in a random selection of 60 per cent of the local authorities in England and Wales about issues relating to the discharge from hospital of elderly people.
2. Monitoring over 2,000 referrals to home-help organizers in four local authorities. Half of these organizers were managing a special 'hospital discharge scheme', which had been set up to provide an intensive service for a limited period after discharge; half were managing a mainstream home-help service.
3. Referrals of people aged 75 years or older who had been in hospital for at least three nights were identified and a sample of 70 selected. A minority of people, suffering from dementia, were not excluded. Interviews were conducted with these old people, their carers, home-help organizers and home-helps 2 and 12 weeks after the old person had been discharged from hospital.

Parts two and three of the research were conducted in four local authorities, each of which had a hospital discharge scheme as well as a mainstream service. These authorities included two London boroughs and one division in two counties. The hospital discharge schemes in these four authorities varied. The scheme provided intensive domiciliary help for between two to six weeks after discharge.

A. Pre-Discharge Planning and Hospital Discharge Schemes

Findings

1. Our research, supported by other studies, suggests that the *hospital discharge schemes studied offered a more timely and integrated service* to elderly people leaving hospital and scored higher on a count of 'good discharge procedures.'

2. Some advantages of schemes:

- they provide a quick and high-quality service to patients for a brief period after discharge;
- the organizer can have personal contact with patient and carers before and after discharge;
- through regular personal contact with ward staff, the organizer can obtain better information, sometimes act as an advocate for the patient, and re-negotiate discharge dates when appropriate.

3. Some disadvantages of schemes:

- there can be a knock-on effect on mainstream home-help services;
- help is time-limited;
- they can become too popular and 'silted-up';
- they can increase inequity of provision;
- they can be expensive, given limited social services resources.

B. The Discharge Process

Findings

In our sample:

- two-fifths had relatives who rallied to provide special help and turned discharge into a family celebration, but *half were not in this fortunate position*;
- most hospital admissions had been *unplanned*;
- most people *lived alone* or with another elderly person;
- one-fifth were *seldom visited* in hospital by relatives or friends;
- the *cumulative repercussions* of the above factors led to some patients returning home to decaying food and unheated rooms;
- delays in *transport* were common. This meant that the day of discharge could be a disappointing and exhausting experience. It was not unusual for a patient to wait on the ward from early morning until evening for an ambulance for the journey home;
- hospital-car-service drivers did not usually see patients indoors, possibly because they were volunteers, might themselves be elderly and were uninsured for this task. Some patients *could not negotiate the steps to their front door* without considerable help;
- essential aids, such as commodes, were usually provided before, or soon after discharge, but patients waited several weeks or even months for other *aids and adaptations*.

C. Care in the Community

Findings

In our sample:

- almost all the elderly people had lived in their present accommodation for many years, wished to remain there, and had roots in the local community;
- almost all were strongly motivated towards recovery and increased independence;

- on dishcarge, most of the elderly people felt ill, were severely disabled, and housebound. Two-fifths were in pain and a third were possibly depressed. Some elderly people had a very poor quality of life;
- although most people did not usually receive help with personal self-care tasks, they expressed satisfaction with home-help with their housework;
- at discharge, the predicted level of home-help required was accurate in less than a third of cases;
- transition from a hospital discharge scheme to a mainstream home-help service meant, for most people, a reduction in home-help provision, a financial reassessment and sometimes a new scale of charges and a change of home-help;
- care networks were comparatively small;
- there was a shortfall in chiropody and bath-aid services.

Researchers

June Neill, Jenny Williams, Peter Gorbach

National Institute for Social Work Research Unit, Mary Ward House, 5–7 Tavistock Place, London WC1H 9SS. (071 387 9681; FAX 071 387 7968)

Publications

Neill, J., and Williams, J. (1991) *Elderly People Leaving Hospital: a Study of Discharge to Community Care*, Report to DH, National Institute for Social Work Research Unit.

Neill, J., and Williams, J. (1992) *Leaving Hospital: a Study of Elderly People and Their Discharge to Community Care*, London, HMSO.

Rehabilitation of Patients after Myocardial Infarction

Objectives

The objectives of this study were:

Quality of life

Counselling

Costs and benefits

- to evaluate the effectiveness – in terms of reduction in mortality and morbidity – of rehabilitation of patients discharged from hospital, and their spouses, following an acute myocardial infarction (MI), using a programme of counselling and psychological therapy.
- to seek characteristics of patients and spouses who respond to counselling and psychological therapy.
- to monitor and evaluate the initiative in terms of patient benefits and good value for money.

All patients discharged from six general hospitals after an MI were entered into the trial. Random allocation to intervention and control groups was done with knowledge only of date of admission to hospital, and fact of discharge.

Patients in the control groups followed normal discharge procedures with no formal rehabilitation. All patients in the intervention groups were invited to attend a seven-week course of rehabilitation once a week at the out-patients department. Partners were also invited to attend the first two sessions. Therapy sessions, led by a clinical psychologist and a health visitor, covered education regarding circulation, the heart, heart disease, MI, treatment of MI, angina and its treatment, and rehabilitation expectations. Relaxation, with bio-feedback, and stress-management techniques were taught, discussed and practised.

Patients and spouses were interviewed independently in their own homes within the first month of MI and again six months later by a second interviewer. The semi-structured patient interviews included questions on: angina, health status, medication, diet, exercise, smoking and drinking, social support, sexual activity, anxiety and depression, and other indications of quality of life. Patients' attitudes towards their MI and their expectations of future life were also explored using standard techniques. The spouse interviews were much shorter and concentrated on measures of health and psychological status. A clinical examination was done at 12 months, and mortality data are being collected from the NHS central register.

Preliminary Results

- of those invited to attend rehabilitation programmes, three-quarters attended one or more sessions; of these, more than half attended four or more, despite the ambulance strikes. Ill-health was the main reason for non-attendance, followed by transport difficulty.
- Three-quarters of attenders found the programmes helpful, as did the spouses.
- Compared with those in the non-intervention group, those in the intervention group, when followed up, were taking fewer medications, suffering fewer angina attacks, less anxiety and less depression.

Full results should be available in 1993.

Acknowledgement

This project is being funded jointly by the British Heart Foundation and the Department of Health (Welsh Office).

Researchers

Dr Dee Jones and Dr Robert West

Research Team for the Care of Elderly People, Department of Geriatric Medicine, University of Wales College of Medicine, Cardiff Royal Infirmary, Cardiff CF2 1SZ. (0222 491000)

Publications

Jones, D. A., and West, R. R. 'A randomised controlled trial of patients after myocardial infarction', First Annual Report 1989, Second Annual Report 1990, Third Annual Report 1991.

Hospital Care and Community After-Care in Patients aged 65 years and Over

PRELIMINARY RESULTS

Hospital discharge

Consumer views

The aims of the research were:

— to study elderly people's satisfaction with hospital care;

— to investigate discharge procedures; and

— to investigate the nature of provision of after-care in the community and consumers' opinion of it.

A random sample of hospital patients discharged during July or August 1990 and aged 65 or over was supplied for each of the three health authorities in South Glamorgan, Mid-Glamorgan and Gwent. Approximately three months after discharge each patient was sent a questionnaire, which covered the patient's opinion of the hospital environment, information and staff communication, discharge procedures and discharge process, and included both closed and open-ended questions. Questions were also asked about the help they received from family, friends and health and social services and their opinion of these services.

Questionnaires and reminders were sent to 1,281 patients and the final response rate was 87 per cent. There were 41 patients (4 per cent) who were discharged to residential care (nursing homes or homes for elderly people). Of these, 23 had been residents before hospital and 18 were new admissions.

Opinions of Hospital

Seventy-two per cent of patients made positive comments, but the majority of these (60 per cent) were of a very general nature – for example commenting on the kindness of nurses, or that they were 'looked after well'. Only 30 per cent made negative comments, but these tended to be more specific, with 26 per cent of complaints relating to poor medical or nursing care. Other complaints related to dirty or inadequate toilets and bathrooms and unpleasant food, with six patients claiming that their diabetes had been adversely affected by incorrect diet. In structured sections relating directly to diet and cleanliness, 8 per cent thought that the cleanliness of lavatories was poor or very poor and 14 per cent thought that the hospital food was poor or very poor.

Discharge Procedures and Process

Patients were asked whether a member of hospital staff had discussed how they would cope at home, and 38 per cent said that no discussion had taken place. Patients most often discussed their return home with the ward sister (21 per cent) or a doctor (20 per cent), followed by a nurse (12 per cent) or social worker (11 per cent). Only 2 per cent of patients were aware of having seen a liaison nurse, and 4 per cent discussed discharge with an occupational therapist. Patients were asked whether anyone had visited their home before discharge, and in 93 per cent of cases no visit had taken place. When a visit was made the usual person was either an occupational therapist or social worker.

Most patients (33 per cent) were told when they would be discharged on the day of leaving and a further 16 per cent were not told until after visiting-time the night before. Twenty-three per cent were told in time for visitors to be informed on the evening before discharge, 21 per cent had up to three days' notice and 5 per cent had more than three days' warning. Despite short notice, 82 per cent said that there had been plenty of warning for making the necessary arrangements. However, 4 per cent said that they had definitely not had enough notice and 1 per cent had their discharge delayed due to inadequate notice. The majority of patients (84 per cent) thought that they had been discharged at about the right time, but 10 per cent thought that it was too soon and 3 per cent thought that they had been kept in too long. On leaving hopsital, 16 per cent were taken home by ambulance or hospital car and 78 per cent by private car with others using a taxi (4 per cent), public transport (1 per cent) or walking (1 per cent).

Help and After-Care

Patients were asked whether they had received help from family or friends since hospital discharge. The main source of help was the spouse (47 per cent) followed by a daughter (31 per cent) and son (16 per cent). Men were more likely to be helped by their wives (67 per cent) and women by their daughters (40 per cent). Other sources of informal care were daughters-in-law (9 per cent), sons-in-law (7 per cent), other relatives (14 per cent) and friends (15 per cent).

Many patients had received help from the health or social services since leaving hospital. Health services received included district nurse or health visitor (32 per cent), chiropodist (16 per cent), day hospital (6 per cent), physiotherapy (5 per cent), occupational therapy (2 per cent) and speech therapy (1 per cent). The social services received were home-help/care aide (27 per cent), social worker (13 per cent), meals-on-wheels (11 per cent), and day-centre (5 per cent). Some of those discharged had received help from Age Concern (2 per cent) and voluntary help such as shopping-girls, self-help and counselling groups (such as the Altzheimers' Society) and other voluntary groups (2 per cent).

In the first week after discharge, 12 per cent of respondents had no help at all. The primary source of help was the spouse (39 per cent) or daughter (21 per cent) followed by other family and friends. Only 7 per cent said that their primary source of help was a formal service. The majority of these were home-helps (3 per cent), health visitor or district nurse (2 per cent), and other services including physio-therapy, occupational therapy, meals-on-wheels or day-centre.

At three months after discharge, the proportion of respondents having no help had risen slightly to 16 per cent, with the main sources of help similar to the first week. The overall proportion of formal help was similar, but more had a home-help (6 per cent).

A repeat of the study commenced in July 1992.

Researchers

Dr Dee Jones, Dr Robert West, Mrs Carolyn Lester

Research Team for the Care of Elderly People, Department of Geriatric Medicine, University of Wales College of Medicine, Cardiff Royal Infirmary, Cardiff CF2 1SZ. (0222 491000)

Publications

Jones, D. A., Lester, C., and West, R. (in press) 'Patient report of hospital care: study of a random sample of discharged elderly people', *European Gerontology and Geriatrics.*

Monitoring and Developing Home-Care Services

Background

Previous inspections conducted by the Social Services Inspectorate had shown that social services departments had little information about their current home-help clients and that information systems were either non-existent or inadequate. Undertaking client-surveys as part of the inspection process would start to bridge the gap in information and provide a firmer basis for policy and service development.

In early 1989, four boroughs in London participated in an inspection of their home-help and home-care services. Two of these authorities had both home-help and separate, but directly-managed, home-care services. As part of the inspections, staff of the 'mainstream' home-help and the special home-care services helped to conduct a survey of their current clients.

FINDINGS

Organizers were able to identify persons who, at referral, were at higher risk of admission to residential care.

Using indicators of risk of admission to residential care developed from previous research, organizers of both home-help and special home-care services had clients who would be at higher risk of admission to residential care. As expected, the special home-care services were more frequently targeted at this group.

The home-help service covered clients at wider levels of disability, and it was the service which appeared to help prevent neglect for large numbers of elderly people. Until now, all the work on indicators of risk of admission to long-stay residential care has been in the context of this fairly pervasive service. If the coverage and intensity of the basic home-help service is reduced, the number of persons at risk of admission to institutional care now or in the future may increase.

Organizers can assess or at least be aware of the clients' major problems and disabilities related to the clients' social functioning.

The health sector, including hospital social workers, was the most frequent source of referrals for both the home-help and special home-care services. In general, home-help and special home-care clients were remarkably similar. *The majority were white women, aged 75 or over, who lived alone in rented accommodation. In both service-groups, about two in three clients had at least four of these five characteristics.*

The great majority of clients of both the home-help and special home-care services had some disabilities which severely limited their own ability to cope with the tasks of daily living.

The special home-care services were more frequently targeted at clients with more severe problems and disabilities. Specific issues for services were also identified:

Home-helps
Targeting
Dementia

for example, in both service-groups, about a third of clients who were regularly incontinent lacked a washing-machine.

Organizers appeared to know the extremes of whether carers and other services are involved and what help they give.

Some organizers were aware of the extent of visits to clients from relatives not living in the same household, friends and neighbours and the practical help they gave. More generally, most organizers appeared to have been aware of two groups of clients:

— those where no one regularly (at least once a week) visits the client;

— those where relatives, friends or neighbours regularly give the client a lot of practical help (for example, with personal care).

Clients of the special home-care services more frequently received other services besides home-care.

Organizers in the special home-care services more frequently assessed clients as requiring personal care and arranged a more intensive service.

Personal care was the most frequently-recorded requirement among special-home-care clients.

- Nine in 10 special-home-care clients were assessed as requiring help with personal care tasks, while 14 per cent of home-help clients were so assessed.
- Although in one authority 33 per cent of home-help clients were assessed as requiring only domestic care, over the four authorities, 8 per cent of the total home-help hours were allocated to clients requiring only domestic care.
- On average, organizers usually allocated about 9.8 hours over 8.9 visits a week to special-home-care clients, while home-help clients were, on average, allocated 3.3 hours over 1.9 visits a week.
- Over 7 in 10 special-home-care clients had two or more home-care workers who visited regularly, while 9 per cent of home-help clients had two or more home-helps who visited regularly.
- The visiting pattern of the home-help services was a 'school day' service, 9 am to 3 pm, while that of special-home-care services was spread more throughout the day, early evenings and at weekends.
- Eight in 10 special-home-care clients, and one in 10 home-help clients, had at least one personal-care task performed by the home-care worker or home-help.
- Home-care workers on average spent 17 per cent of contact time on domestic tasks, while home-helps spent 62 per cent of contact time on domestic tasks. In both services, however, about two hours a week were on average used on domestic tasks.

Overlap of Target Groups, and Relative Coverage

Home-help and special home-care services overlapped in their target groups. Special home-care services more frequently targeted their services at those who apparently were at risk of admission to residential care and those in need of help with personal care. However, the home-help service covered many more people even in the most severe risk groups.

The targeting of the special home-care services was appropriate, but the coverage was limited.

One general indicator of dependency – the time a client could be left alone without risk – did show an overall association with hours of help received. Analyses of this indicator suggested that at similar levels of dependency on this indicator, clients of the home-help services received a less intensive service.

Key Gaps in Targeting

- Very few clients of either type of service lived in households with three or more persons. Comparison with a national survey of home-help clients conducted over 20 years ago suggests that, regardless of the rhetoric about carers and the personal care needs of those elderly persons living with families, *there has not been an extension of home-care services to elderly persons living with families.*

- *All four authorities had significant minority ethnic elderly populations even by the 1981 Census classification, but in three of these authorities the cover was markedly lower than for the white elderly populations.*

- *The third gap in targeting home-care services was to clients with mental illnesses such as dementia, and their carers.* This is a key group of potential applicants for residential care whose carers, whether or not they live with the client, may need help with providing personal and other types of care, which could be made available through the home-help and home-care services.

Researchers

Peter Gorbach, Jenny Williams

National Institute for Social Work, Mary Ward House, 5–7 Tavistock Place, London WC1H 9SS. (071 387 9681; FAX 071 387 7968)

Publications

Social Services Inspectorate (1990) *Inspecting Home Care Services: a Guide to the SSI Method,* London, HMSO.

Home Help and Health Care Services in 4 London Authorities: developing client-based indicators of quality assurance, in preparation, NISW.

Domiciliary Care: Innovations in the social care of elderly people which improve efficiency

The research was based on two rounds of data collection about innovations which aimed to improve efficiency, conducted from the late 1970s to the late 1980s. Managers were asked to describe them using a checklist which focused firstly on symptoms of efficiency improvement, and secondly on the nature of the organizational processes involved in the innovation. A *Sourcebook of Efficiency-Improving Innovations* was based on the responses to the first set of questions; and *A Guide to Efficiency-Improving Innovations in the Care of the Frail Elderly* from the second. The research as a whole was reviewed in *Efficiency-Improving Innovations in Social Care of the Elderly* (1989).

The analysis:

◆ isolated those elements which the innovators expected would cause their innovations to have beneficial outcomes;
◆ analysed the organizational processes;
◆ investigated how contextual variations affected the nature and frequency of innovations;
◆ developed a typology of innovations; and
◆ investigated whether policy devices increased the frequency, and affected the nature of the innovations.

The findings of the research are as follows:

— The work of the late 1970s showed that innovations were in general geographically very localized; they were seldom directed towards a specific clientele; and they represented piecemeal, rather than coordinated, system-wide change. Greater clarity was needed in defining the core functions of government and department in order to improve the cost-effectiveness of outcomes, and to provide individuals with the right context for carrying out essential responsibilities with increasing resourcefulness.

— Statistical analysis of the information showed how the frequency of innovations reflected the characteristics and circumstances of authorities. For instance, in the late 1970s and early 1980s, authorities conducting service reviews tended to raise resources for innovations from outside agencies – particularly joint finance from health authorities. It also showed that the frequency was higher in larger authorities, and that authorities with high expenditures and continuing growth were less likely to make innovations financed from their own funds. Many of the early innovations were almost panic responses to cuts. However, the analysis of the second sweep showed a changed pattern. Some innovations introduced during the previous period had become fairly common, and fewer innovations were made in response to cuts. The development of community services as the basis for a more efficient pattern of care had become a major feature, reflecting long-term trends in arguments about systems development.

— The statistical analysis of information from the second sweep showed how types of innovation reflected their institutional sponsorship – sponsors' interests

Process
Structures

and assumptions – and structural features, which created incentives, opportunities and constraints. There were some which were centrally concerned with improving the performance of case-management tasks. One type was based on inter-professional cooperation, often led by geriatricians but involving social workers as case managers. There was a clear contrast between schemes based on joint finance and other funding sources.

— The special analysis of innovations in the mid-1980s, conducted as part of the study of resources, needs and outcomes showed:

- the prevalence of augmented home-care schemes;
- new forms of residential care, blurring the boundary between community-based and residential care; and
- boarding out for short-term and rotating care.

The analysis of the relationship between resources and outcomes failed to show that the schemes produced more outcomes given their levels of inputs, and did not appear to reduce the probability that users would have been admitted to institutions for long-term care within 6 months and 2.5 years.

Researcher

Professor Bleddyn Davies

Personal Social Services Research Unit, Cornwallis Building, The University, Canterbury, Kent CT2 7NF. (0227 764000 x 7587)

Publications

Davies, B. (1981) 'Strategic goals and piecemeal innovations: Adjusting to the new balance of needs and resources', in E. M. Goldberg (ed.), *A new look at the social services*, London, Heinemann for Policy Studies Institute, 96–121.

Davies, B., and Coles, O. (1981) 'Towards a territorial cost function for the home help service', *Social Policy and Administration*, **15**, 1: 32–42.

Davies, B., and Ferlie, E. (1982) 'Efficiency-improving innovations in social care', *Policy and Politics*, **10**, 2: 181–203.

Ferlie, E., Challis, D., and Davies, B. (1984) 'Models of innovation in the social care of the elderly', *Local Government Studies*, **10**, 6: 67–82.

Ferlie, E., Challis, D., and Davies, B. (1985) 'Innovation in the care of the elderly: the role of joint finance', in A. Butler (ed.), *Ageing: recent advances and creative responses*, Beckenham, Croom Helm, 137–159.

Ferlie, E., Challis, D., and Davies, B. (1989) *Efficiency-improving innovations in social care of the elderly*, Aldershot, Gower.

Ferlie, E., and Davies, B. (1984) 'Patterns of efficiency-improving innovations: Social care and the elderly', *Policy and Politics*, **12**, 3: 281–296.

A Survey of Nursing Homes and Hospices

INTRODUCTION

Service planning
Private sector
Charges

This survey of nursing homes and hospices was commissioned by the Department of Health in January 1990. In view of the proposed changes in funding arrangements for long-term care in the independent sector, up-to-date information was needed about nursing homes and hospices, and their patients. The Department was particularly interested in levels of fees, sources of financial support for patients, and locational issues.

The survey was conducted by means of a questionnaire posted to proprietors in advance, and collected personally by field-workers; and was carried out in ten local authority areas in England and Wales.

RESEARCH FINDINGS

Eight hospices were registered to take patients with terminal illnesses. The registrations for the 100 nursing homes were divided into three main categories of Old Age, Mental Disorder and Mental/Physical Handicap. The majority (88 per cent) fell within the 'Old Age' category. Seventy-eight of the 96 nursing homes which responded to the questionnaire were first registered less than five years ago.

Number of Patients and Vacancies as at 1st May, 1990

The number of patients accommodated in the nursing homes at 1st May 1990 is shown in table 2.1 and the number of vacancies in table 2.2.

Vacancies were greatest in homes which had been opened more recently. Of the eight nursing homes which had 11 or more vacancies, three had been opened in 1990 and one in the summer of 1989. The survey did not ascertain the reasons for the relatively large number of vacancies in the other four homes.

Table 2.1: *Number of Patients in the Nursing Home or Hospice on 1st May, 1990*

	Number of	
Patients	Nursing Homes	Hospices
0–5	0	0
6–10	4	3
11–20	28	2
21–30	41	2
31–40	13	1
41–50	11	0
51–60	2	0
61–70	1	0
TOTAL	100	8

Table 2.2: *Number of Vacancies at 1st May 1990 (Excluding Day-Care)*

Vacancies	Number of	
	Nursing Homes	Hospices
None	2	2
1–5	56	2
6–10	8	1
11–20	6	3
21 or more	2	0
TOTAL	100	8

The hospices tended to have a smaller capacity (average 13 places) and had more vacancies (average 7 places).

Charges

The hospices did not charge patients.

Charges for nursing-home accommodation varied considerably, from less than £200 per week to more than £300. As well as variations between individual homes, charges depended on the type of accommodation, with patients paying more for a single room than for a shared room.

The Provision of Extra Services and Charges Made for Them

The extra services provided are shown in table 2.3, together with the number of homes making extra charges for them.

All homes and hospices provided laundry and incontinence services. While only one per cent made extra charges for laundry services, 15 per cent made extra charges for incontinence supplies.

Almost all homes (98 per cent) provided wheelchairs, but none made an extra charge for this service. The most common extra services provided, for which the

Table 2.3: *Percentage of Homes Providing Extra Services and Percentage Making Extra Charges*

Service	Percentage of Homes	
	Providing Services	Making Extra Charges
Laundry	100	1
Incontinence Supplies	100	15
Wheelchairs	98	0
Hairdressing	97	78
Chiropody	96	73
Medical Equipment	90	3
Occupational Therapy	79	7
Physiotherapy	72	27

majority of homes make charges, are two that are usually brought into the home: hairdressing (available in 97 per cent of homes with 78 per cent levying extra charges) and chiropody (available in 96 per cent of homes with 73 per cent levying charges).

A minority of homes (11 per cent) made extra charges to patients with higher dependency nursing needs.

Patient Characteristics

The mean age of patients in the hospices was 68 years. Most patients were women (77 per cent), although in the hospices 49 patients were men compared with 52 women.

Most patients in the nursing homes (98 per cent) were long-stay and 2 per cent were short-stay.

The most common source of admission to the nursing home was from a hospital (50 per cent), followed by the patient's own home (31 per cent).

Movement Across Local Authority Boundaries

Two-hundred and seventy-eight long-stay patients (13 per cent) moved from one English local authority area to a home in another English local authority area, while 17 patients (less than 1 per cent) moved from a Welsh local authority area to a home in England. By comparison, 23 out of 463 patients (5 per cent) moved from an English local authority area to a home in Wales.

Only three people moved from Scotland to a home in England.

Length of Stay

Most patients (49 per cent) had been admitted in the last year, 34 per cent in the last six months. As would be expected, most (57 per cent) of the patients with a terminal illness had been admitted within the previous six months.

Table 2.4: *Source of Finance for Patients in the Nursing Homes – Numbers*

Source of Finance	Old Age	Mental Disorder	Mental/ Physical Handicap	Terminal Illness	Other	Total
No Charge	1	0	0	38	1	40
Private	642	37	25	47	1	752
Social Security Only	1035	197	158	148	0	1538
Social Security & Top-up	204	9	8	12	1	234
Health Authority	2	0	7	0	6	15
Other	1	0	0	6	0	7
Total	**1885**	**243**	**198**	**251**	**9**	**2586**

Sources of Finance

Social security was a major source of finance for many patients. The care of 60 per cent of all patients was funded by income support alone, with a further 9 per cent funded by income support with a top-up.

CONCLUSION

The study found that the nursing-home sector was a thriving, developing industry. The recent expansion of the sector was clearly illustrated: more than half of the homes were first registered as nursing homes in 1988 or more recently.

The data on charges suggest that people seeking places in May 1990 and entirely dependent on income support, with no access to additional resources, were likely to be restricted in their access to nursing homes. The findings suggested wide-spread dependence on using the income support personal allowance towards basic fees, using up savings, or relying on contributions from relatives or charities.

Researchers

Sally Baldwin, Anne Corden (SPRU)

Social Policy Research Unit, University of York, Heslington, York YO1 5DD. (0904 433608; FAX 0904 433618)

Eileen Sutcliffe, Ken Wright (CHE)

Centre for Health Economics, University of York, Heslington, York YO1 5DD. (0904 433646; FAX 0904 433644)

Survey of Private and Voluntary Residential Care and Nursing Homes

In 1986/7, the PSSRU at the University of Kent and the CHE at the University of York jointly undertook a survey of private and voluntary registered residential care and nursing homes.

The balance between private and voluntary residential provision, and the overall level of provision changed significantly during the early 1980s; and the aim of the survey was to draw together information about the different types of homes as a contribution to assessing the implications of these changes.

Dependency levels

Charges

FINDINGS

Overlaps in disability levels for individuals in residential and nursing homes have been reported from a number of studies, and similar overlaps were found in the 1986/7 survey.

Table 2.5: *Characteristics of Residents and Patients*

Information	Residential homes			Nursing homes	
	Local authority	Private	Voluntary	Private	Voluntary
Mean age	83	82	83	83	70
% females	74	79	81	84	70
% walk with aids or help/ cannot walk	52	45	39	70	62
% need assistance to use WC	22	25	16	51	44
% need assistance to feed self	5	6	5	19	25
% incontinent	24	19	16	38	38
% mildly/ severely confused	59	48	38	63	43
% midly/ severely disruptive	38	23	12	25	22
Total number of individuals	1683	3048	1926	1206	456

Sources: *Department of Health Social Services Inspectorate; PSSRU/CHE survey.*

However, overall levels of dependency were substantially higher among patients in nursing homes than among residents in independent residential homes; and residents in voluntary homes tended to be less dependent than residents in private homes, particularly in the residential home sector. Differences between nursing homes and residential homes were greater for levels of physical disability, incapacity in self-care tasks and levels of incontinence than for levels of mental confusion or anti-social behaviour. But levels of confusion were significantly higher among patients in private nursing homes than among residents of private residential homes, and anti-social behaviour was significantly more prevalent in voluntary nursing homes than in voluntary residential homes.

Levels of physical disability, incontinence and confusion among residents of the local authority homes in a study undertaken by the Social Services Inspectorate in 1988 were intermediate to those recorded for private residential and private nursing homes, while the levels of anti-social behaviour reported were substantially higher than in private residential or nursing homes. However, the proportions of individuals in local authority homes recorded as requiring assistance with self-care tasks were generally similar to those recorded for private residential homes. In an earlier study of residential homes, in 1981, residents in private homes and local authority homes had similar levels of dependency in terms of physical abilities, continence and mental state, and were more dependent than residents in voluntary homes.

The relationship between variations in the fees charged by homes and factors relating to the characteristics of homes, the characteristics of residents and the characteristics of the areas in which the homes were situated were also examined in the 1986/7 survey.

For private residential homes, mean charges were positively related to resident dependency and to the proportion of residents supported by private means; and were higher in areas with lower rates of unemployment and lower levels of car ownership (which is negatively related to unemployment), and in Scotland. Mean charges were negatively related to the proportion of residents supported by supplementary benefit without topping up by other organizations or individuals, and were lower in homes with a high proportion of proprietors relative to the total number of staff, or which had been in operation under the current management for longer.

For voluntary residential homes, mean charges were higher for homes which accommodated a higher proportion of residents supported by supplementary benefit with topping up and for dual registered homes, and were lower in homes in Wales and in the South East, outside London.

For private nursing homes, mean charges were higher in areas of low unemployment, and were lower for dual-registered homes than for homes registered as nursing homes only. Unlike in private residential-care homes, mean charges were not related to the aggregate levels of dependency among patients.

Researchers

Robin Darton

PSSRU, University of Kent, Cornwallis Building, Canterbury, Kent CT2 7NF. (0227 764000; FAX 0227 764327)

Sheila Jefferson, Eileen Sutcliffe, Ken Wright

CHE, University of York, Heslington, York YO1 5DD. (0904 433646; FAX 0904 433644)

Publications

Darton, R. A., Jefferson, S. F., Sutcliffe, E. M., and Wright, K. G. (1987) 'The PSSRU/CHE Survey of Residential and Nursing Homes: Postal Questionnaire Coding Manual', March 1987, PSSRU Discussion Paper No. 485.

Darton, R. A., Jefferson, S. F., Sutcliffe, E. M., and Wright, K. G. (1987) 'The PSSRU/CHE Survey of Residential and Nursing Homes: Interview Questionnaire Coding Manual', March 1987, DP490.

Darton, R. A., Jefferson, S. F., Sutcliffe, E. M., and Wright, K. G. (1987) 'The PSSRU/CHE Survey of Residential and Nursing Homes: Preliminary Tables', January 1987, DP491.

Darton, R. A., Jefferson, S. F., Sutcliffe, E. M., and Wright, K. G. (1987) 'The PSSRU/CHE Survey of Residential and Nursing Homes: Descriptive Statistical Report', September 1987, corrected October 1987, DP523.

Darton, R. A., Jefferson, S. F., Sutcliffe, E. M., and Wright, K. G. (1987) 'The PSSRU/CHE Survey of Residential and Nursing Homes: Descriptive Statistical Report Commentary', September 1987, DP536.

Darton, R. A., Jefferson, S. F., Sutcliffe, E. M., and Wright, K. G. (1987) 'The PSSRU/CHE Survey of Residential and Nursing Homes: Tables of Charges', December 1987, DP549.

Darton, R. A., Jefferson, S. F., Sutcliffe, E. M., and Wright, K. G. (1988) 'The PSSRU/CHE Survey of Residential and Nursing Homes: The Costs and Charges of the Surveyed Homes', June 1988, corrected September 1988, DP563/3.

Darton, R. A., Jefferson, S. F., Sutcliffe, E. M., and Wright, K. G. (1988) 'The PSSRU/CHE Survey of Residential and Nursing Homes: Interview Questionnaire Descriptive Statistics', August 1988, corrected July 1989, DP573.

Darton, R. A., Jefferson, S. F., Sutcliffe, E. M., and Wright, K. G. (1989) 'The PSSRU/CHE Survey of Residential and Nursing Homes: Interview Questionnaire Descriptive Report Commentary', April 1989, DP601.

Darton, R. A., Sutcliffe, E. M., and Wright, K. G. (1989) 'The PSSRU/CHE Survey of Residential and Nursing Homes: General Report', DP654.

Darton, R. A., and Wright, K. G. (1989) 'The PSSRU/CHE Survey of Residential and Nursing Homes: Tabulations of the Characteristics of Residents and Patients', December 1989, DP678.

Darton, R. A., and Wright, K. G. (1990) 'The characteristics of Non-Statutory Residential and Nursing Homes', in R. Parry (ed.), *Research Highlights in Social Work 18. Privatisation*, London, Jessica Kingsley Publishers.

Darton, R. A., and Wright, K. G. (1992) 'Residential and Nursing Homes for Elderly People: One Sector or Two?', in F. Laczko and C. Victor (eds), *Social Policy and Elderly People*, Aldershot, Avebury.

An Evaluation of Continuing-Care Accommodation for Elderly People

In 1983, the DHSS commissioned the then Health Care Research Unit to undertake an evaluation, by means of a range of studies which had the following policy objectives:

1. To provide a sound basis for judging the relative efficiency of care given in experimental NHS nursing homes and conventional geriatric wards. This objective is concerned solely with a decision as to whether to implement a policy which in the long term replaces continuing-care geriatric beds with places in NHS nursing homes.

2. To identify variations in the process of care between different kinds of physical and social environments providing continuing care for very frail elderly people. This objective has implications not only for the implementation of a policy to introduce NHS nursing homes but also in relation to the way care is provided in a variety of existing facilities.

3. To provide an understanding of the factors which might explain variations in the process and outcome of care provided in the facilities studied.

This summary report focuses on the first objective. Further reports of the evaluation will consider the other two objectives.

Consumer views
Costs
Private sector

FINDINGS FROM THE STUDIES

A Randomized Controlled Trial of Continuing-Care Accommodation for Very Frail Elderly People

Which mode of care is most appropriate for future use? The results of the analyses of survival are inconclusive in two of the centres, although in the third there is evidence of lengthier survival among people selected for an NHS nursing home (the 'home'-group). The results of the analyses of personal well-being are also inconclusive for one of the centres, but suggest that personal well-being in the other two centres was greater among the home-group. Consumer views indicated greater satisfaction among the home-group in all three centres. Changes in behavioural ability showed no relative disadvantages in either the home-group or controls. The results suggest a decision in favour of NHS nursing homes.

A Multiple-Case Study of Six NHS Hospital Wards and the Three Experimental NHS Nursing Homes

One finding of this study is that, in terms of patient and resident activity, the NHS nursing homes provide a more positive environment than conventional NHS hospital wards. However, differences in the type and level of activity show that differences also exist between nursing homes.

The case studies show that there are substantial differences in the physical environment of the homes and wards. The provision of single rooms for most residents is the most significant feature of the physical environment of the homes, but their size, greater variety of spaces, spatial organization and greater prosthetic quality are also important.

The three NHS nursing homes were better endowed with nursing staff than all but one of the hospital wards. All had more unqualified staff and only in one of the homes was there a higher level of qualified staff than in hospital wards.

Surveys (1984 and 1987) of Continuing-Care Accommodation in Six Health Authorities

The surveys show marked variation between health authorities in the provision of continuing-care accommodation for elderly people. They also show that different types of accommodation care for elderly people with broadly similar behavioural characteristics. However, the hospital geriatric wards and NHS nursing homes had a higher proportion of very frail elderly people than private nursing homes and private and local authority residential homes. These data suggest the need for health authorities to monitor carefully the expansion in the private sector and the characteristics of occupants entering all continuing-care institutions, in order to make effective and equitable use of the available scarce resources.

A Cost-Study of NHS Hospital and Nursing-Home Accommodation

The conclusion of the cost study is that NHS nursing homes are no more costly than NHS hospital accommodation. In most scenarios, using different assumptions about factors affecting costs, it is likely that NHS nursing-home accommodation will be less costly than continuing-care hospital accommodation. In revenue terms alone, according to various assumptions, a 30-bed NHS nursing home running at 100 per cent occupancy would cost a health authority between £72,000 less and £33,000 more per annum than its hospital equivalent. At an average cost of £260 per patient per week, this is more costly than some estimates of the costs in private nursing homes. However, a judgement about the relative efficiency of public and private nursing-home care would require data on the case-mix of residents, quality of care and the outcomes associated with each type of environment.

Surveys of Relatives and Volunteers

The conclusion of the relatives' survey is that relatives favour NHS nursing-home care over NHS hospital care. Both relatives and volunteers have positive views about the physical and social environments of the nursing homes.

POLICY CONCLUSION

On the basis of outcome data, we have no evidence to suggest that nurse-managed NHS nursing homes should not be introduced in other health authorities. A second report on the process of care will inform policy-makers about the features of the homes which lead to better outcomes.

The conclusion of this report is that an authority considering developing new accommodation for elderly continuing-care patients should opt to build NHS nursing homes rather than new continuing-care hospital wards. If high occupancy is maintained, the cost per patient per week is unlikely to be higher than existing hospital costs, and improved outcomes in relation to activity levels and resident views should be the benefit.

Researchers

John Bond, Senga Bond, Cam Donaldson, Barbara Gregson, Ann Atkinson

Centre for Health Services Research, University of Newcastle upon Tyne, 21 Claremont Place, Newcastle upon Tyne NE22 4AA. (091 222 6000; FAX 091 222 6043)

Publications

Copies of the full report of individual volumes – *Evaluation of Continuing-Care Accommodation for Elderly People*, HCRU Report No 38 – are available from the Centre. The cost of individual volumes and the full report include postage and packing. Cheques should be made payable to the University of Newcastle upon Tyne.

Complete Set:

Evaluation of Continuing-Care Accommodation for Elderly People. 7 volumes ISBN: 1–870399–26–9 £45.00 incl. p&p –

Vol. 1:   *Evaluating Continuing Care for Very Frail Elderly People.* ISBN: 1–870399–27–7 £5.00 incl. p&p

Vol. 2:   *The Randomised Controlled Trial of the Experimental NHS Nursing Homes and Conventional Continuing-Care Wards in NHS Hospitals.* ISBN: 1–870399–28–5 £11.00 incl. p&p

Vol. 3:   *A Multiple-Case Study of NHS Hospital Wards and Nursing Homes: Some Aspects of Structure and Outcome.* ISBN: 1–870399–29–3 £13.00 incl. p&p

Vol. 4:   *The 1984 and 1987 surveys of Continuing-Care Institutions in Six Health Authorities.* ISBN: 1–870399–30–7 £8.00 incl. p&p

Vol. 5:   *A Cost Study of Continuing-Care Institutions for Very Frail Elderly People.* ISBN: 1–870399–31–5 £5.00 incl. p&p

Vol. 6:   *Surveys of NHS Hospital Wards and Nursing Homes: Views of Relatives and Volunteers.* ISBN: 1–870399–32–3 £6.00 incl. p&p

Vol. 7:   *Overview of and Evaluation of Continuing-Care Accommodation for Elderly People.* ISBN: 1–870399–33–1 £5.00 incl. p&p

Reports:

Bond, J., Atkinson, A., Gregson, B. A., Hughes, P., and Jeffries, L. (1989) 'Evaluation of Continuing-care Accommodation for Elderly People: the 1984 and 1987 surveys of continuing-care institutions in six health authorities', University of Newcastle upon Tyne: Health Care Research Unit, Report No 38, Vol. 4.

Bond, S., and Bond, J. (1989) 'Evaluation of Continuing-care Accommodation for Elderly People: a multiple-case study of NHS hospital wards and nursing homes: some aspects of structure and outcome', Newcastle upon Tyne: Health Care Research Unit, Report No 38, Vol. 3.

Bond, J., Bond, S., Donaldson, C., Gregson, B. A., and Atkinson, A. (1989) 'Evaluating Continuing Care Accommodation for Elderly People. Evaluating continuing care of very frail elderly people', University of Newcastle upon Tyne: Health Care Research Unit, Report No 38, Vol. 1.

Bond, J., Bond, S., Donaldson, C., Gregson, B. A., and Atkinson, A. (1989) 'Evaluation of Continuing-Care Accommodation for Elderly People: Overview of an Evaluation of Continuing-Care Accommodation for Elderly People', Newcastle upon Tyne: Health Care Research Unit, Report No 38, Vol. 7.

Bond, J., Gregson, B. A., Atkinson, A., and Hally, M. R. (1989) 'Evaluation of Continuing-Care Accommodation for Elderly People: The randomised controlled trial of the experimental NHS nursing homes and conventional continuing-care in NHS hospitals', University of Newcastle upon Tyne: Health Care Research Unit, Report No 38, Vol. 2.

Donaldson, C., and Bond, J. (1989) 'Evaluation of Continuing-care Accommodation for Elderly People: a cost study of continuing-care institutions for very frail elderly people', Newcastle upon Tyne: Health Care Research Unit, Report No 38, Vol. 5.

Donaldson, C., and Bond, J. (1989) 'Evaluation of Continuing-care Accommodation for Elderly People: surveys of NHS hospital wards and nursing homes: views of relatives and volunteers', Newcastle upon Tyne: Health Care Research Unit, Report No 38, Vol. 6.

Published papers:

Atkinson, D. A., Bond, J., and Gregson, B. A. (1986) 'The dependency characteristics of older people in long-term institutional care', *Dependency and inter-dependency in old age – theoretical perspectives and policy alternatives,* in C. Phillipson, M. Bernard and P. Strang (eds), London, Croom Helm, 257–269.

Bond, J. (1984) 'Evaluation of long-stay accommodation for elderly people', *Gerontology: social and behavioural perspectives,* in D. B. Bromley (ed.), London, Croom Helm, 88–101.

Bond, J. (1990) 'The cost of quality in nursing homes', *This Caring Business,* **16**, July/Aug.

Bond, J. (1991) 'National Health Service Nursing Homes Again', *Age and Ageing,* **20**: 313–315.

Bond, J., Atkinson, D. A., Bond, S., Donaldson, C. R., Gregson, B. A., and Hally, M. R. (1986) 'Evaluation of Long-Stay Accommodation for Elderly People: First Interim Report', University of Newcastle upon Tyne: Health Care Research Unit, Report No 29.

Bond, J., Atkinson, A., Gregson, B. A., and Newell, D. J. (1989) 'Pragmatic and explanatory trials in the evaluation of the experimental National Health Service nursing homes', *Age and Ageing,* **18**: 89–95.

Bond, J., and Bond, S. (1987) 'Development in the Provision and Evaluation of Long-term Care for Dependent Old People', *Research in the Nursing Care of Elderly People,* in P. Fielding (ed.), London, Wiley, 47–85.

Bond, S., and Bond, J. (1990) 'Outcome of care within a multiple-case study in the evaluation of the experimental National Health Service nursing homes', *Age and Ageing,* **19**: 11–18.

Bond, J., Bond, S., Donaldson, C., Gregson, B. A., and Atkinson, A. (1989) 'Evaluation of an innovation in the continuing care of very frail elderly people in the United Kingdom', *Ageing and Society,* **9**: 347–381.

Bond, J., Bond, S., and Gregson, B. A. (1990) 'Nursing Homes and Continuing Care, Part I', *Nursing Standard,* **4**, 36: 38–60.

Bond, J., Bond, S., and Gregson, B. A. (1990) 'Nursing Homes and Continuing Care, Part III. The Future Role of NHS Nursing Homes', *Nursing Standard,* **4**, 38: 35–37.

Bond, J., Bond, S., Gregson, B. A., Donaldson, C., and Atkinson, A. (1990) 'Evaluating continuing care in NHS Nursing Homes and Hospital Wards', *Generations Bulletin of the British Society of Gerontology,* **13**: 19–21.

Bond, S., Bond, J., Gregson, B. A., Donaldson, C., and Atkinson, A. (1990) 'Nursing Homes and Continuing Care, Part II', *Nursing Standard,* **4**, 37: 21–23.

Bond, J., Gregson, B. A., and Atkinson, A. (1989) 'Evaluation of continuing-care accommodation for elderly people. Analysis of final and intermediate outcomes', *Tijdschrift Voor Sociale Gezondneidszorg,* **67**: 5.

Bond, J., Gregson, B. A., and Atkinson, A. (1989) 'Measurement of Outcomes within a Multicentred Randomised Controlled Trial in the Evaluation of the Experimental NHS Nursing Homes', *Age and Ageing,* **18**: 292–302.

Bond, J., Gregson, B. A., Atkinson, A., and Newell, D. J. (1989) 'The implementation of a multi-centred randomised controlled trial in the evaluation of the experimental National Health Service nursing homes', *Age and Ageing*, **18**: 96–102.

Donaldson, C., and Bond, J. (1991) 'Cost of continuing-care facilities in the evaluation of experimental National Health Service nursing homes', *Age and Ageing*, **20**: 160–168.

Multi-Purpose Homes for Elderly People

This project was designed to assess the development of multi-purpose homes – Part III homes offering more than one substantive community-support service for elderly people living in their own homes in the community.

There were three main components to the study. The first was a postal survey of Directors of Social Services in England and Wales, with a telephone follow-up, to establish the number of existing and planned multi-purpose homes. The second was a postal questionnaire to a sample of managers of multi-purpose homes, to establish the extent and type of community support services offered. The third component was a set of case studies involving six multi-purpose homes in different areas of England and Wales.

FINDINGS

The survey of Directors of Social Services showed that by April 1990, 268 Part III homes in England and Wales provided more than one substantive community-support service and that there are plans to develop a further 233 such homes in the near future. It also showed that although 2 out of 5 local authorities use the term 'resource centre' in the name of the home, the reaction against the term was so strong in some authorities that it seemed preferable to use a neutral term – 'multi-purpose' home.

In the survey of a sample of managers of multi-purpose homes, it was found that 4 out of 5 multi-purpose homes had small group-living units. The main pattern of provision in 75 per cent of the homes was long-stay, short-stay, day-care, and additional community-support services. One in 5 homes in the sample had sheltered housing attached.

In the multi-purpose homes studied, in detail, a substantial proportion of the residents, 1 in 4, was unaware of the existence of a day-centre in the home. Few residents, an average of two or three at each home, actually went to the day-centre during the week. One in 3 had used the day-centre or the short-stay facilities before becoming a permanent resident. There is concern about possible intrusions into the residential part of multi-purpose homes: such intrusions were reported in one home by day-centre users and in another home by sheltered housing tenants. In a third home, intrusions occurred because home-help organizers and social workers had to go through the residential part of the home to reach their offices, and members of the public similarly had to take the same route to reach the appropriate offices. Because of the absence of a receptionist at the main entrance of any of the six homes, intrusion by members of the public seeking information about community support services was always a possibility.

Day-centre users potentially gained access to additional services, such as help with bathing or hairdressing. But there was evidence of needs not being met by the multi-purpose homes. Although 1 in 5 users was helped to take a bath, as many

Day-centres
Carers

people again wanted such help but were not getting it. Almost half the day-centre users had used the short-stay beds in the homes.

Three out of 4 informal carers were themselves elderly, and the majority were spouses of the day-centre users. These elderly spouses were particularly vulnerable, since they not only had a heavier caring burden than the daughters and sons who were carers, but were also less likely to be given advice on coping with particular problems, such as the dependent person's incontinence. Few carers had talked to anybody at the home or a social worker about their own needs for support in continuing to care for the dependent person.

CONCLUSION

Since so few residents attended the day-centre, it is difficult to see what positive long-term advantages they gained from living in a multi-purpose home, except that the 1 in 3 residents who had used either the day-centre or short-stay beds before permanent admission had gained some familiarity with at least part of the building. The advantages to day-centre users and to informal carers of basing community-support services in a multi-purpose home were much more obvious. Not only were the homes' facilities usually of a high standard, but also there was a possibility of a flexible, swift response to crises because of the range of facilities under one roof.

A particular problem in this type of home is the possibility of intrusion, not only in the actual lounges but in the main corridors of the residential part of the home. There are two ways of minimizing the possibilities of these types of intrusions. The residential part of the home could be clearly separated from the day-centre and the offices used by social services staff; or a receptionist could be positioned at the main entrance to the home, who could deal with public referrals.

If elderly people in the community are to be encouraged to refer themselves, or others, for community-support services in multi-purpose homes, then local authorities should consider indicating the existence of the services in the building with a noticeboard.

Researcher

Dr Fay Wright

Age Concern Institute of Gerontology, King's College London, Cornwall House Annexe, Waterloo Road, London SE1 8TX. (071 872 3035; FAX 071 872 3235)

Publications

Wright, F. (1991) *Multi-Purpose Homes for Elderly People*, Report to the Department of Health.

Wright, F. (1991) 'Home from Home', *Social Work Today*, 25 April.

Wright, F. (1992) 'Multi-purpose homes. Some issues arising from the research', in J. Morton (ed.), *Multi-purpose homes for elderly people*, King's College London, Age Concern Institute of Gerontology.

Evaluation of the Welsh Office Elderly Initiative

Progress Report

The Welsh Office Elderly Initiative is a programme of grant aid to promote innovative forms of community care for elderly people. Fifty-four projects across Wales have been supported. Projects began between 1987 and 1991, to run for up to five years. This study is designed to evaluate the Initiative and is funded for three years from mid-1990.

Early work in this project is based upon an examination and analysis of secondary sources of information. These comprise: Welsh Office policy statements; grant applications from projects; Welsh Office summaries of projects; and annual reports from project leaders. So far, analysis has been based on an overview of funded projects, their major characteristics and relationship to the stated aims of the Initiative.

It was found that the criteria for applications were essentially based on a consultation document, *A Good Old Age: An Initiative in the Care of the Elderly in Wales*. The criteria could be divided into the following categories: specific tasks; specific targets; particular ways of working and underlying principles.

The projects varied considerably in terms of the number and type of criteria met. There have also been shifts over the course of the Initiative. The use of assessment procedures and the use of existing resources were the most commonly met task-oriented criteria. Almost two-thirds of the projects provided services for elderly people with specialist needs, such as elderly mentally ill people. Half of the projects involved collaboration between voluntary and statutory agencies and over half involved health and local authority collaboration. These aspects of the Initiative are particularly welcome in light of current and planned changes in community care. Two-thirds of the projects claimed to have the underlying principle of retaining elderly people in the community. However, those criteria which one might expect to be the most important for elderly people at the threshold of residential care – such as respite-care, day hospital provision and day-care facilities – are less evident.

Over the course of the four years in which projects were approved, there has been an observable trend towards voluntary sector projects and a reduced emphasis on the use of service packaging.

Projects have been funded in all eight counties in Wales. However, the concentration of projects in parts of South Wales is unrelated to the proportions of elderly people living in these areas. If this distribution of projects reflects more and better-drafted applications from these areas it may be appropriate to provide more support or training in drafting grant applications for those authorities who require it.

Continuing research on the Elderly Initiative will focus on those aspects which are potentially the most important in terms both of future central funding of develop-

Collaboration

Multi-disciplinary working

Voluntary sector

ment projects and of the implementation of the 1990 NHS and Community Care Act – namely: internal monitoring and evaluation, and multi-disciplinary working.

The study of multi-disciplinary working in the Initiative has involved site visits to a selection of the Initiative's projects and will be the focus of more detailed research. It will involve the investigation of differences between projects with multi-disciplinary staff working together as a discrete and identifiable team and multi-disciplinary staff working together loosely, not identifiable as a specific team. This will include an investigation of awareness of the role of other workers, power relations, training, lines of accountability, team-building, and the decision-making process. The area of multi-disciplinary working is being looked at in the context of the forthcoming community care plans and the changes heralded by the White Paper. The work will continue to involve interviews, observation, analysis of project documents and reference to both Department of Health and Welsh Office policy documents.

Researcher

Ms Catherine Robinson

Centre for Social Policy Research and Development, University of Wales, Bangor, Gwynedd LL57 2DG (0248 351151)

Publications

Robinson, C. A., and Wenger, G. C. (1992) *An Overview of Projects funded under the Welsh Office Elderly Initiative 1987–91.* Bangor, Centre for Social Policy Research and Development, University of Wales.

Robinson, C. A., and Wenger, G. C. (1992) *Welsh Office Elderly Initiative: Organisation and Impact,* Bangor, Centre for Social Policy Research and Development, University of Wales.

Robinson, C. A., and Wenger, G. C. (1992) *Internal monitoring and evaluation: The projects' perspective,* Bangor, Centre for Social Policy Research and Development, University of Wales.

Monitoring and Evaluation of Selected Projects under the Initiative for the Care of the Elderly in Wales

PROGRESS REPORT

Costs
Effectiveness
Outcomes

Introduction

The purpose of this research is to monitor and evaluate two of the projects financed under the Initiative on the Care of the Elderly in Wales, concentrating attention on:

(a) value for money;
(b) quality of service;
(c) effectiveness of preventing hospitalization/residential care;
(d) effectiveness of multi-disciplinary working.

The two projects identified for evaluation were:

1. The Staying at Home Initiative (SAHI), established by West Glamorgan Social Services Department. The aim of the scheme is to explore ways of improving community services and, in particular, to enable elderly people, who would otherwise have required residential care, to remain in their own homes.

2. The Ruddlan Elderly Mentally Infirm Team (REMIT), set up by Clwyd Health Authority. This scheme aims to enable people to remain at home who
   — are suffering from functional or organic psychiatric illness;
   — are over the age of 65 on referral; or
   — whose carers are under great stress.

The total costs for the schemes are shown in figures 2.1 and 2.2.

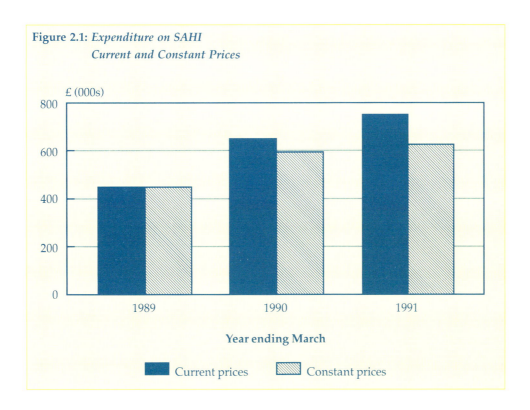

Figure 2.1: *Expenditure on SAHI*
Current and Constant Prices

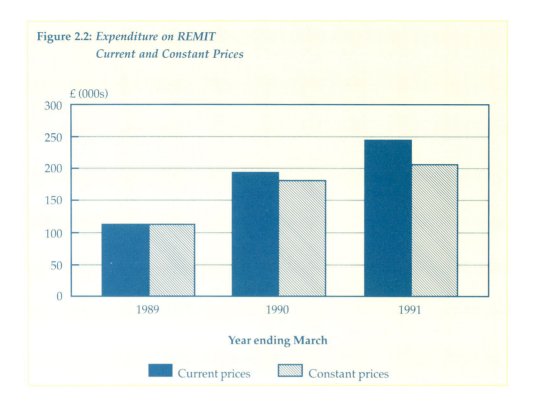

Figure 2.2: *Expenditure on REMIT*
Current and Constant Prices

Year ending March

Current prices   Constant prices

With both schemes, the increase in costs has been in excess of inflation and the growth of the schemes. These increases have led to restrictions in the numbers of people who have been taken on to the schemes – SAHI achieved only about half its original target figure.

Other non-financial costs which have emerged from REMIT include inconvenience to neighbours, wandering, and carer stress; loneliness, unrealistic expectations and costs to families have occurred in SAHI.

Output

The number of clients who have been provided with care by REMIT has ranged from seven at its inception, to a maximum of 24 in January 1990. The scheme currently has 21 clients as a caseload, with 17 receiving the full package of care and four receiving more limited 'sessional' care. The average age of the clients when they start on the REMIT scheme is 81, while the average age of those who have been discharged and who die was 83.

There is no evidence to indicate that gender, marital status or living alone affects the likelihood of discharge into hospital or private nursing-home care. The number of deaths and discharges from the scheme is 27; 14 of these entered hospital and five a nursing home.

The two major factors contributing to the discharge of clients are requests by the family or carer for the client to be admitted to hospital or a nursing home, and the assessment of the supervisor that the client can no longer be cared for within the community.

The number of elderly people who have been taken on by SAHI is 123. The numbers who have died and been discharged amount to 75, 57 of whom have died at home.

The scheme coordinators have reported that the decision to discharge clients to residential or nursing-home care is taken only after much discussion with the service user, carer(s) and family. Discharge from SAHI does not mean that clients are forgotten: care is taken to find suitable accommodation, and clients are given time to get accustomed to their new environment and receive visits from the home care assistants. The family is also supported during the intermediate period following admission.

Outcomes

REMIT

Data collected so far does not suggest that REMIT clients or their carers are anything other than satisfied with the services provided. Other findings measured in terms of the 'dimensions of quality of life' suggested by Challis (1981)[9], include:

1. REMIT ensures that all clients' homes are sound, warm, draught-free and in an acceptable decorative state, while negotiations with builders etc., are undertaken by REMIT on the client's behalf.
2. Services are provided on a regular basis, but it is only on rare occasions that services are provided after mid-evening, with no put-to-bed service and late-evening checks to ensure that clients are safe.
3. Services are provided in two- and three-hour blocks of time, which may not be the most efficient and effective use of the home-support workers, given that one of the objectives of REMIT is to enable users to carry out as many tasks for themselves as they can manage. There also appears to be little scope for a reduction in input if the client (or carer) requests it.
4. Another of REMIT's objectives is to increase awareness about mental illness in the community, and avoid unnecessary admissions to residential care.

SAHI

Data relating to outcomes on the SAHI scheme were collected by administering a questionnaire on two separate occasions over a 12-month period, to SAHI clients and clients receiving mainstream home-care support.

Over time, SAHI clients were more mobile, whilst the opposite was the case in the comparison group. In addition, SAHI clients demonstrated an improvement in ability to undertake household tasks and care for themselves, with no difference recorded in the comparison group.

The evidence to date suggests that SAHI clients are very content with the services provided. Measured against Challis' 'dimensions of quality of life', the following observations may be made:

1. The homes of clients are sound, warm, draught-free and in a reasonable decorative state with additional advice and assistance available from the local Care and Repair representative and from the Disablement Assessment Officer.
2. Assistance is available, if necessary, around the clock, and at short notice in emergencies, via the Community Alarm System, although initial findings suggest wide variations in usage between areas.
3. Physical security is provided through the installation of remote-control door systems for those who have difficulty reaching their doors.
4. SAHI has sought to ensure that daily needs are met – for example, by encouraging clients to eat properly and regularly.
5. There have been attempts to increase awareness within the community.

---

[9] Challis, D. (1981) 'The Measurement of Outcome in Social Care of the Elderly; *Journal of Social Policy*, **10**, 2: 179–208.

Processes

A. Referral Procedures

REMIT has adopted a range of methods for providing information, improving contacts with professionals and the community, generating referrals and finding clients.

The majority of referrals have come from the Community Psychiatric Nurses (45 per cent) and day hospitals (24 per cent).

The 'marketing' activities adopted by SAHI range from the production of Information Packs, to the establishment of networks of representatives of the scheme and other professionals and agency representatives. The location of the scheme's bases in Area Social Service Offices also enables more regular (and informal) contact between the staff involved with the scheme and other social service department staff.

The major proportion of referrals to SAHI comes from social workers (including hospital social workers).

B. Assessment of Needs, Care Planning and Provision of Services

The REMIT *assessment process* seeks to determine

> (1) the eligibility of the client for admission on to the scheme, and
> (2) the mix and degree of service provision to meet their assessed needs.

If a vacancy exists, selection is based on whether

— the person has behavioural problems that other services have failed to cope with and whether they have been referred to REMIT 'as a last resort'; and

— the neighbours are supportive, or at least not hostile, to the person remaining at home.

The process of *care planning* in REMIT has three components: an initial visit, in which the carer and client may discuss the care-package with the CPN; a monthly care-planning meeting; and – when necessary – changes to plans in response to requests from carers and/or families.

In SAHI, one of the coordinators visits prospective service-users and undertakes an *assessment* based on criteria listed on an assessment form. The *care planning* process involves a multi-disciplinary meeting during which a care plan is drawn up in consultation with the client and carer, followed by a review meeting within two weeks. Further monthly reviews are undertaken for the first six months with regular, but less frequent, reviews thereafter. Clients are also visited regularly by the coordinator and the home-care organizer. Service-users can choose from a range of services which are available to all other clients of social services in the County, including home-care, access to day-centres and respite-care, aids and adaptations, the community alarm system, use of the night mobile-service and the services of the coordinator(s) and health visitors.

CONCLUSIONS

Although there is no clear statement of the target number of REMIT clients, the current total of about 20 seems low. Both schemes have failed to meet the efficiency criteria chosen for the evaluation because of an under-estimate of the costs needed to achieve their respective objectives. Although both schemes are demonstration projects which may incur 'additional' costs, this is balanced by the fact that a proportion of management time has been devoted to the schemes without any costs being incurred.

There is not much evidence of inter-organizational cooperation in the schemes. REMIT is very much a scheme run by a team housed within the health authority, while SAHI – although it has forged strong links with Age Concern – has sought to handle the inter-disciplinary working arrangements by appointing a health visitor to the scheme, thereby avoiding recourse to the Health Authority. The evidence also suggests that professional disciplines tend to influence the source of referral and therefore the approach to care-management adopted. In comparing the clients on both schemes it is clear that the vast majority have been referred via traditional, professional routes and reflect the institutional origins of each scheme.

Researchers

C. J. Phillips, C. F. Palfrey, H. N. Harding, S. Pickard, R. J. Urquhart

Policy Studies Unit, Gwent College of Higher Education, Allt-yr-yn Avenue, Newport, Gwent NP9 5XA. (0633 430088)

Abuse of Elderly People

The research was an exploratory study of existing data, literature and innovatory schemes. It provided a new perception of the questions involved and a clear view of possible future research directions.

Inter-agency cooperation

US research

BACKGROUND

Despite concern expressed in this country about the problem of abuse of elderly people, over a period of nearly 15 years almost no systematic or reliable research has been carried out. In contrast, in North America a considerable amount of research has been undertaken and it is this work that provides the most up-to-date and reliable insights into the problem of what is now generally referred to as 'elder abuse'.

DEFINITION

There is an unresolved question over whether elder abuse has characteristics which distinguish it from abuse of other adults, for example with learning disabilities or physical handicaps. There is no standard definition. Definition varies according to the purpose for which it is needed. Research definitions in the USA have generally focused on the domestic setting of abuse and have included physical abuse, psychological abuse, neglect and sometimes financial abuse. The operational meaning given to the definitions varies. There has been little research on specific incidents of abuse in institutions although the existence of such incidents is well-documented here. A distinct, although possibly related phenomenon, is institutional abuse. This occurs when the ethos and regulations governing daily life in institutions lead the residents to be treated in a dehumanizing and demeaning way.

RECENT RESEARCH

The problem of abuse, particularly in this country, has invariably been framed in the context of the stress imposed by caring for an elderly relative. Recent research suggests that there are problems about this formulation. It is not always clear what kind of abuse is being referred to. Secondly, the kinds of abusive situations identified and reported by professionals may not accurately reflect the total picture of abuse. Thirdly, the view that physical abuse results from the stress of caring has been challenged by research. What emerges clearly is the complexity of elder abuse and the pitfalls of generalization. While psychological abuse may, it appears, be linked to other kinds of abuse and to neglect, physical abuse, financial abuse and neglect of an elderly person appear to display distinct patterns of their own.

PREVALENCE

Nothing is known in this country about the prevalence of abuse – how much of what kind of abuse there is throughout the elderly population. The most reliable information in the USA came from a random-sample survey of Boston residents in 1986. This suggested a figure of 32 cases per 1,000 elderly people. The researchers excluded financial abuse and their definitions were strictly geared to the purposes of the research. A Canadian national survey which included financial abuse suggested a figure of 40 per 1,000 elderly, of which 25 were cases of financial abuse.

DEVELOPMENTS IN THIS COUNTRY

Various largely un-coordinated initiatives are occurring in health authorities, social services departments, voluntary organizations, professional associations and training bodies. A comprehensive review of relevant legislation is being under-taken by the Law Commission. This surge of activity is a reflection of professional concern about the problem. Few authorities have policies or procedures to guide their workers, although an increasing number are working on them. Guidelines are not always connected to an adequate or informed understanding of the problem. There is awareness that inter-agency coordination between health, social services, police and housing is fundamental but even fewer authorities have developed *joint* guidelines. The complexity of boundaries does not help.

THE NEXT STEPS

It cannot be assumed that American research findings are valid here. The findings are heavily dependent on the definitions used, the underlying research and the methodology. Research is needed here, some of which could build on the American experience. There is also a case for central guidance on the development of policy and procedures, and on inter-agency coordination.

Researchers

Claudine McCreadie and Anthea Tinker

Age Concern Institute of Gerontology, King's College London, Cornwall House Annexe, Waterloo Road, London SE1 8TX. (071 872 3035; FAX 071 872 3235)

Publications

McCreadie, C. (1991) *Elder Abuse: an exploratory study,* King's College London, Age Concern Institute of Gerontology.

McCreadie, C., and Tinker, A. (forthcoming) 'Abuse of Elderly People in the Domestic Setting: a UK perspective', *Age and Ageing.*

Health and Social Care Provision for Older People from Ethnic Minorities

A decade of research has consistently demonstrated low uptake of statutory social and community health services by black and minority ethnic older people. There is no evidence of less need among these groups, and it has become increasingly apparent that traditional attitudes and methods of service delivery, misunderstanding of cultural and socio-economic factors, and language differences place major barriers to service access.

There is an urgent need to tackle these problems. Older people from black and minority ethnic groups in certain areas are particularly vulnerable because of low incomes, poor housing, isolation and higher health risks. Coupled with this is the growth in both the size and proportion of the older black and ethnic population which means that service providers must increasingly find ways of reaching this group.

Voluntary and statutory service innovations have developed in response to some of these needs, but these have generally been on a patchy or *ad hoc* basis, often with short-term funding. We still have little information about general trends in statutory service development to older people, or of the perceptions or preferences of older people.

To fill this gap, the Age Concern Institute of Gerontology is carrying out a review of existing statutory service provision to black and ethnic minority older people. The study consists of a survey of current services and a consumer survey.

Survey of Current Service Provision

Trends in service delivery to groups of black and ethnic minority people are being addressed, from social service departments, district health authorities and family health service authorities in areas with significant black and minority ethnic populations. To complete the picture of primary health care provision, a survey of GPs is also being carried out in a sub-sample of areas.

Information has been collected by postal surveys and interviews with a wide range of staff involved with older people. A particular focus has been on the development of any specific provision in relation to black and ethnic minority older people, and the extent to which this has taken place inside or outside mainstream services.

Survey of Older People

A survey of groups of older people from black and ethnic minority communities in six areas is currently being carried out. Interviewers have been recruited from within the communities in each area, and speak a range of languages. Questionnaires have been translated into a number of different languages and explore perceptions, use and experiences of services, as well as satisfaction and preferences.

Consumer views

Innovation

The result of the research will enable us to build up a comprehensive picture of the extent to which health and social services are attempting to meet the specific needs of older people from black and minority ethnic communities, and make an assessment of the success with which they are doing this as perceived by older people themselves. It should provide information about successful service development, highlight gaps in service delivery and indicate the priorities for service managers as they draw up the contracts which will determine the quality of care of older people in the multi-racial society.

Researchers

Dr Janet Askham and Cathy Pharoah

Age Concern Institute of Gerontology, Cornwall House Annexe, Waterloo Road, London SE1 8TX. (071 872 3035; FAX 071 872 3235)

Publications

Pharoah, C. (1991) 'Health and social care provision for older people', *Share Newsletter*, Issue 1, November 1991, 5.

NOTE: We are grateful to the Editor of the *Share Newsletter* for permission to print a version of Ms Pharoah's article.

Weaning Elderly People off Psychotropic Medication: a Randomized Controlled Trial

Objectives

1. To investigate the use of psychotropic medication in the community.

2. To evaluate a policy of weaning elderly people on long-term psychotropic medication (sedatives, hypnotics, anxiolytics and anti-depressants) off their medication.

Counselling Nurse's role

The study was undertaken in two large urban practices in South Wales, in a town that has been classified as 'average' for urban areas for England and Wales. A register was compiled of all elderly patients (65 years and over) who had been taking psychotropic medication for at least three months. Each elderly person was interviewed in his/her own home. They were asked questions about their health and their medication, including details about their psychotropic medication, and all medication was checked personally by the interviewer. Each patient was interviewed for a second time nine months later in his/her own home. The second questionnaire investigated the changes in medication and also whether patients had attempted to reduce their psychtropic medication and their experiences of attempting to reduce medication, if they had attempted so to do.

Patients with epilepsy and those under long-term psychiatric care were excluded from the study. Patients allocated to the intervention group were invited for a consultation with the GP and the practice nurse. Those unable to come to surgery were visited by the GP and nurse at home on separate occasions. Patients who agreed to attempt this withdrawal of medication were provided with an agreed strategy of gradual reduction, leading to ultimate withdrawal. A practice nurse provided relaxation and counselling sessions for as long as was thought necessary by the patient.

MAIN RESULTS

- Eight per cent of older people were taking psychotropic medication.
- The most commonly consumed long-term psychotropic medications were nitrazepam (28 per cent), diazepam (15 per cent), chlorazepate potassium (8 per cent), chlordiazepoxide (6 per cent) and fluorazepam (6 per cent).
- Elderly people taking psychotropic medication tended to be older, more likely to be female and widowed than a 'normal' population. They were more disabled, more anxious, more depressed, experienced more minor symptoms, for example, confusion, lack of energy, nausea and insomnia. They also reported a worse health status.

    The finding that this group of people had experienced significantly more falls in the previous six months was particularly important.

- Fourteen per cent of respondents had been taking long-term psychtropic medication for less than 2 years, 19 per cent for less than five years, 25 per cent for less than ten years and 34 per cent for more than ten years.

- The vast majority of the sample (79 per cent) were female and half were aged over 75 years.
- The majority of patients, when approached, were keen to attempt to discontinue or reduce their psychotropic medication. Those who were not keen felt they 'needed their medication' or that they would not be able to sleep.
- Most of those attempting discontinuation (60 per cent) experienced no difficulties; only 10 per cent found it moderately difficult and 10 per cent very difficult; sleep problems were the most frequently reported problems.
- Of those who attempted reduction, 41 per cent completely discontinued and 43 per cent significantly reduced their medication; 16 per cent failed completely. Twice as many people in the intervention group reduced medication as in the non-intervention group.
- Of those who reduced or stopped, 39 per cent felt the same as before, 42 per cent better than before and 11 per cent worse than before. Those who reported feeling better when they reduced their medication indicated that they felt 'less drowsy and more clear-headed'.
- Many patients found the support of the nurse very helpful. It seems unlikely that such a policy would have met with the same success without the provision of counselling, support and relaxation therapy by the practice nurse.
- GPs involved in the study did not feel that the policy had significantly increased their workload.

In the light of these results, it is clear that the introduction of a policy to reduce the number of elderly people on unnecessary long-term psychotropic medication would improve the health and well-being of many people, and significantly reduce the cost of GPs' prescribing.

Researcher

Dr Dee Jones

Research Team for the Care of Elderly People, Department of Geriatric Medicine, University of Wales College of Medicine, Cardiff Royal Infirmary, Cardiff CF2 1SZ. (0222 491000)

Publications

(1990) *Weaning elderly people off psychotropic medication: a randomised controlled trial,* Research Team, Cardiff, ISBN 869923–05–1.

Jones, D. A. (1991) 'Weaning elderly patients off psychotropics in general practice: a randomised controlled trial', *Health Trends, 22,* 4: 164–166.

Jones, D. A. (in press) 'Characteristics of elderly people taking psychotropic medication', *Drugs and Ageing.*

Chapter 3

Informal Care and Carers

Informal Care and Carers

The work described in this Chapter represents a body of evidence about the extent of informal caring: who are the carers, and for whom do they care. Again, much of the work is concerned with elderly people, but there are also a number of studies – some described in subsequent Chapters – which centre on the carers of people with mental illness, dementia or learning disabilities. Two studies described here focus on families caring for children who are physically frail or have learning disabilities.

The research provides data about the extent and nature of caring; evaluates services and demonstration districts designed to support carers or offer respite; and analyses the needs of particular groups of informal carers. One project in particular focuses on their financial circumstances: others deal with the coping strategies employed by families and individuals.

Several linked projects examine the support networks available to elderly people, document how they change over time, suggest a typology of support patterns, and propose a practical technique for their identification and analysis. Two other studies have looked at the ways in which support networks are relevant to the needs of people with dementia and learning disabilities.

Analysis of 1985 General Household Survey Data on Informal Care

The aim of this project was to carry out secondary analysis of data from the 1985 General Household Survey (GHS) which had generated the first-ever, nationally representative data-set on informal care.

The analysis was in two main stages; first, the development of a typology of caring and second, a number of papers on specific topics: the consequences of caring, service receipt and substitution, and male carers.

Typology of carers

Costs of caring

Services

Typology of Carers

By dividing up the six million people identified in the 1985 GHS as 'carers' on the basis of the tasks they were carrying out, we constructed a framework for a more sophisticated understanding of the nature of informal caring activity.

We identified around 1.8 million people involved in substantial levels of caring activity, providing personal and/or physical care for long hours and over relatively long periods of time. These carers are often quite elderly themselves and are most likely to be caring for close relatives who live in the same household. The remainder were people involved in activities which might more accurately be termed 'informal helping'. They provide practical help to friends, neighbours and less close relatives, who do not live in the same household, for relatively few hours, but may do so over long periods of time. These 'helpers' seem to fall into two main sub-groups: those who are the only or main source of help for the other individual and, more commonly, those who are part of a network where others, presumably, take major responsibility.

These differences have implications both for the type of services that might be required to support informal care in the community and for the number of carers that might need support.

The Consequences of Caring

In order to examine the consequences of caring, carers were compared with a matched group of non-carers. Matching was done by age and sex. The most significant steps forward in understanding the impact of caring lie in the areas of *finance and health*.

First, the analysis showed that carers – particularly those providing the most intense forms of care and caring for someone in the same household – suffer effects on their labour market participation and, therefore, on their personal earnings and income. Even when in paid work, carers earn less than their non-carer peers, regardless of whether they are male or female, or whether they provide care in the same household or elsewhere. These effects carry through into household income, indicating that other household members' incomes (if any) are not able to make up the 'deficit' caused by carers' depressed earnings and incomes. Carers are far less likely than their peers to have income from savings, indicating that depressed incomes are likely to have a life-long effect. The income effect of caring appears to carry over into housing tenure and conditions for some groups of carers, meaning that they have less access to owner-occupation and are more likely to be in overcrowded conditions.

Secondly, the analysis suggested that previous research, which has argued a causal relationship between caring and current physical ill-health, may have confused the effects of caring with those of age and sex, both of which also influence health status. Female carers were slightly more likely than their peers to report a long-standing illness or disability, but this was among the *least* involved carers.

Service Receipt

The original GHS report revealed substantial differences in service receipt between people whose carers lived in the same household and those whose carers lived elsewhere. This analysis, however, left a number of issues to be explored: the effect of service substitutability; the effect of the sex of the carer; her or his relationship to the cared-for person and whether or not s/he lived in the same household; and the effect of services, in general, going to those who live alone rather than those who live with others.

Fewer than half the people being cared for were receiving any service at all. Among those who were, visits from a home-help or doctor were the most common, followed by a community or district nurse. Very few people received more than one service.

With the exception of meals-on-wheels, all services appeared to be relatively well-targeted in relation to the level of disability of the person being cared for. By contrast, there was very substantial variation in service receipt across different caring relationships and situations, **regardless** of the level of disability of the person being cared for. Those being cared for by relatives in the same household were, across the board, less likely to be receiving services than others. Some services appeared to discriminate against some people even more than others. The home-help service was the one least likely to be received by those cared for by relatives in the same household, regardless of level of disability.

Some services distinguish between different caring relationships and circum-stances much more sharply than others. Community nursing services, for example, appear to be delivered more equitably than visits from doctors and the meals-on-wheels service.

The findings support the idea that a hierarchy of service substitution exists, in that carers in the same household are less likely to provide nursing or medical care than to cook or to do housework for the cared-for person.

Once dependence levels and the caring relationship and circumstances were taken into account, there were no differences in service receipt between those with male and female carers. There was some evidence that sex and marital status together influenced service receipt. For example, those cared for by male, unmarried, carers were around two-thirds more likely to receive home-help services than those cared for by female, unmarried, carers. However, regardless of level of disability or the caring relationship and circumstances, home-help services were much more likely to be going to women cared for by men than to men being cared for by women. As in previous research, this suggests that home-help services act to replace disabled or frail women's domestic labour rather than to support women who have caring responsibilities.

Among those people with carers living elsewhere, the only service which those who lived alone were more likely to receive was the home-help service. In all other cases, those living with others (not their carers) were more likely to receive services. This finding questions the suggestion that those without resident carers get more services because they are more likely to be living alone. It also leads to the conclusion that, all other things being equal, service provision is generally biased against those who have resident carers, and those whose carers are relatives.

Male Carers

Three different sorts of questions were asked in relation to male carers. What is the incidence of caring activities as between men and women? What is the nature of caring activities that men carry out compared to women? What impact does caring have on men as compared with women?

Among all men, those with the highest likelihood of being carers were single men aged 45–64, while those with the lowest were single men aged 19–29. However, across all ages, married men were more likely to report caring responsibilities than single or ever-married men.

While similar proportions of men and women in the population-at-large identify themselves as carers, the 'risk' of becoming a carer is much smaller for men than for women, particularly in some age/marital status groups.

Controlling for the nature of the relationship between carer and cared-for person, and for the carer's level of responsibility, removes most differences between men and women in terms of the nature of their caring activities. A major difference which does remain is in the type of care provided. Except when they have main responsibility for the care of a spouse, men are less likely than women to be providing personal care (such as washing or bathing). However, overall, the carer's relationship to the cared-for person has more influence in determining the type of care provided than does sex of the carer.

Caring responsibilities appear to have a much more significant effect on male carers' employment patterns (and consequently their earnings) than on women's. This is explained to a large degree by the fact that labour-market activity among women is already depressed by marriage and having dependent children. When in some form of paid employment, male carers are substantially more likely to be in part-time work than their age/sex peers. A similar, but not so pronounced, effect is evident among women where, again, marital status and having dependent children are more influential.

The only remaining major difference in the apparent impact of caring on men and women is in relation to long-standing illness or disability. Male carers are less likely than female carers to report such problems. However, it is difficult to tease out cause and effect here. Those involved in the greatest caring responsibilities are not the same as those who report a long-standing illness or disability – a finding which militates against a direct causal link.

Researchers

Dot Lawton and Gillian Parker

Social Policy Research Unit, University of York, Heslington, York YO1 5DD. (0904 433608; FAX 0904 433618)

Publications

Parker, G., and Lawton, D. (1990) 'Further analysis of the 1985 General Household Survey data on informal care. Report 1: A typology of Caring', University of York, Social Policy Research Unit, Working Paper DHSS 715.

Parker, G., and Lawton D. (1990) 'Further Analysis of the 1985 General Household Survey data on informal care. Report 2: The consequences of caring', University of York, Social Policy Research Unit, Working Paper DHSS 716.

Parker, G., and Lawton, D. (1991) 'Further analysis of the 1985 General Household Survey data on informal care. Report 3: Carers and services', University of York, Social Policy Research Unit, Working Paper DHSS 789.

Parker, G., and Lawton, D. (1991) 'Further analysis of the 1985 General Household Survey data on informal care. Report 4: Male carers', University of York, Social Policy Research Unit, Working Paper DHSS 849.

Parker, G., and Lawton, D. (1992) *Different types of caring, different types of carers: evidence from the General Household Survey*, London, HMSO.

Evaluating Support to Informal Carers

The purpose of the study was to evaluate the effectiveness of formal service-provision in supporting informal carers. The study covered the carers of adults with learning disabilities, adults diagnosed as mentally ill, adults with physical disabilities, older people with physical disabilities, and older people with mental infirmity.

Services

Carers' views

'Normaliza-tion'

The study was not confined to services provided exclusively for the carer, but looked at the ways in which the care system as a whole – health services, social services and the voluntary sector – relates to and supports informal carers. There were two main areas of interest: first, the carers – their situation, needs, judgements and perceptions of formal services; and secondly, service provision and its models of policy and practice in relation to informal carers. The study explores the judgements and attitudes of service providers to carers, and the negotiation that takes place between these two perspectives.

The main conclusions are:

► Carers are rarely the direct subjects of service provision, and are often helped only on the margins by services that are primarily aimed at the cared-for person. The attitudes of mainstream services are, therefore, of greater overall significance than those of small-scale, carer-orientated services.

► The relationship between informal carers and their social care agencies is an uncertain and ill-defined one. Agencies shift between approaching carers as a kind of resource to be maximized, and a response which appears to focus on their well-being. The chosen approach depends on a variety of factors: the professional training of the service provider; their location in the organization; whether their practice is focused around medical or social care; and pressure on resources.

► The carers' perceptions of their role and their response to caring are vital in determining the relevance of service provision. Relationship and gender play an important part in this. Some carers subordinate their lives to the cared-for person in ways that make it difficult for them to distance themselves from the situation. As a result, they are reluctant to seek help from services, and remain invisible to service providers, hidden behind the needs of the person they look after. Other carers detach themselves from their caring in ways which make it easier for them to cope with the burden of caring, and allow them to seek and accept service help.

► A number of factors affect the relationship between carers and service provision. These include the role of the cared-for person and the role of other family members; the nature of the relationship between carer and cared-for person; the presence or otherwise of a future for the cared-for person beyond the life of the carer; as well as more structural factors such as gender, age, race and class.

► Services are limited in the problems they cover. Having a need which fits within the normal range of service provision is obviously central to getting any help. Service practitioners find it easier to help where there is a clear task to be done, and when paid workers can be substituted for unpaid ones. This is particularly true of activities for which there is a tradition of provision within the formal economy – for example, domestic tasks and meal provision. It is harder to design and supply services which replace the carer's role in 'being responsible' for the cared-for person.

► A service may be one-off or continuing, and this can have important consequences for carers. One-off service contact, such as the provision of aids and adaptations or a visit to a GP, by definition ends once the specific 'problem' is dealt with. Onward referral from such a contact is rare. Service contact that is continuing – such as with mental handicap teams or services for older, mentally infirm people which centre on a day hospital – makes it more likely that the carer's needs will be noticed and referred on to other services. Continuing contact also means that changes in the carer's situation can be identified.

► The way in which practitioners see their role can have repercussions for the carer. Some service providers adopt a proactive attitude towards carers, encouraging them to accept help and offering information. Others are more passive and wait for carers to make demands on them. Not all carers appreciated these differences: some imagined that if they had not been offered help, it did not exist.

► The concept of 'normalization' underpins much provision of services for people with a learning disability. This philosophy – although bringing many benefits for clients – creates tensions between some carers and service providers. Normalization necessarily undermines the carer's assumption that he/she will remain responsible for the situation and in control of the main decisions regarding care, and can cause considerable anxiety. Service providers, although generally recognizing these tensions, tend to give priority to developing the autonomy of the person with a learning disability.

► Caring for someone with mental health problems has not traditionally been included in accounts of care-giving. The report explores the differences posed by mental health problems, but concludes that there are sufficient similarities to make the application of a 'carer' perspective useful.

Implications for Further Development

The research shows that the major issue for policy-makers and managers is whether informal carers should be incorporated into mainstream provision, and – if so – in what way. There needs to be much greater clarity of aims in relation to carers among policy-makers and service providers. Substantial improvement in the situation of carers is likely to require either an injection of further resources or a re-targeting of provision from current recipients towards carers.

A second issue of importance for policy-makers and service providers is that a commitment to support for service users will sometimes lead to conflicts of interest. While guidance on the NHS and Community Care Act acknowledges that such conflicts may arise, clear advice is needed on how they might be resolved.

Researchers

Karl Atkin, Christina Perring and Julia Twigg

Social Policy Research Unit, University of York, Heslington, York YO1 5DD. (0904 433608)

Publications

Perring, C., Twigg, J., and Atkin, K. (1990), *Families Caring for Those Diagnosed as Mentally Ill: The Literature Re-examined*, London, HMSO.

Twigg, J. (1989) 'Models of Carers: How do Social Care Agencies Conceptualise Their Relationship with Informal Carers?', *Journal of Social Policy*, **18**, 1: 53–66.

Twigg, J., and Atkin, K. (1991) 'Evaluating Support to Informal Carers (Part 2): Final Report', University of York, Social Policy Research Unit, Working Paper DHSS 809.

Twigg, J., and Atkin, K. (1991) 'Evaluating Support to Informal Carers: Summary Report', York, SPRU.

Twigg, J., and Atkin, K. (1991) 'Providing service support to carers', *Benefits*, **2**: 31.

Twigg, J., Atkin, K., and Perring, C. (1990) *Carers and Services: A Review of the Literature*, London, HMSO.

Twigg, J., Atkin, K., with Perring C. (1990) 'Evaluating Support to Informal Carers (Part 1) Final Report', University of York, Social Policy Research Unit, Working Paper DHSS 709.

Demonstration Districts for Informal Carers – An Evaluation

In 1986, as part of the 'Helping the Community to Care' programme, the Department of Health funded three 'demonstration districts' to explore ways in which voluntary organizations could provide support to carers. The programme was set up at a time when carers were barely on the policy agenda and services were still quite rare; but by 1991, the NHS and Community Care Act had given carers a central place in the overall provision of community care.

Voluntary sector

Volunteers

Costs

The evaluation by the Tavistock Institute comprised support for self-evaluation, as well as external evaluation activities. The project team worked alongside district consortia of voluntary organizations, monitoring their activities, reviewing the lessons emerging, and preparing reports on their work. External evaluation involved observation of activities over the three years, and a survey of consortia members and development workers. The team also designed a questionnaire for carers, which was used to evaluate services in two of the districts.

What Kind of Services Work for Carers?

A review of the needs of carers at the start of the study confirmed the findings from elsewhere: while many carers are committed to the continuing support to their dependants, the costs are frequently high – loss of employment, of freedom, of contact with other family members and friends, and poor health. Support from other family members, friends and neighbours is variable and only within very clear limits. We considered the needs of carers in the context of an ideal, overall care-system for someone with a severe disability living in the community, and how the various elements in such a system might be separately or jointly provided.

The services developed within the three districts fell into three broad categories: alternative care for people being cared for in the home; alternative care away from home; and services that provided support, information and advice for carers themselves. In addition to the direct services, the workers employed by consortia in the three districts also undertook developmental work to establish new groups and new services, and campaigning and educational work to raise the profile of carers within their areas.

The balance between the carer and the person s/he is looking after has constantly to be considered in the design and implementation of services. Although needs may be inter-dependent, they are also potentially in conflict; carers can reach the point where the pressure on their lives is no longer tolerable. The carers' response to most of the services set up was a positive one. They welcomed provision which took account of their needs, rather than being entirely focused on the needs of their dependents. However, it was also clear that the services had to provide acceptable and reliable care: the more the service is able to provide positive support and enjoyment for the person with disabilities, the more acceptable it is to their carer as well.

The range of services offered within the three districts appeared to provide potential for comparisons to be made between different kinds of provision. In practice, however, services provided by the voluntary sector were found to be **complementary** rather than providing alternatives. This was because they had been set up in a situation where little had existed at all before for carers. Many of the care systems they were supporting needed a range of different kinds of visits from the district nurse, a home-help, a regular care-attendant, an occasional longer break involving residential care for the person they were looking after, and perhaps a worker or group to provide emotional support and advice. Even when the needs of carers were similar, one kind of service might be more suitable than another.

It was clear that any support services for carers and their dependants must be offered with sensitivity if they were not to increase the feelings of guilt and stigma that carers generally experience. Workers attached to services for people with disabilities were often in a good position to establish a contact with carers and to provide support, information and advice. But they also needed sufficient **time** to be able to respond to carers individually, and sufficient **information and training** to be able to provide appropriate help.

The Role of Voluntary Organizations in Provision of Support to Carers

The consortium in each district provided an important context for discussion and assessment of carers' needs by local agencies. As a result, in all three districts, carers moved up in the list of policy priorities, and the majority of services established during the three years were refunded from local sources when the Department of Health funding came to an end. However, the representation of carers in consortium decisions was not easily achieved: meetings were quite formal, and could be intimidating if only a small number of carers were present. Arranging for carer attendance at meetings also involved making arrangements for alternative care for the people they were looking after.

A number of innovative approaches to carer support were tried, including helplines, carer-centres, and a range of different kinds of 'carer support workers' attached to existing services. Most of the services were staffed primarily by paid workers: volunteers had a role, but this was often a supplementary one. The provision of services through volunteers (who needed a paid coordinator) was not a great deal cheaper to run than a service provided by paid staff, and the range of activities that could be provided, and level of dependency catered for, was limited.

In some cases, the apparently low cost of services concealed subsidies in the form of premises, management help, and services from other agencies – statutory and voluntary. All management was provided by 'volunteers', but many of these were paid workers from other organizations.

Very few of the services set up during the three-year period were self-financing by the end of it. The implication of this is that local authorities that wish to see the growth of services in the voluntary sector for carers will have to assume a major responsibility for funding them. They will also need to offer practical help. Some of the voluntary organizations which came forward to set up services were quite small and inexperienced; some found it difficult to manage the transition to a new way of working, particularly when this involved employing staff for the first time. With help, most of these agencies were able to learn from their mistakes and eventually become established. Others did not, and a potentially useful service therefore disappeared.

Researcher

Dione Hills, with Dr Eric Miller

The Tavistock Centre, 120 Belsize Lane, London NW3 5BA. (071 435 7111; FAX 071 794 4661)

Publications

Haffenden, S. (1991) *Getting it Right for Carers*, London, HMSO.

Hills, D. (1991) *Carer Support in the Community*, London, HMSO.

Hills, D., and Miller, E. (1992) *Demonstration Districts Final Research Report*, Tavistock Occasional Paper.

Sandwell Child Carers Report (1989), available from Sandwell Carers Centre, 2 Bearwood Lane, Smethwick, W. Midlands.

East Sussex Evaluation Report (1989), available from Carers' Council, 143 High St., Lewes, East Sussex.

The Financial Circumstances of Informal Carers

This research explored in detail the financial impact of providing help and support to a severely disabled or infirm elderly person. There were four main areas of interest:

- the impact of caring on paid employment opportunities, hours of work and earnings;
- the impact of caring on income and living standards – taking into account social security benefits which were received, the extra expenditure incurred in the course of giving care, and changes in carers' use of savings, credit and other potential resources;
- transfers of resources and their impact on carers' material circumstances; and
- carers' receipt of statutory, private and voluntary sector services, and the costs and gains of service receipt.

**Costs of caring
Employment
Substitute care**

The research focused on people of working age who were living in the same household as, and caring for, someone who needed considerable personal attention or supervision. Carers of children and of spouses with disabilities were excluded, as they were the focus of other past or current studies.

The carers were interviewed using a semi-structured schedule. The interviews were tape-recorded and subsequently analysed to yield both facts and opinions about the financial consequences of care-giving.

The 30 people interviewed were the primary carers of 29 disabled or older people – mainly a parent/parent-in-law (one sister and brother lived with and shared equally in their father's care). For most, their current substantial care-giving responsibilities had arisen in the past few years. Seven of the carers were male, 23 were female. Fourteen were married, 14 single, 2 widowed and 2 divorced.

Findings and Recommendations

Nearly half the carers (mainly unmarried sons and daughters) had always lived with the person being cared for. A similar proportion had formed new joint households because of the cared-for person's substantial care needs. Thirteen carers lived alone with the cared-for person; the remainder lived in larger households with a spouse or unmarried sibling, and sometimes children of different ages as well.

Six carers had full-time, paid employment. Most had lost disposable income through loss of pay and/or substantial extra spending on private substitute care while at work. Eight carers had part-time or casual employment. All felt restricted to their current jobs and hours of work, and most of these part-timers had also lost or foregone earnings. Eight carers had stopped work since beginning to give care; most had also experienced interruptions and loss of earnings before this. Five carers had been out of work at the time they began giving care and had to delay or forego re-entry to the labour market. Only three carers were economically inactive when they began giving care and would have remained so in any case.

The 13 carers living alone with the cared-for person were much less likely than those in the three adult households to have earnings from employment. Almost all had very low incomes, from invalid care allowance, supplementary benefit, unemployment benefit and their own savings. Their living standards therefore tended to be partially maintained by the resources of the cared-for person, particularly where s/he had additional income from disability benefits, occupational pensions or savings. Further economic dependency was created through the linking of carers' benefit entitlements to the cared-for person's receipt of benefit and their householder status. Despite their own very low incomes, the carers in two-adult households were still likely to have contributed towards the purchase of extra aids and equipment to ease the work of care-giving. Moreover they were experiencing longer-term costs by drawing regularly on savings which, because of their high rate of withdrawal from the labour market, they risked being unable to replenish before their own retirement.

The carers in three-adult households were much more likely to have some earnings of their own, as well as being able to benefit from the earnings of a full-time employed spouse or sibling. These carers therefore tended to subsidize the cared-for person because her/his income was insufficient to pay for an equal share of the commodities (including housing costs) and level of comfort enjoyed by the rest of the household. Half of these carers also regularly had to meet some additional disability or care-giving-related costs which the cared-for person's contribution did not fully cover.

The three-adult households also tended to have experienced additional capital costs associated with the formation of a new joint household, as well as those arising from the purchase of extra aids and equipment to ease the work of caring. They were also more likely to anticipate further deferred spending in the future. However, they did not draw on the cared-for person's savings to maintain their own living standards, and they also stood a greater chance of being able to replenish their own savings in the longer term because of their household's continuing economic activity.

Helping carers to retain – or acquire – paid employment while giving care appears to be the clearest way of avoiding their immediate and longer-term impoverishment. Improvements in the level and variety of substitute care services are necessary, as well as labour market developments which would make paid work and care-giving easier.

A cross-sectional study such as this can provide only limited information on the long-term financial effects of caring. Longitudinal research is needed to trace in more detail the impact over caring 'careers'. Nothing is yet known about the financial circumstances of elderly carers, including those who begin providing care after retirement and those whose withdrawal from the labour market is preceded (and perhaps influenced) by an earlier period of caring.

Researcher

Caroline Glendinning

Social Policy Research Unit, University of York, Heslington, York YO1 5DD. (0904 433608; FAX 0904 433618)

Publications

Glendinning, C. (1986) 'The costs of caring', *Community Outlook, Nursing Times*, **82**, 37: 11–14.

Glendinning, C. (1988) 'The cost of caring' *Poverty*, **73**: 11–13.

Glendinning, C. (1988) 'Dependency and interdependency: the incomes of informal carers and the impact of social security', in S. M. Baldwin, G. M. Parker, and R. Walker (eds.), *Social Security and Community Care*, Aldershot, Avebury.

Glendinning, C. (1988) 'The invisible carers', *New Society*, **84**, 1324: 26–27.

Glendinning, C. (1989) 'The financial circumstances of informal carers', *Department of Health Yearbook of Research and Development*, 33–34, London, HMSO.

Glendinning, C. (1989) 'The financial needs and circumstances of informal carers: final report', University of York, Social Policy Research Unit, Working Paper DHSS 529.

Glendinning, C. (1989) 'The financial needs and circumstances of informal carers: summary', University of York, Social Policy Research Unit, Working Paper DHSS 554.

Glendinning, C. (1990) 'Dependency and inter-dependency: the incomes of informal carers and the impact of social security', *Journal of Social Policy*, **19**, 4: 469–497.

Glendinning, C. (1992) *The costs of informal care: looking inside the household*, London, HMSO.

A Study of Non-Elderly Spouse Carers

The aims of this research were:

Continuity of care

Services

Informal networks

► to explore the experiences and views of younger people (under pension age) caring for a disabled or chronically ill spouse – previously neglected in research on informal care;

► to examine the impact of the presence of dependent children in the household, the sex of the carer, the nature of the spouse's impairment and condition (progressive vs sudden onset, stable vs deteriorating), the ages of the partners, and the time since onset of the spouse's disability; and

► to compare and contrast the views and experiences of the carer with those of the cared-for person.

The study used qualitative methods to explore the experiences of 21 couples where one of the partners had become disabled since marriage. Spouses and carers were interviewed separately but at the same time, using two interviewers.

In 13 couples, it was the husband who was disabled and in eight it was the wife. The average age of female carers was 50 years and of their spouses, 54 years. The average age of male carers was 46 years and of their spouses, 45 years. All but one couple had children and seven had dependent children still at home. The most common disabling conditions were arthritis and back injuries. Seven of the 13 male spouses had been injured at work or had a condition known to be a hazard of the work they had done.

The range of impairment in the spouses was wide, from a woman who had previously suffered from epileptic fits, but who had not actually had one for 18 months, to a man who was a double amputee, had a paralysed arm, was doubly incontinent and usually unable to feed himself.

Spouse carers carry multiple burdens because they have *no one with whom to share responsibility*. This is particularly the case for those with dependent children: they received very little help – either from informal or formal sources – with the tasks of caring, although adult children, if living nearby, did sometimes help with domestic tasks or household maintenance. Few respondents had extensive kinship networks and the limitations imposed by disability and the demands of caring weakened the networks still further.

Neither friends nor neighbours provided help with caring tasks and the interviews identified strong constraints against their ever becoming involved. The desire for privacy made help from these sources unacceptable to many spouses and carers.

What little help couples did receive tended to be the *one-off provisions of aids and adaptations*. Only two received any home-help or day-care service, and several had substantial unmet needs which local authority provision could have met. In most of these cases there was clear evidence of a lack of communication between health service providers, who were aware of couples' needs, and social service providers who, had they known about the needs, might have been able to help.

Failures in communication **within** the health service – between hospital-based and community services – led to *serious gaps in continuity of care*, particularly after early discharge from hospital. Carers who had been in hospital were sent home without adequate help and support for convalescence, and spouses were sent home while still very ill and requiring substantial care. There was no evidence of preparation for their care in the community after they had first become disabled.

General practitioners played little part in the majority of spouses' lives and even less in those of carers. Young and/or female GPs were most likely to have played a supportive role for spouses, but even these few tended to overlook carers' needs.

Age and lifecycle effects, combined with caring, meant that *female carers had more variable patterns of labour market participation* than male carers. Male carers were more likely to undergo a once-and-for-all change at the point at which their wives' need for care passed a threshold. Beyond this, the men were unable to maintain full-time jobs and had few options for part-time work.

Household incomes varied substantially between the couples, influenced by the receipt of invalidity benefit, occupational pensions, mobility and/or attendance allowance, compensation payments and industrial disablement benefit, and by the carer's paid work. Singly or in combination, these factors *disadvantaged* couples where the *spouse had become disabled while young*, and couples where the wife was disabled.

The study challenged the assumption implicit in other work on caring that it might be easier to provide care for a spouse than for other kin. Regardless of the couple's ages or the length of the marriage, the *provision of personal care to a spouse created problems*, both because it breached 'normal' expectations about what spouses do or should do for one another and also because it was seen as challenging the cared-for partner's status as an adult.

Marriages had often been under the greatest strain at the time when the spouse's disability had started or become substantially worse. Many couples were unsupported at this time, and had made many psychological and practical adjustments to their lives with little help or advice.

Sudden onset or deterioration of a parent's condition when children were between the ages of 6 to 12 or 13 seemed most likely to affect the *children*, and these effects were exacerbated if the second parent also became ill. However, it was clear that a lack of financial and practical support for couples at the time around onset was a major contributory factor.

Couples who were relatively young at onset suffered most in terms of immediate financial and emotional effects. Further, because of the financial and practical demands of child-rearing, younger carers were more likely to be attempting to carry out several roles at once. By contrast, couples who had been older at onset were more likely to experience difficulties because of the carer's own ill-health, and the longer term financial effects. Obviously younger couples would eventually suffer both types of effects. Other things being equal, then, *the negative impact of disability is likely to be the greater the younger the couple are at onset.*

Degree of disability, suddenness of onset, and fluctuations in the spouse's condition were all more important than the type of condition or 'diagnosis'. *A high level of disability* had the greatest effects on carers' labour market participation, regardless of their sex, and was most likely to be associated with high levels of reported stress in the carers and the inability of the carer to get a break. Couples with the most-disabled spouses were more likely to have contemplated separation or divorce.

The differences between female and male carers were not as large as other research on caring has suggested. *However, there were some differences.* Women had more difficulty than men in recognizing what they did as caring. Male carers found receiving or asking for services less difficult, while women saw available services as inappropriate to their needs. Female and male carers appeared to feel the same about caring for their partners. They expressed similar notions of duty and reciprocity in talking about why they continued to care, and experienced similar levels of sadness and hurt at their partners' condition.

The research suggests the need for reviews of policy/practice in a number of areas including: hospital discharge of disabled people and their carers; the role of GPs in supporting carers; hospital-based respite-care for younger disabled people; the appropriateness and usefulness of services for younger disabled people and carers, especially those which might help them to remain in paid work; and the equalization of disablement and carers' benefits between men and women, across different age-groups, and in relation to different 'causes' of disability.

The research raised very serious questions about the likely role of *informal networks* **in supporting disabled people and carers. It cannot be assumed that untapped reserves of help within kinship, neighbourhood and friendship networks can be drawn on for this support.**

Researcher

Gillian Parker

Social Policy Research Unit, University of York, Heslington, York YO1 5DD. (0904 433608)

Publications

Parker, G. (1989), 'A study of non-elderly spouse carers: final report', University of York, Social Policy Research Unit, Working Paper DHSS 501.

Parker, G. (1989) 'A study of non-elderly spouse carers: summary of the final report', University of York, Social Policy Research Unit, Working Paper DHSS 523.

Parker, G. (1990) 'Spouse carers: whose quality of life?', in S. Baldwin, C. Godfrey and C. Propper (eds.), *Quality of life, perspectives and policy*, London, Routledge.

Parker, G. (1991) 'They've got their own lives to lead': carers and dependent people talking about family and neighbourhood help', in J. Hutton, S. Hutton, T. Pinch, and A. Shiell (eds.), *Dependency to Enterprise*, London, Routledge.

Parker, G. (1992) *'With this body: caring and disability in marriage'*, Buckingham, Open University Press.

Respite Services for the Carers of Confused Elderly People

Background: In 1988, the Department of Health funded the National Institute for Social Work Research Unit to take forward earlier work[10] by setting up a programme concentrating on respite services for carers who were resident with the elderly person for whom they cared.

Consumer views

Outcomes

Mixed Economy

- *Definition*: The term 'respite' currently has no universally accepted meaning. We use the word to refer in broad terms to means by which carers are given a temporary break from their caring responsibilities. The respite services examined in this study are day-care, sitting and carers' support services, and relief-care in homes, hospitals or in a family-based environment.
- *Aims*: Undertaken in collaboration with staff in health and social services and voluntary organizations, the study had three aims:

  (1) to establish and compare the characteristics and problems of elderly people and their carers with a range of mixes and types of break;

  (2) to elicit their views of such breaks; and

  (3) to examine the effectiveness of differing types and mixes of break.

- *Methods*: A sample of elderly people living with carers was obtained through systematic and repeated contact with services across three study areas. Two hundred and eighty-seven elderly people and their carers were interviewed. The carers were re-interviewed one year later.

Carers and elderly people: The elderly people formed a very old and dependent group of whom most were cared for by spouses or daughters. They required high levels of supervision and help with personal care. While carers received help from family and services, most care was provided by just *one* person, the carer. Most of the carers were themselves elderly and 40 per cent reported health problems of their own. Most carers reported a high degree of restriction. On the basis of the measures we used, there was evidence pointing to a level of psychological ill-health in a substantial group of carers.

Introduction to services: New information was obtained on the people using packages of services, both respite and non-respite, which will provide a basis for 1993 community care plans. A clear link was found between an elderly person's dependency in the widest sense and his or her use of services. The role of social workers, doctors and nurses as gatekeepers is vital. For a group whose health and social needs are blurred, collaborative working becomes particularly essential.

Day-care: Day-care was provided by a variety of sources through health and social services, and voluntary organizations. The amount of day-care an elderly person received and its source was dependent upon where he or she lived. Weekend and evening day-care were rarities. Given that day-care was the major source of respite

---

[10] Levin, E., Sinclair, I., and Gorbach, P. (1989) *Families, services and confusion in old age*, Aldershot, Avebury.

currently available to carers, under-provision was obvious. Users of day-care only, or day-care and sitting form an intermediate group in terms of their dependency.

Sitting and carers' support services: This relatively recent form of respite service offers the advantage of providing care within the elderly person's home. Such services are under-provided nationally and, as with day-care, receipt of the service was dependent upon the study area where the elderly person lived. These services are suitable for elderly people with very varying degrees of dependency.

Relief-care: Relief-care was provided in a number of settings. Relief care most usually takes place in an institutional setting and the NHS and local authorities were the prime providers of relief-care. This service is clearly targeted at the most dependent elderly people. In this sense it occupies an intermediate position between remaining within the community and permanent residential care.

Outcome: Outcome was established for all the elderly people in the sample. On follow up, 35 per cent had died. Of those who were still alive, over 70 per cent were still at home. To give some idea of the essential role of the carers, of the 13 elderly people whose *carer* had died, just one was still at home. Of those who entered permanent residential care, the predictors of institutionalization included: the mental health of the carer; his or her willingness to accept permanent care, and the use of relief-care. The study provided evidence to suggest that respite services had a positive effect.

Conclusion: The key findings from the study are that respite-care services are needed and valued; and that elderly people with dementia are heavy users of community and residential services. Taken together, the evidence suggests that they are a priority group in terms of their needs for community care. The 1993 community care arrangements offer both a challenge and an opportunity in developing services for this group.

Researchers

Enid Levin, Joanna Moriarty and Peter Gorbach

National Institute for Social Work, Mary Ward House, 5–7 Tavistock Place, London WC1H 9SS. (071 387 9681; FAX 071 387 7968)

Publications

Levin, E. (1991) 'Carers – problems, strains and services', in R. Jacoby, and C. Oppenheimer (eds), *Psychiatry in the Elderly*, London, Oxford University Press, 301–312.

Levin, E., and Moriarty, J. (1990) 'Ready to Cope Again: Sitting, Day and Relief Care for the Carers of Confused Elderly People', National Institute for Social Work Research Unit.

Levin, E., Moriarty, J., and Gorbach, P. (1992) ' "I couldn't manage without the breaks": respite services for the carers of confused elderly people', National Institute for Social Work Research Unit.

Moriarty, J. (1991) 'Time Off for Carers of Elderly Infirm People', *Social Work and Social Sciences Review*, **2**, 3, supplement: 52–58.

Longitudinal Study of Ageing

Background

This study was conducted in the rural areas of North Wales and was primarily concerned with the access of elderly people to services; with establishing the nature of the help available to them; and in comparing the situation of elderly people in rural areas with those in urban locations.

The aim was to study the same people over a period of time: interview surveys were carried out in 1979, 1983, 1987 and 1991, and an intensive study of 30 of the older subjects took place over four years from 1983 to 1987. The study was based on a sample of people who were representative of the general population aged 65 or over, and who were living independently in the community. In 1979, they were all interviewed in their own homes.

The first survey in 1979 included 534 people. In 1983, 1987 and 1991, all members of the sample were traced who had been alive when the last interview had been conducted. Most were still living in the same community. Some had moved to another address and some of these had moved out of the area. Some had entered institutional care and some had died.

In 1983, the survivors of those who had been aged 75 or over in 1979 were re-interviewed. Thirty of them were selected for the intensive study. This sample was chosen to ensure that representative numbers of men and women, married and widowed people, and people living alone, with a spouse, or with an adult child were selected.

In 1987 and 1991 as many survivors as possible of the original sample, aged 65 or over in 1979, were re-interviewed. In 1983 and 1987, questionnaires were designed so that interviewers could check some answers against the previous response. Where change had occurred this was then explored with the respondent.

KEY FINDINGS

The Lives of Elderly People

The first survey showed that most elderly people are well, happy and able to handle the day-to-day activities of life competently. They did not see members of their families any more often than elderly people in urban areas, but they were more satisfied with the level of contact. They were more likely than those in urban areas to belong to churches and voluntary organizations and it was suggested that because they were more involved with their communities, they were more satisfied generally.

More elderly people in this rural study lived in households with cars and telephones than in urban areas. A substantial minority were dependent on private transport for access to shops and other services. Use of public transport was low, probably because services were rudimentary, fares were high and concessions minimal. (Services have deteriorated further since 1979.)

Most elderly people received help as needed from members of their families, but a minority relied on friends and neighbours. Use of domiciliary statutory services was comparable with urban areas, but even those receiving these services relied for most help on informal sources. Nearly all immediate emergency help was informal.

The study covered most aspects of the lives of elderly people. However, the main focus of the study was the 'support network' on which elderly people could rely. **The support network is defined as: all those people with whom an elderly person living in the community is in regular contact and who provide practical help, emotional support or companionship or advice.** As well as survival, each later survey looked at the changes which occurred in the support networks.

Survival was found to be related most closely to self-assessed health as good/ excellent. For those over 75, apart from age itself, survival was related to:

◆ being middle-class;
◆ an owner–occupier;
◆ spending several hours alone during the day (i.e. not needing supervision);
◆ self-assessed health; and
◆ the absence of physical limitations at previous interview.

No social or quality-of-life factors were associated with survival. Those who moved away from the area tended to be those who had come to the rural community at or around retirement. When widowed, they tended to return to where they had come from. Those entering local authority residential homes tended to be long-term residents of the area.

Networks

Within support networks it was found that elderly people expect different things from different types of relationships. These expectations follow a hierarchy in relation to care and support. Most is expected of spouses, followed by adult children. Only these two categories are expected to provide personal care, and adult children only when such care does not interfere with their other responsibilities. After children come brothers and sisters: if they have no children elderly people expect more of their brothers and sisters. Expectations as regards friends are mainly for companionship and expressive support, and they come after brothers and sisters. Neighbours follow friends, but expectations of neighbours are mainly for practical and emergency help. Grandchildren come after neighbours, but expectations are minimal unless a grandparent has brought them up, when the expectations of children apply. Usually grandchildren help their own parents to care for a grandparent, if they are involved at all. Grandchildren are followed by nieces and nephews, where expectations are minimal unless the old person is childless. Expectations of cousins are for purely symbolic recognition, unless the relationship is also one of friendship.

Expectations for all relationships may be exceeded under certain conditions. They are also affected by gender, health and distance. Expectations are almost always met, but rarely exceeded, **unless** extenuating circumstances occur, such as an older sister acting as a parent when a younger brother or sister was young and being cared for as if she were a parent in old age.

Most elderly people had support networks of 5–7 members. Small networks were often the result of poor health or of a 'loner' lifestyle. Few people were isolated, lonely or suffered from low morale. Loneliness was not necessarily associated with isolation. Networks tended to be either very local with all members within five miles; or to be dispersed with at least one member living more than 25 miles away. Long-distance support-links tended to be mainly adult children or sisters. The support networks of elderly people tend to have a high proportion of other people aged 60 or more. Perhaps because of the greater survival of women, a high proportion of the network members are female.

Over time, networks tended to remain at about the same size. Large networks remained large and small networks remained small even when other changes occurred. On average they lost or gained one or two members. This was surprising because old people have a lot of old people in their support networks; those who dropped out of networks did so mostly because they died or became ill or infirm. Those who joined networks were usually people who were already known to the old person previously but had not been providing any form of support. On the whole, networks tended to adjust to the needs of elderly people as they became more dependent.

Within networks, some tasks were done only by family members. These tended to be those tasks involving intimacy or privacy, including personal care or financial matters. Some support came mainly from friends or neighbours. This tended to be support based on companionship or dependent on proximity, such as talking things over, lifts or borrowing small items. Over time, family substituted for family *and* non-family members, but non-family *only* substituted for other non-family members so that some support networks became more family-based with the passage of time.

> Five different types of support networks were identified. The main differences between them are associated with: the availability of local close family; the frequency of interaction within the network; and the degree of involvement in the community. Some types of networks are better able to support vulnerable elderly people in the community than others. In one type of network, almost no informal sources of help are available. Different types of networks are associated with different patterns of behaviour in terms of: self-help; mutual assistance; help-seeking; response to dependency and so on.

Statistically, network type is related to age, marital status, household composition, parenthood, length of residence in the community, community type and most other demographic variables. Use of statutory health and social services is also related to network type. Some networks are more likely to ask for formal help than others. Some networks use some services more than others.

Within the population generally, more people have networks which provide good support than those which are unable to provide support, but this differs from one community/neighbourhood to another. High population turnover results in higher proportions of less supportive network types. As a result, more elderly people in some neighbourhoods may seek and need formal services than in others. In communities/neighbourhoods the distribution of network types tends to remain stable over time unless, for example, the turnover of population increases or decreases.

Over time, as elderly people become more frail and need help, those with some types of networks rely increasingly on family members, and those with other types rely increasingly on friends or neighbours. Those with the types of networks which imply that there is no informal help available seek help from statutory services *at lower levels of dependency*. For *these* people, needs not met by formal services (such as companionship) often remain unmet. As a result of these changes, network type may change over time. The types of changes which occur are related to the type of network and some are more common than others. Shifts are mainly to a less independent network type and result from deterioration of physical or mental health: shifts are more likely as people get older.

Researcher

Professor Clare Wenger

Centre for Social Policy Research and Development, University of Wales, Bangor, Gwynedd LL57 2DG. (0248 351151)

Publications

Grant, G., and Wenger, G. C. (1989) 'Working with networks: implications of network change', in *Networks, Solidarity, Reciprocity*, Marcinelle, Belgium, European Regional Clearing House for Community Work.

Grant, G., and Wenger, G. C. (1991) 'Dynamics of Support Networks: differences and similarities between vulnerable groups', (submitted) *Ageing and Society*.

Shahtahmasebi, S., Davies, R., and Wenger, G. C. (1989) 'Factors Influencing the Probability of Survival in Old Age', Conference Paper (BSG, September).

Shahtahmasebi, S., Davies, R., and Wenger, G. C. (1989) *Modelling the Probability of Survival in Old Age using GLIM*, Bangor, Centre for Social Policy Research and Development, University of Wales.

Shahtahmasebi, S., Davies, R., and Wenger, G. C. (1991) *Morale in Old Age: A Cross-sectional Analysis*, Bangor, Centre for Social Policy Research and Development, University of Wales.

Shahtahmasebi, S., Davies, R., and Wenger, G. C. (1991) *Morale in Old Age: A Longitudinal Analysis*, Bangor, Centre for Social Policy Research and Development, University of Wales.

Shahtahmasebi, S., Davies, R., and Wenger, G. C. (Forthcoming) 'A Longitudinal Analysis of factors Related to Survival in old age', *The Gerontologist*.

Wenger, G. C. (1986) 'A Longitudinal Study of Changes and Adaptations in the Support Networks of Welsh Elderly over 75', *Journal of Cross-Cultural Gerontology*, **1**, 277–304.

Wenger, G. C. (1986) 'What do Dependency Measures Measure? Challenging Assumptions', in C. Phillipson, M. Bernard, and P. Strang (eds), *Dependency and Interdependency in old Age: theoretical perspectives on policy alternatives*, London, Croom Helm, 69–84.

Wenger, G. C. (1987) 'Dependence, Interdependence and Reciprocity after 80', *Journal of Ageing Studies*, **1**, 4: 355–377.

Wenger, G. C. (1987) *Relationships in Old Age – Inside Support Networks: a third report of a follow up study of the old elderly in North Wales, United Kingdom*, Bangor, Centre for Social Policy Research and Development, University of Wales.

Wenger, G. C. (1987) *Support Networks: Change and Stability: a second report of a follow up study of the old elderly in North Wales, United Kingdom*, Bangor, Centre for Social Policy Research and Development, University of Wales.

Wenger, G. C. (1988) *Help in Old Age: Facing up to Change: Fourth Report on a Follow-up Study of Old People in North Wales*, Bangor, Centre for Social Policy Research and Development, University of Wales.

Wenger, G. C. (1988) *Old People's Health and Experiences of the Caring Services: accounts from rural communities in North Wales*, Institute of Human Ageing, Liverpool, Liverpool University Press, 117.

Wenger, G. C. (1988) *Relationships of Old People 80+ with their Children and Grandchildren in North Wales, United Kingdom*, Bangor, Centre for Social Policy Research and Development, University of Wales.

Wenger, G. C. (1989) *Research Methodology of Longitudinal Study of Elderly People in Rural North Wales 1978–1987*, Bangor, Centre for Social Policy Research and Development, University of Wales.

Wenger, G. C. (1989) 'Support Networks in Old Age – Constructing a Typology', in M. Jefferys (ed.) *Growing Old in the 20th Century*, London, Routledge, 166–185.

Wenger G. C. (1990) 'Change and adaptation in Informal Support Networks of Elderly People in Wales 1979–1987', *Journal of Ageing Studies*, **4**, 4: 375–389.

Wenger, G. C. (1990) 'Elderly Carers: the need for appropriate intervention', *Ageing and Society*, **10**, 2: 197–219.

Wenger, G. C. (1990) 'Personal Care: variation in network type, style and capacity', in J. F. Gubrium, and A. Sankare (eds), *The Home Care Experience: ethnography and policy*, Newbury Park, CT, USA, Sage Publications Inc., 145–171.

Wenger G. C. (1990) 'The Special Role of Friends and Neighbours', *Journal of Aging Studies*, **4**, 2: 149 *et seq.*

Wenger, G. C. (1991) 'A Network Typology: from theory to practice', *Journal of Ageing Studies*, **5**, 1: 147–162.

Wenger, G. C. (1991) 'Informal Care – the bedrock of care in the Community', paper to *II European Congress of Gerontology*, Madrid, 11–14th September.

Wenger, G. C. (1992) 'Bangor longitudinal study of ageing', *Generations Review, Journal of the British Society of Gerontology*, **2**, 2: 6–8.

Wenger, G. C. (1992) 'Family Support in the Major English-speaking Countries', in H. Kendig, A. Hashimoto, and L. Coppard (eds), *Family Support to the Elderly: the International Experience*, Oxford, Oxford University Press.

Wenger, G. C. (1992) *Help in Old Age: Facing up to Change: A Longitudinal Network Study*, Institute of Human Ageing, Liverpool, Liverpool University Press.

Wenger G. C. (1992) *Keeping in Touch: access to cars and telephones*, paper presented, *International Conference on the Marginalisation of the Elderly*, Liverpool, May 1992.

Wenger, G. C. (in press) 'Morale in Old Age: a review of the evidence; *International Journal of Geriatric Psychiatry.*

Wenger, G. C. (in press) 'Support Networks', in J. R. M. Copeland, M. T. Abu Salah, and D. G. Blazer (eds), *The Psychiatry of Old Age: An International Textbook*, Chichester, John Wiley and Sons.

Wenger, G. C. (in press) 'The Formation of Social Networks: self-help, mutual aid and old people in contemporary Britain', *Journal of Aging Studies.*

Wenger, G. C., and Shahtahmasebi, S. (1989) *Network Variation: demographic correlates of network type*, Bangor, Centre for Social Policy Research and Development, University of Wales.

Wenger, G. C., and Shahtahmasebi, S. (1990) *Ageing and dependency in Rural Areas: eight years of domiciliary visiting of the old elderly*, Bangor, Centre for Social Policy Research and Development, University of Wales.

Wenger, G. C., and Shahtahmasebi, S. (1990) 'Variations in Support Networks: some social policy implications', in J. Mogey (ed.), *Aiding and Ageing: the coming crisis*, Westport, CT, Greenwood Press 255–277.

Wenger, G. C., and Shahtahmasebi, S. (1991) 'Survivors: Support of Network Variation and Sources of Help in Rural Communities', *Journal of Cross-cultural Gerontology*, **6**, 1: 41–82.

Wenger, G. C., and St. Leger, F. (1992) 'Community Structure and Support Network Variation', *Ageing and Society*, **12**, 2: 213–236.

Development of a Support Network Typology for Practitioner Use

BACKGROUND

This study grew out of earlier phases of the **Longitudinal Study of Ageing**, which had identified considerable variation in the support networks of elderly people living in the community; it had been shown that people with different types of networks used formal services differently. The aim of the study was to design a short questionnaire which could be used by community-care workers to identify network type, and to use this knowledge in practice in designing appropriate packages of care.

The study involved working with a range of community care teams. Data collected by workers were analysed to see if there were any connections between presenting problems and network type. Discussions of this work and specific cases were used to extend understanding of the implications of network type for practice.

'PANT' instrument

Identifying networks

KEY FINDINGS

Using the five support network types identified in the **Longitudinal Study**, the following findings emerged:

- Elderly people with different support network types make different levels of demand on statutory domiciliary services. This means that the distribution of network types on caseloads is distinctively different from that in the general population. In particular, the most vulnerable network type is 3–4 times more common on caseloads than in the population. Other types of networks are under-represented on caseloads.

- As a result of this, communities/neighbourhoods/catchment areas with high proportions of vulnerable support networks in the general population will make heavier demands on stautory services.

- Clients with different types of networks make different types of demands on statutory (and voluntary) services, because some types of problems are more likely to occur in some types of networks than others. Also, situations which are not a problem in some types of networks may be so in others.

- All problems can occur in all types of networks, although they may be more common in some than others; but clients with different types of support networks respond differently to the same intervention. This means that the solution for a problem existing in one type of network may not work, or may make a similar situation worse in a different network type.

- Understanding network variation and using knowledge of network type in making decisions can result in more appropriate interventions.

- Introducing change into practice is not easy. Some resistance to change is to be expected. However, innovation is likely to be more difficult where workers are already being subjected to change in other areas of their work. Too much change leads to insecurity and demoralization, which results in an inability to make decisions or to assimilate new working methods.

- Social workers' disinclination to take notes during (assessment) interviews with clients or potential clients leads to inaccuracies in recording. This practice is likely to be dysfunctional in the context of care in the community. Multi-disciplinary teamwork will need to rely on shared records and the quality of response will be affected by the quality of information collected by other workers.
- The support network typology is a useful tool for community-care workers, but it does have training implications.

The project developed the Practitioner Assessment of Network Type (PANT) instrument. On the basis of answers to eight interviewer-administered questions, this instrument makes it possible to identify the support network of the respondent.

Researcher

Professor Clare Wenger

Centre for Social Policy Research and Development, University of Wales, Bangor, Gwynedd LL57 2DG. (0248 351151)

Publications

Wenger, G. C. (1991) *Support Network Variation and Community Care*, Bangor, Centre for Social Policy Research and Development, University of Wales.

Wenger, G. C. (1991) *Introducing a Support Network Typology in Social Work Practice*, Bangor, Centre for Social Policy Research and Development, University of Wales.

Dementia and Adaptation in Support Networks – Interim Report

The dementia and support network project was designed to:

(1) study the impact of dementia on support networks, and

(2) to replicate the rural network study in an urban area.

The study has been conducted in Liverpool in conjunction with the Institute of Human Ageing, as part of a larger study concerned with the prevalence and incidence of dementia in the population.

The larger dementia study is based on a screening sample of approximately 6,000 elderly people living in Liverpool. Subjects are interviewed twice, two years apart. The network assessment instrument (PANT) was used in the screening interviews to determine network type for the entire sample.

In addition to the screening interviews, approximately 600 subjects have been interviewed in detail about the extent of their support network, sources of informal help and use of formal services. All carers of identified cases of dementia have also been interviewed. Re-interviewing commenced in April 1992.

The elderly population of Liverpool has been found to be very stable. Approximately 95 per cent have lived in the city for 30 years or more. This is in contrast with the rural Welsh Study, where approximately 25 per cent were retirement migrants. This meant that 25 per cent had come to their present community from more than 15 miles away after the age of 60. As a result, the distribution of support networks in Liverpool was slightly different from that in the rural sample. More old people had those types of networks able to support dependent elderly people at home. This finding was contrary to expectations. We cannot assume that rural elderly populations are more stable or better supported than urban ones: the opposite may be the case.

Most cases of dementia were found to be in residential care. The prevalence of dementia amongst those living in the community was approximately five per cent. Early analysis indicates that the networks of those dementia sufferers who remain in the community are concentrated in two types. The distribution of support networks of those suffering from dementia is distinctively different from that of the general elderly population.

Researcher

Professor Clare Wenger

Centre for Social Policy Research and Development, University of Wales, Bangor, Gwynedd LL57 2DG. (0248 351151)

Publications

Wenger, G. C. (in press) 'The Impact on the Family of Chronic Mental Illness in Old Age', *Archives of Public Health*.

Urban/rural comparison

'PANT' instrument

Residential care

Support Networks, Transitions and People with Learning Disabilities

Background

Services

Assessment

This study was carried out in two North Wales districts. **Its primary aim was to describe and account for patterns of change and stability in the support networks of people with learning disabilities**.

In 1983/4, 100 family carers were interviewed in order to establish baseline data about the membership, structure and internal dynamics of their informal support networks. This helped to establish the boundaries to the community's capacity to support people with learning disabilities, and also to shed some light on the unwritten rules and norms of informal support. Seventy-eight survivors of the 1983/4 sample were followed up two years later, in 1985/6, in order to elicit information about change and stability in informal support. This longitudinal study was based on a sample of young to middle-aged adults and their families. However, comparable data were also gathered in 1985/6 on young children, older adults and their families, as part of related work on the impact of mental handicap policy in Wales.

OUTCOMES

Over the two-year fieldwork period, support networks reduced only slightly in membership from 7.5 (range 1–22) at baseline to 7 (range 1–9) at follow-up. However, these crude figures conceal considerable change and attrition within different membership groups.

The dominant presence within the support networks of this group was close kin, but within the space of two years, their average membership had dropped from 5.8 to 4.3. These network losses affected all social groups, but were noticeably higher in families supporting the most physically incapacitated individuals, and in families where subjective loneliness amongst the primary carers was much in evidence. Kinship losses were associated with life-cycle changes within families, particularly moves of siblings from the family home, deaths and the reduced capacity of individuals to offer support. Hence, these losses reflect not so much the active withdrawal of network members, but natural attrition within the informal support network.

Despite these losses, close family members continued to provide the central and most enduring role in the support of people with learning disabilities. At baseline and follow-up stages, 90 per cent of the primary carers were mothers, and it was they who anchored and orchestrated the management of care, often at considerable personal costs to themselves, confirming the findings of other studies.

At baseline, less than 6 out of 10 persons with learning disabilities had any friends or neighbours in their support network, and at follow-up this had only slightly increased. However, there was a considerable ebb and flow of friends and neighbours into and out of the network over time; although the average number of friends and neighbours within networks remained about the same, they were not always the same people. They played less central support roles and were rarely involved or expected to be involved in personal-care tasks requiring privacy or intimacy. Sometimes they assisted with occasional homemaking tasks or at times of crisis or need, often when kinship carers were looking for someone to talk to.

Over time, the involvement of frontline professional workers within support networks grew significantly, as a result of Welsh policy emphasizing the development of multi-disciplinary teamwork and the release of resources for new services.

The radius of support networks was typically local, and orientated around the household. For many of the individuals concerned, the household is the nearest they get to the community. This is especially the case amongst women with learning disabilities, and amongst those with severe physical incapacities or challenging behaviours. Their support networks were so embedded in the family that – in effect – they insulated the person with learning disabilities from the local community. The drive towards the integration of people into communities around them will have to contend with this protective culture of family care.

The impacts of support network changes on the lives of persons with learning disabilities lay outside the scope of the study, but some important indicators were identified. Firstly, deaths of family supporters were described as having profound, long-lasting, but not well-understood effects on the individuals concerned. Secondly, where the loss of a person from the network affected the structure or routines for managing individuals at home, this presented a severe test of practical and emotional adaptation, which formal support services did not always fully appreciate. Thirdly, the increasing frailty or incapacity of familial supporters presented severe tests to their own determination to maintain support at all costs for relatives with learning disabilities. However, when such circumstances arose, individuals within support networks were often without the counselling and practical help they required.

Over the two-year study period, major swings in the attitudes of informal supporters about the appropriate arrangements for long-term support were very clear. Qualitative information from interviews also illustrated the range of beliefs and values which underpinned people's hopes and aspirations. These were usually rooted in expectations about help from family, perceptions about personal survival, the history of personal experience with services, and attitudes towards state and local welfare.

Evidence explaining the varied attitudes of informal supporters towards long-term support was also derived from quantitative data from the same study. The findings suggested that family supporters looking for long-term support primarily from statutory agencies were more likely to be lonely, with fewer kinship supporters but more friends, living in a non-manual-occupation household and supporting someone with learning disabilities with rather less challenging behaviour. The analysis points to the importance of factors in the social context of care rather than the personal characteristics of the person with learning disabilities as key influences in decision-making. By contrast, informal supporters seeking reliance on continued care by the family typically had more kinship supporters but fewer friends and neighbours available to them. They generally experienced less loneliness in their lives, even though they were more likely to be presented with problems of challenging behaviour from their relative.

The findings of the study help to throw into relief a number of potential conflicts of interest for policy: the rights of individuals to lead independent lives as opposed to the maintenance of essential reciprocities and inter-dependencies between family members; the instinctive desire of many mothers to carry on nurturing sons and daughters with disabilities as against letting siblings take over responsibilities for support; the rights and wishes of the person with learning disabilities as against those of informal supporters; and the known costs and benefits of persisting with informal support against the unknown costs and benefits of future services.

More information, opportunities to ask probing questions, and time to reflect on the implications of these issues are required both by people with learning disabilities and their family supporters. This places a high premium on arrangements for assessment and care-management, which need to take more fully into account the social context of support and the informal rules which appear to govern it.

Researcher

Dr Gordon Grant

Centre for Social Policy Research and Development, University of Wales, Bangor, Gwynedd LL57 2DG. (0248 351151)

Publications

Grant, G. (1986) 'Older carers, interdependence and the care of mentally handicapped adults', *Ageing and Society*, **6**: 333–351.

Grant, G. (1987) 'The structure of care networks in families with mentally handicapped adult dependants', in P. Gutridge (ed.), *Social Work in Action in the 1980s*, Occasional Paper, Bangor, Department of Social Theory and Institutions, University of Wales.

Grant, G. (1988) *Stability and Change in the Care Networks of Mentally Handicapped Adults Living at Home: First Report*, Bangor, Centre for Social Policy Research and Development, University of Wales.

Grant, G. (1990) 'Elderly Parents and Handicapped Children: anticipating the future', *Journal of Aging Studies*, **4**, 4: 359–374.

Grant, G. (1990) 'Letting go: decision-making among family carers of people with a mental handicap', *Australia and New Zealand Journal of Developmental Disabilities*, **15**, 3 and 4: 189–200.

Grant, G. (in press) 'Support Networks and transitions over two years among adults with a mental handicap', *Mental Handicap Research*.

Grant, G., and Wenger, G. C. (1989) 'Working with networks, implications of network change', in *Networks, Solidarity, Reciprocity*, Marcinelle, Belgium, European Regional Clearing House for Community Work.

Grant, G., and Wenger, G. C. (1992) 'Dynamics of Support Networks: differences and similarities between vulnerable groups', submitted to *Irish Journal of Pyschology*.

McGrath, M., and Grant, G. (in press) 'The life-cycle and support networks of families with a mentally handicapped member', *Disability, Handicap and Society*.

Informal Carers and their Elderly Dependants: a Community-Based Longitudinal Study

INTRODUCTION

The objectives of the study were:

1. To examine the roles of formal and informal carers in the support of elderly people living in the community.
2. To define those factors which are important to the maintenance or breakdown of the caring relationship between informal carers and their dependent friends or relatives.
3. To identify the factors associated with stress amongst informal carers.
4. To examine the extent to which statutory services could alleviate the burden on informal carers.
5. To investigate the changes over a 12-month period which occur among elderly people and their carers.
6. To make recommendations concerning the future policies of Health and Social Services for maintaining both elderly people in the community and the integrity of families.

A population of 1,079 people aged 70 years and over was drawn from the age/sex registers of two large general practices. The sample was community-based, not one drawn from service providers, and should be generalizable to other areas of England and Wales. It included people of different mental and physical disabilities, and people with no contact with statutory services. Almost all of these were interviewed in their own homes, and topics covered in the interview included: physical and mental health, quality of life, social networks, contact with voluntary, health and social services; and the standard demographic information.

The amount of help received from informal carers was investigated and the names and addresses of the main carers were obtained if the elderly person received assistance at least once a week with one or more of 15 tasks basic to daily living. Main carers were then interviewed and the topics covered included: physical and mental health of the carers; quality of life of the carers; nature and quantity of assistance given to and received from elderly dependants; statutory, voluntary and informal sources of support available to carers; nature and amount of support received; impact of their caring activities on their own health and quality of life; and their attitudes to their caring role. Both elderly people and carers were interviewed 12 months later to assess changes that had taken place – in particular, the effects on carers of changes in the elderly people. By this means, we planned to identify predictors of improvement or deterioration in the quality of life of carers, institutionalization and the increase in use of services.

MAIN RESULTS

1. The main carer was almost invariably identifiable.
2. Carers were mostly women (80 per cent): most of the carers were either daughters (45 per cent) or spouses (26 per cent); 8 per cent were sons, 11 per cent were other relatives, and 10 per cent were unrelated to the dependant.

Stress

Costs of caring

Respite care

Two-thirds of the carers shared the same household as their elderly dependant. Half were aged 45–64 years but one in five were themselves aged 75 years or over.

3. Families undertook by far the majority of regular, committed informal care, and caring usually fell to one person.

4. Lack of privacy (in particular for resident carers) and loss of freedom (being tied to the home) were the factors that upset carers most frequently. Female carers in particular felt a conflict of interest between their varied caring roles: wife, daughter and mother.

5. Most carers were wanting to continue their caring role, and very few sought residential care.

6. Many carers were caring at great cost to themselves in terms of their own quality of life and health.

7. Many carers had been forced to cease employment, reduce hours or forego employment opportunities. The effects of caring upon their social life and family life were the major predictors of stress in carers: self-reported loneliness was the main predictor of anxiety and depression. Female carers were more likely to suffer from stress and anxiety, as were daughters when other variables were controlled. Carers were more likely to suffer from depression if their elderly dependant suffered from depression.

8. Half of the carers reported that they received no support from informal or statutory sources, and most reported receiving little support from other family members.

9. Most carers felt that they needed and would like more support, and that their needs had not been assessed, identified or satisfactorily responded to.

10. Most carers (90 per cent) were resistant to the idea of their elderly dependant entering institutional care. Those experiencing high levels of stress were more likely to be seeking institutional care. Daughters were more likely to consider institutional care than were spouses, as well as those caring for highly dependent people.

    Carers in social classes 1 and 2 more often considered that the family rather than the state should be responsible for provision of general and financial assistance and accommodation.

11. The most frequently-mentioned assistance that carers would like was *respite-care*. They wanted respite-care to be well planned in advance, and not only consequent upon crises; to be for long periods – a week or more – for holidays, and also to be available for a few hours on a regular basis. Some reported that they would prefer respite-care to be provided outside the home (but not in geriatric wards) and others said that they would prefer respite-care to be provided in their own homes. Many elderly spouses would like to be enabled to have holidays or breaks *with* their elderly dependant, rather than separately.

Researcher

Dr Dee Jones

Research Team for the Care of Elderly People, Department of Geriatric Medicine, University of Wales College of Medicine, Cardiff Royal Infirmary, Cardiff CF2 1SZ. (0222 491000)

Publications

Jones, D. A. (1985) 'A carer's work is never done', *Community Care*, **569**: 22–23.

Jones, D. A. (1986) 'A survey of carers of elderly dependants living in the community', *Report – Research Team for the Care of the Elderly*, Cardiff, St David's Hospital.

Jones, D. A. (1986) 'The role of community nurses in supporting informal carers', in Social Services Inspectorate Development Group (ed.), *Supporting the Informal Carers: The Role of the Nurse in the Community*, London, DHSS, 19–21.

Jones, D. A. (1990) 'Informal care and community care', Occasional paper no. 4, Research Team for the Care of Elderly People.

Jones, D. A. (in press) 'Problems of Carers: the United Kingdom view', in Evans, J. G. (ed.), *Oxford Textbook of Geriatrics*, Oxford University Press.

Jones, D. A., and Peters, T. (in press) 'Caring for elderly dependants – effects on the carer's quality of life', *Age and Ageing*.

Jones, D. A., and Salvage, A. V. (1992) 'Attitudes to caring among a group of informal carers of elderly dependants', *Archives of Gerontology and Geriatrics*, **14**: 155–165.

Jones, D. A., and Vetter, N. J. (1984) 'A survey of those who care for the elderly at home: their problems and their needs', *Social Science and Medicine*, **19**: 511–514.

Jones, D. A., and Vetter, N. J. (1985) 'Formal and informal support received by carers of elderly dependants' *British Medical Journal*, **291**: 643–645.

Jones, D. A., Victor, C. R., and Vetter, N. J. (1983) 'Carers of the elderly in the community', *Journal of the Royal College of General Practitioners*, **33**: 707–710.

Stress and Coping in Families Caring for a Child with Severe Learning Disabilities: a Longitudinal Study

SUMMARY

This longitudinal study of 200 children with severe learning disabilities and their families found that:

- Mothers of children with severe learning disabilities have more health problems and consult their doctors more frequently than do mothers in the general population.
- Mothers of the children have high stress levels which remain remarkably stable over time.
- Having a child who is younger and who has behaviour problems makes mothers more vulnerable to stress.
- Certain coping resources are able to mediate the harmful effects of stressful behaviour for mothers. These are being middle-class, having no financial worries, having good coping skills, having no recent illness, and being well-adjusted to the child.
- Child behaviour problems show considerable persistence over time.
- Child characteristics predicting *change* in behaviour over time were age, academic skills, self-help skills, communication skills, and mobility. Family characteristics predicting change in behaviour were marital discord, maternal stress and low household income. It is likely that these factors act as antecedent risk factors for behaviour disorder.
- Mothers who had a felt need for additional services were those whose children had multiple impairments, poor communication skills, severe medical problems, high levels of dependency, challenging behaviour and sleep problems.
- Family characteristics associated with high felt need were having money worries, poor social support, high impact scores, greater maternal stress, extra work because of the child, and additional social problems.

Introduction and Methodology

The project extends previous work with 200 families caring for a child with severe learning disabilities (Pahl and Quine, 1984[11]), forming the second phase of a longitudinal study. The families provide a representative sample of children with severe learning disabilities and their carers from two health districts in south-east England. The first phase of the study was funded by the South East Thames Regional Health Authority, and the second phase by the Department of Health. The families were interviewed in 1982 and 1985.

The two phases of the study produced a set of longitudinal descriptive data on a very wide range of child and family variables, which enabled us to examine the antecedent risk factors for poor family and child outcomes, the ways families coped with the task of bringing up a child with severe learning disabilities, sleep problems, and the factors predicting the need for additional services.

---

[11] For details, see *Publications*, page 187.

Findings

Maternal Health

Women caring for a child with severe learning disabilities were more likely to report that their health was not good or only fairly good than were women of comparable age in the general population (see figure 3.1). Additionally, a higher proportion of mothers in our sample were suffering from symptoms of psychological distress. Fifty-four per cent of mothers in the sample at Time 1, and 51 per cent at Time 2 had a score of six or more on the Malaise Inventory, compared with 20 per cent of mothers in a general population survey of mothers with young children. The stressed women in the sample had consulted their doctors more than twice as many times over the previous year as those who were not stressed. Nearly 30 per cent of women in our sample reported consulting their doctor in the 14 days before interview, a figure almost double that found in women of similar age in the general population in the 1985 General Household Survey.

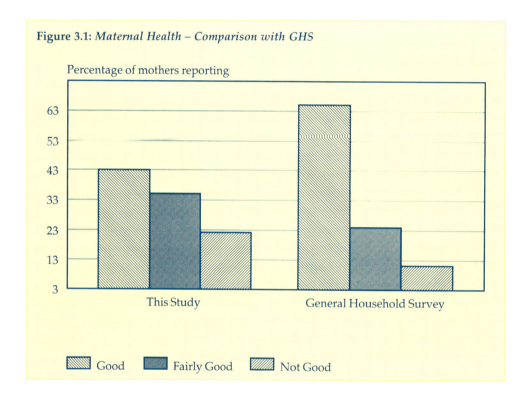

Figure 3.1: *Maternal Health – Comparison with GHS*

Percentage of mothers reporting

Stress and Coping in Mothers of Children with Learning Disabilities

The study investigated the factors affecting how mothers cope with caring for a child with learning disabilities. The Malaise Inventory was used to measure symptoms of psychological distress (see figure 3.2). The most important *child variables* affecting mothers' stress were behaviour problems and the child's age. *Coping resource* variables predicting stress were lower social class, financial worries, negative assessment of coping skills, poor acceptance of and adjustment to the child, and recent maternal ill-health. There was evidence that being middle-class with few financial worries and good health was able to buffer the effect of stressful behaviour for mothers.

Figure 3.2: *Most Frequently-Occurring Symptoms of Maternal Stress*

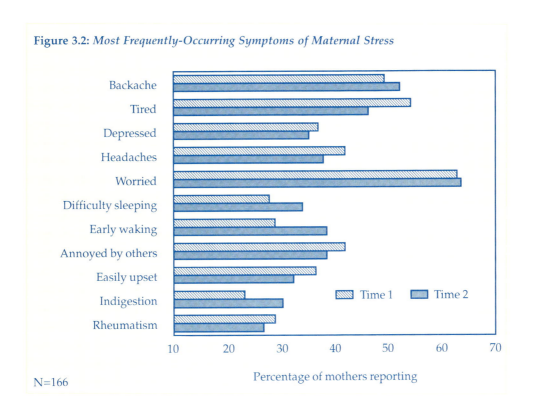

N=166

Child Behaviour Problems

The study presents the prevalence of behaviour problems in the sample of children and their continuities and discontinuities. Significant numbers of children exhibited behaviour problems. Rates of behaviour problems showed remarkable similarity in prevalence between Time 1 and Time 2. There was also continuity in the *persistence* of behaviour problems; 71 per cent of the sample remained unchanged between Time 1 and Time 2, while 29 per cent of children moved into or out of the behaviour problem group (see figure 3.3). It was possible to predict group membership, in 80 per cent of cases, from factors concerned with the child's and family's characteristics. Marital discord was a significant predictor of behaviour disorder, as was maternal stress and family income. It is likely that these factors are *causally* related to the risk of poor outcome in terms of behaviour disorder. Child characteristics predicting change in behaviour were academic skills, self-help skills, communication skills, mobility and age.

Figure 3.3: *Persistence of Behaviour Problems*

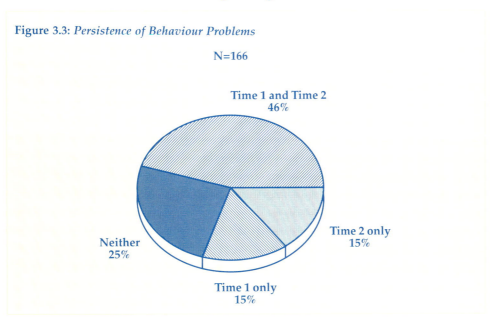

Sleep Problems in Children with Learning Disabilities

Children with learning disabilities are more likely to present problems of night-settling, night-waking and sleeping in their parents' bed than are non-handicapped children. This study found that large numbers of children had such problems (see figure 3.4). Sleep problems were related to age, though significant numbers of young people aged 15 or over still had irregular sleeping patterns. Sleep problems were very strongly associated with maternal stress. A path model showed that communication skills are a key factor and this may reflect the difficulty parents experience in trying to train children with limited communication skills to present more socially appropriate behaviour.

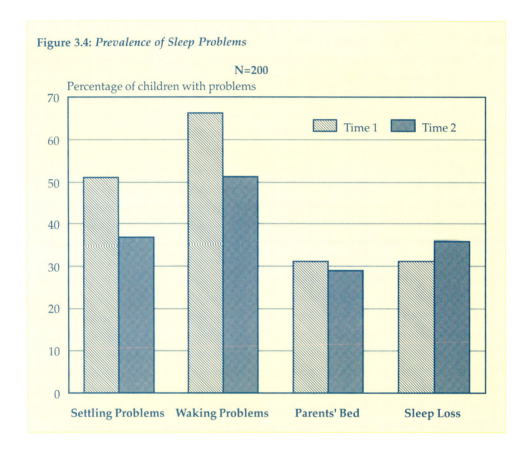

Figure 3.4: *Prevalence of Sleep Problems*

Felt Need for Additional Services

The study investigated the factors that predicted the families' greatest felt needs for additional services in order to provide information about the families that services should target. Felt need was highest in parents whose children were younger, had challenging behaviour, sleep problems, multiple impairments, poor communication skills, severe medical problems, or lack of mobility. Family characteristics associated with high felt need were money worries, poor social support, a greater burden of extra work, high maternal stress, many stressful life events, and many other social problems. The parents with high felt need made greater use of the services.

Researchers

Lyn Quine and Jan Pahl

Centre for Health Service Studies, University of Kent, Canterbury. (0227 764000)

Publications

Bebbington, A., and Quine, L. (1987) 'Evaluating the Malaise Inventory', *Social Psychiatry*, **22**: 5–7.

Ferlie, E., Pahl, J., and Quine, L. (1984) 'Professional collaboration in services for mentally handicapped people', *Journal of Social Policy*, **13**, 2: 185–210.

Manley, M. C. G., and Pahl, J. M. (1989) 'Dental services for children with mental handicaps: policy changes and parental choices', *British Dental Journal*, **167**, 5: 163–7.

Pahl, J., and Quine, L. (1984) 'Families with Mentally Handicapped Children: a Study of Stress and of Service Response', Centre for Health Service Studies, University of Kent at Canterbury. Second edition 1985. Price £3.50.

Pahl, J., and Quine, L. (1987) 'Families with mentally handicapped children', in J. Orford (ed.), *Coping with Disorder in the Family*, Croom Helm, 39–61.

Quine, L. (1986) 'Behaviour problems in severely mentally handicapped children', *Psychological Medicine*, **16**, 895–907.

Quine, L. (1987) 'Encounters between doctors and parents: first diagnosis of severe mental handicap', in H. R. Dent (ed.), *Clinical Psychology: Research and Development*, London, Croom Helm.

Quine, L., and Chornley, H. (1987) 'The Malaise Inventory as a measure of stress in carers', in J. Twigg (ed.) *Evaluating Support to Informal Carers*, Social Policy Research Unit, University of York.

Quine, L., and Lawton, D. (1990) 'Patterns of take-up of the family fund: the characteristics of eligible non-claimants and reasons for not claiming', *Child: Care, Health and Development*, **16**: 35–53.

Quine, L., and Pahl, J. (1985) 'Examining the causes of stress in families with severely mentally handicapped children', *British Journal of Social Work*, **15**: 501–510.

Quine, L., and Pahl, J. (1986) 'Parents with severely mentally handicapped children: marriage and the stress of caring', in R. Chester, and P. Divall (eds.), *Mental Illness and Handicap in Marriage*, National Marriage Guidance Council, Report No. 5, 62–81.

Quine, L., and Pahl, J. (1986) 'First diagnosis of severe mental handicap: characteristics of unsatisfactory encounters between doctors and parents', *Social Science and Medicine*, **22**, 1: 53–62.

Quine, L., and Pahl, J. (1986) 'First diagnosis of severe handicap: a study of parental reactions', *Developmental Medicine and Child Neurology*, **29**: 232–242.

Quine, L., and Pahl, J. (1989) 'First diagnosis of severe mental handicap: characteristics of unsatisfactory encounters between doctors and parents', in F. Uski and J. Stockman (eds.), *1989 Year Book of Paediatrics*, Chicago, Yearbook Medical Publishers.

Quine, L., and Pahl, J. (1989) 'Stress and Coping in Families Caring for Children with Severe Mental Handicaps', University of Kent at Canterbury.

Quine, L., and Pahl, J. (1991) 'Stress and coping in mothers caring for a child with severe learning difficulties: a test of Lazarus' transactional model of coping', *Journal of Community and Applied Social Psychology*, **1**: 57–70.

Quine, L., and Pahl, J. (1992) 'Growing up with severe learning difficulties: a longitudinal study of young people and their families', *Journal of Community and Applied Social Psychology*, **2**: 1–16.

Adaptation and Help-Seeking Strategies in Families of Children with Physical Disabilities

AIMS AND STUDY DESIGN

The aims of the two-part study were:

(1) to identify factors related to good and poor adaptation in families of children with major physical disabilities;

(2) to investigate contacts between the families and voluntary and statutory services, and how help received related to family adaptation;

(3) to identify how paediatricians provide support and information to families following the diagnosis of disability, factors which affect these practices, and how practice relates to parents' views of their own needs.

The family study used a model of family adaptation, based on a theoretical model of stress and coping, and developed in studies with the Manchester Down's Syndrome Cohort. This model maintains that parental adaptation is related both to risk factors concerning the child's characteristics and recent events in the parents' lives, as well as to personal and family resources. Those include family relationships, psychological resources, informal social support, socio-economic factors, service support and coping strategies. Data were collected on a wide range of factors which the literature suggests may be relevant to how well the family adapts to living with the child's disability. The sources of help available to and used by families were also investigated.

In order to achieve a comprehensive view of parental adaptation, positive as well as negative outcome measures were collected from both mothers and fathers. The three outcome measures were: adaptation to the child; parental psychological distress; and satisfaction with life. In addition, two factors derived from interviews with mothers – perceived need for services, and satisfaction with how the news of their child's disability was disclosed to them – were used as outcome measures. Data were collected using both self-completed questionnaires and interviews.

The study of paediatric practice aimed to identify current practice for providing support and information to families of children with physical disability after the disability had been diagnosed. By comparing the paediatricians' descriptions of policy and practice and their need for help and information, the study investigated how services operated, and how they may be improved. Twenty-four consultant paediatricians in 13 hospitals in the area were interviewed.

THE FAMILIES IN THE STUDY

The study adopted three criteria for inclusion of families in the study: residence in the Greater Manchester area; severity of the child's physical disability (defined as a likely prognosis of inability to walk unaided); and duration since disclosure of diagnosis or school-entry being two years or less. The final sample was 107 families, with characteristics broadly representative of families in the general

Outcomes
Coping
Unmet need

population. Interviews were completed with 105 mothers and 2 fathers (where the mother spoke no English); questionnaires were returned by 98 mothers (92 per cent) and 72 fathers (86 per cent of the 84 families where the father was present).

Forty per cent of children had cerebral palsy; 16 per cent, spina bifida; 13 per cent, degenerative disorders; and 31 per cent, other conditions. The mothers of 48 per cent of the children reported that some learning disability had been diagnosed.

MAIN FINDINGS

The results indicated the most significant factors associated with good or poor outcome for the parents. In this summary, the results will be described for each outcome measure from the point of view of **risk of poor outcome**.

1. Adaptation to the Child

Low levels of mothers' adaptation to the child, in terms of their emotional adjustment and attitudes towards the child, were found to be related to their own personality (high scores on neuroticism and low scores on extroversion); high use of 'wishful thinking' as a strategy for coping with child problems; problems in communication with the child; and high levels of unmet need for help from services. For fathers, high use of 'wishful thinking' as a coping strategy was also important, but their personality traits were not. Poor adaptation by the fathers was also related to poor family relationships; the child having feeding problems; and the child being a girl.

2. Psychological Distress

Many mothers in the study showed high levels of psychological distress, and these were related to personality (high scores on neuroticism); lack of financial resources; the mother not being employed outside the home; and high levels of unmet service needs. High levels of distress among fathers were linked to poor family relationships as well as personality (neuroticism), and lack of material resources.

3. Satisfaction with Life

For both mothers and fathers, low satisfaction with life was linked to high levels of strain from recent life-events. For mothers, ways of coping with problems (high use of 'wishful thinking'); failure to seek help from informal sources for early emotional support; a high level of physical disability of the child; and lack of financial resources were also important. For fathers, family relationships were particularly important.

4. Unmet Need for Services

Despite high levels of contact with services for most of this sample, there was still evidence of considerable unmet need, particularly in relation to the provision of information. Families with high levels of unmet service needs were likely to have experienced a high level of strain from recent stressful life events, to have a child with learning disabilities, an unemployed father, and to cope with problems in ways characterized by passive optimism.

5. Satisfaction with Disclosure

Mothers were asked a series of questions about how they were told the news of their child's disability. Only 37 per cent indicated they were satisfied with the handling of disclosure. The most important factors related to satisfaction were the manner of the professional involved, the adequacy of information, and opportunities to ask questions. Mothers from families of non-manual social class backgrounds were less likely to be satisfied with how disclosure was made.

6. Paediatric Practice and Policy

The study of paediatric practice on disclosure revealed considerable variation between paediatricians. None said they were aware of any written guidelines in hospital policy regarding disclosure. There was widespread recognition of the problems involved in communicating such a diagnosis, and of the need for a broader training, involving counselling or communication skills. The paediatricians' responses suggest that few were able to operate within the kind of team structure which would support families in the period following disclosure.

Overall, the factors which were identified as relevant to parental adaptation in this study support the theoretical model of stress and coping: some child characteristics, life events, parental and family resources, and coping strategies were all found to be significantly related to good or poor outcome. The high level of distress identified in the study underlines the value of defining the resources – both psychological and material – which may be reinforced through formal or informal channels. For example, factors related to the child were found to be important potential sources of stress, and relevant to the mothers' satisfaction with life and both parents' adaptation to the child; the use of 'wishful thinking' as a response to these problems was associated with poorer outcome. This might well be a productive area for intervention in helping parents.

The results in relation to service needs, satisfaction with disclosure, and the significance of unmet service needs in relation to poor outcome suggest that *improvements in information* to families are necessary. Information must be comprehensible, easily accessible, appropriate and sensitive to the problems faced by the most vulnerable families. Finally, the finding that the manner of the professional involved in the disclosure of the diagnosis was the most important factor relating to satisfaction at this point has implications for the inclusion of *communication skills* in medical training.

Researchers

Patricia Sloper and Stephen Turner

Hester Adrian Research Centre, University of Manchester, Manchester M13 9PL. (061 275 3340; FAX 061 275 3333)

Publications

Sloper, P., and Turner, S. (1991) 'Parental and professional views of the need of families with a child with severe physical disability', *Counselling Psychology Quarterly*, **4**, 4: 323–330.

Sloper, P., and Turner, S. (in press) 'Risk and resistance factors in the adaptation of parents of children with severe physical disability', *Journal of Child Psychology and Psychiatry*.

Sloper, P., and Turner, S. (in press) 'Service needs of families of children with severe physical disability', *Child: Care, Health and Development*.

Turner, S., and Sloper, P. (in press) 'Paediatricians' practice in disclosure and follow-up of the diagnosis of severe physical disability in young children', *Developmental Medicine and Child Neurology*.

Chapter 4

Mental Health

Mental Health

This Chapter covers research which has approached mental health, and services to prevent or cure mental illness, from a number of different starting-points. Elderly people suffering from mental illnesses are the subject of a number of studies, while other projects have focused on younger patients, carers and families, social workers' clients, and the needs of ethnic minority service users.

The move from hospital to community care including the costs and quality of life associated with hospital discharge, has been investigated. One group of studies deals with the relationship between primary care and social services departments, the interface between specialist and generic services, and questions of inter-professional and inter-agency collaboration. Another group focuses on the organization of community care, and – in particular – evaluates community mental health centres, and compares the day and in-patient treatment for psychotic illness.

The effectiveness of particular kinds of intervention – for example, to prevent the relapse of schizophrenia, to manage depression in elderly people, or to provide inter-culture therapy – are also dealt with by projects included in this Chapter.

Team for the Assessment of Psychiatric Services – Summary of Results So Far

Follow-Up Results for Leavers, 1985–1989

Costs
Hospital
discharge
Quality of life

This is a summary of the results of following up 350 patients one year after leaving hospital. In the period 1985–1989, during the first four years of the 'reprovision' programme at Friern and Claybury hospitals, 44, 117, 117 and 79 patients were discharged (357 in total). Significant findings include the fact that of patients discharged in the fourth year, none died in the following year, compared with three in the comparison group of patients remaining in hospital. Of the leavers, 16 (20 per cent) were readmitted to hospital during the first year.

There are clear and significant differences in the quality of the residential environ-ments of patients in hospital and community settings. There are many more opportunities for autonomy and choice for discharged patients. In particular, they enjoy far fewer restrictions on their everyday activities. When asked whether they wished to return to hospital or remain in their current setting, patients decisively preferred their new homes in the community.

Costs of Provision in the Community

The Personal Social Services Research Unit of the University of Kent at Canterbury (PSSRU) has been examining the costs of hospital and community services for people leaving the two hospitals and the relationship between these costs, client characteristics, service and client outcomes, and other relevant factors. Findings are now available for 254 clients who had been living in the community for one year. The average comprehensive cost of community care was £390 per week (1991 prices). Accommodation costs account for 82 per cent of the total cost. Sixty-five per cent of the clients live in high-support residential homes or hostels. A wide range of services is used but those provided by the health sector predominate in terms of funding, absorbing half the total cost of care packages. Clients bear a further third of the cost from their social security receipts, which can fund accommodation, car and living expenses. Local authorities and the voluntary sector are the main providers of social care (15 per cent of total costs). Family Health Services Authorities, despite the high rate of use of primary care services, fund only 1 per cent of the total cost of care. Although virtually all these resources come originally from public sources, the *route* which the money takes is of importance in planning a 'mixed economy of care'.

The PSSRU study runs in parallel with the TAPS research. Together they show that within a cost-effectiveness framework, *higher cost* is associated with *greater client needs* and *better outcomes*.

Researcher

Professor Julian Leff

Research Unit, Friern Hospital, Friern Barnet Road, London N11 3BP. (081 368 1288)

Publications

Books:

Tomlinson, D. (1991) *Utopia, community care and the retreat from the asylums*, Milton Keynes, Open University Press.

Reports:

Margolius, O. (1989) *Friern Hospital 1985–1988: Movement and Accumulation of the Long-stay Population*, London, North East Thames Regional Health Authority.

Team for the Assessment of Psychiatric Services (1988) *Preliminary Report on Baseline Data from Friern and Claybury Hospitals*, London, North East Thames Regional Health Authority.

Team for the Assessment of Psychiatric Services (1990) *Moving Long-stay Psychiatric Patients into the Community: First Results*, London, North East Thames Regional Health Authority.

Team for the Assessment of Psychiatric Services (1990) *Better out than in?*, London, North East Thames Regional Health Authority.

Tomlinson, D. (1988) *The Administrative Process of Claybury and Friern Reprovision*, London, North East Thames Regional Health Authority.

Chapters:

Anderson, J. N. (1991) 'User satisfaction, user participation, and evaluation of mental health services', in J. Orley (ed.), *Quality Assurance in Community Health Services*, Geneva, World Health Organisation.

Leff, J. P. (1988) 'Community Care v hospital care', in T. R. E. Barnes (ed.), *Depot Neuroleptics: A Consensus*, London, Mediscript.

Leff, J. (1988) 'Special needs and their assessment', in P. Bebbington, and P. McGuffin (eds), *Schizophrenia: The Main Issues*, Oxford, Heinemann.

Leff, J. (1990) 'Maintenance (management) of people with long-term psychotic illness', in I. M. Marks, and R. A. Scott (eds), *Mental Health Care Delivery: Innovations, Impediments and Implementation*, Cambridge, Cambridge University Press.

Leff, J. P. (1991) 'Do long-stay patients benefit from community placement?', In H. Freeman, and J. Henderson (eds), *Evaluation of Comprehensive Care of the Mentally Ill*, London, Gaskell.

Leff, J. (1991) 'Evaluation of the closure of mental hospitals', in P. Hall, and I. F. Brockington (eds), *The Closure of Mental Hospitals*, London, Gaskell.

Articles:

Anderson, J. (1989) 'Patient power in mental health – working for users?', *British Medical Journal*, 16 Dec., 1477–1478.

Anderson, J. (1990) 'The TAPS Project, I: Previous diagnosis and current disability of long-stay psychogeriatric patients: A pilot study', *British Journal of Psychiatry*, **156**: 661–666.

Beecham, J., Knapp, M., and Fenyo, A. (1991) 'Costs, needs and outcomes', *Schizophrenia Bulletin*, **17**, 3: 427–439.

Dayson, D. (1990) 'The TAPS Project 2: Challenges and Pitfalls of Community Interviewing', *The Psychiatric Bulletin of the Royal College of Psychiatrists*, **14**, 651–653.

Dayson, D., and Anderson, J. (1991) 'Conference presentation techniques', *The Psychiatric Bulletin of the Royal College of Psychiatrists*, **15**: 676–678.

Dunn, M., O'Driscoll, C., Dayson, D., Wills, W., and Leff, J. (1990) 'The TAPS Project. 4: An Observational Study of the Social Life of Long-stay Patients', *The British Journal of Psychiatry*, **157**: 842–848.

Jones, D. W., Tomlinson, D., and Anderson, J. (1991) 'Community and asylum care: *plus ça change*', *Journal of the Royal Society of Medicine*, **84**, 5, May, 252–254.

Knapp, M., Beecham, J., Anderson, J., Dayson, D., O'Driscoll, C., Leff, J., Margolius, O., and Wills, W. (1990) 'The TAPS Project 3: Predicting the community costs of closing psychiatric hospitals', *The British Journal of Psychiatry*, **157**: 661–670.

Knapp, M. R. J., and Beecham, J. (1990) 'Costing mental health services', *Psychological Medicine*, **20**: 893–908.

Leff, J., O'Driscoll, C., Dayson, D., Wills, W., Anderson, J. (1990) 'The TAPS Project. 5: The Structure of Social-Network Data Obtained from Long-Stay Patients', *The British Journal of Psychiatry*, **157**: 848–852.

Nocon, A., and Tomlinson, D. (1990) 'Inter-agency collaboration in the closure of psychiatric hospitals', *Psychiatric Bulletin of the Royal College of Psychiatrists*, **14**, 11, November.

O'Driscoll, C., Marshall, J., and Reed, J. (1990) 'Chronically Ill Psychiatric Patients in a District General Hospital: a Survey and Two Year Follow-up in an Inner London Health District', *British Journal of Psychiatry*, **157**, 694–702.

Tomlinson, D. (1988) 'Let the Mental Hospitals Close . . .', *Policy and Politics*, **16**, 3; 179–195.

Tomlinson, D. (1988) 'Community Service for the Mentally Ill: What is the Community?', *Health Service Management*, Oct., 120–123.

Tomlinson, D. (1990) 'Stick to the Agenda', *The Health Service Journal*, 15 March, 392–394.

Tomlinson, D. (1991) 'Seeing patients through', *Nursing Times*, **87**, 8, February 20.

Tomlinson, D. (1991) 'Which way to haven?', *The Health Service Journal*, 11 March, 20–21.

Tomlinson, D. (1991) 'Home truths of community care', *The Health Service Journal*, 21 March, 20–21.

Tomlinson, D. (1991) 'Freedom for living', *The Health Service Journal*, 28 March, 20–21.

Tomlinson, D. (1991) 'Life on the outside', *Health Matters*, **7**: 14–15.

Tomlinson, D., and Nocon, A. (1990) 'Joint planning: the day of reckoning draws nigh', *Health Services Management*, **86**, 4, August.

Psychiatric Rehabilitation in North Wales

INTERIM REPORT

This is a long-term study of psychiatric patients resettled from North Wales Hospital, Denbigh, into various community settings and care schemes. The study aims to assess changes in behavioural functioning, psychiatric state, quality of life and the costs of care. The method used is to take repeated measures while in hospital and then in the community, in order to assess changes. This report is based on information from the first six months from when patients were resettled.

Costs
Quality of life
Consumer views

There were 63 clients in the group, 34 of whom have been resettled to date: 79 per cent of the people resettled had a primary diagnosis of schizophrenia. Their age-range was 27 to 77 years.

The younger clients were more positive about leaving hospital than were the older clients, but once resettled, older clients become more positive about community care. Of those resettled, 65 per cent wanted to leave hospital, but 93 per cent now find their lives better in the initial period of community care.

There is no significant change in clients' psychiatric state, although levels of social and behavioural functioning show marked improvements. Clients are significantly more satisfied with living situations and a number of improvements in quality of life have been reported.

Seventy-eight per cent reported more independence and greater freedom to do the things they want to.

Some of the Snags

Some forms of care – especially 24-hour care for small groups in domestic houses – are expensive compared with other forms of community care. The advantages of preferred forms of community care have to be weighed against costs.

These results are based on assessments after only six months in the community: changes may occur in the longer term.

Some Detailed Findings

Attitudes to discharge while in hospital were found not to be correlated with attitudes to the new community settings. A number of clients who had earlier expressed a desire to remain in hospital later described their life in the community as being much better, compared with hospital.

In describing the areas of their life most affected by the move from hospital, clients say that the community settings are less restrictive and point to the greater freedom and independence they offer:

> 'A lot better altogether, my whole life feels better here. I have freedom, I go out and meet people and sing in the choir and I just feel I'm enjoying life like never before.'

'I'm able to do a lot more for myself here, more freedom . . . I feel I can develop here, it was all negative in the hospital . . . Got the privacy, don't have to sleep in a dormitory, can cook my own food, can watch TV and radio, can go shopping. I get the money and more contact with staff.'

Overall, the clients appear to have reacted well to the changes in their living situation and care regime, and are responding positively to the increased opportunities for a more independent lifestyle.

These encouraging preliminary results give some insight into the intermediate outcomes for long-stay clients involved in the resettlement process to date. However it is important to stress the tentative nature of these findings, as true outcome results will not be available until at least 12 months after discharge from hospital.

Researcher

Dr Charles Crosby

Health Services Research Unit, Department of Psychology, University College of North Wales, Bangor LL57 2DG. (0248 382040)

Publications

Reports:

Barry, M. M., Crosby, C., Bogg, J., and Carter, M. F. (1992) 'Evaluation of Resettlement from North Wales Hospital: Brief Report on Client Outcomes at Six Months post-Discharge', Health Services Research Unit, Department of Psychology, University College of North Wales.

Carter, M. F., Bogg, J., Crosby, C., and Barry, M. M., (1992) 'Evaluation of Resettlement from North Wales Hospital: Report of Staff Attitudes and Management Practices in Two Community Residential Care Schemes in North Wales Hospital, Denbigh', Health Services Research Unit, Department of Psychology, University College of North Wales.

Crosby, C., Barry, M. M., Carter, M. F., and Bogg, J. (1992) 'Evaluation of Resettlement from North Wales Hospital: Brief Report on the Care Process in Two Community Care Schemes', Health Services Research Unit, Department of Psychology, University College of North Wales.

Crosby, C., Barry, M. M., Mitchell, D. A., Horrocks, F., and Littlejohns, C. (1990) 'Evaluation of the Clwyd Mental Health Community Service: An Interim Report', Health Services Research Unit, Department of Psychology, University College of North Wales.

Crosby, C., Barry, M. M., Vick, S., and Garrod, N. (1991) 'The Costs of Community Care – Three months after Discharge from North Wales Hospital', Health Services Research Unit, Department of Psychology, University College of North Wales.

Accepted for publication:

Barry, M. M., Crosby, C., and Mitchell, D. A. (1992) 'Quality of Life Issues in the Evaluation of Mental Health Services', in D. R. Trent (ed.), *Promotion of Mental Health*, Vol. 1, Aldershot, Avebury.

Barry, M. M., Crosby, C., and Bogg, J. (in press) 'Quality of Life and Mental Health', in I. Markova, and R. M. Farr (eds), *Representations of Health, Illness and Handicap. Qualitative Health Research.*

Three Experimental Homes for the Elderly Mentally Ill

Against a background of increasing numbers of elderly mentally-ill people, the Department of Health established an initiative to develop and evaluate alternative ways of caring for this client-group. Three experimental schemes were established, with the Department providing 50 per cent funding for five years. All three units aim to provide a homely and domestic living environment, and provide individualized care for clients.

Costs
'Positve' care
Quality of life

> *Highgrove House, High Wycombe, opened 1985:* Highgrove provides residential care for 17 residents and assessment and relief-care for a further three. It is a joint scheme between High Wycombe Health Authority and Buckinghamshire Social Services, but is run on a social services model. Highgrove caters primarily for people who have been classed as managerial problems and is set up to provide an alternative to long-term psychogeriatric care.

> *Redcourt, Liverpool, opened 1986:* Redcourt provides permanent residential care for 23 elderly people with severe dementia, but not suffering from other significant physical illness. Older people suffering primarily from functional psychiatric illness are catered for by other local psychogeriatric services. Redcourt functions as an independent nursing home within Liverpool Health Authority.

> *Seward Lodge, Hertford, opened 1987:* Seward Lodge contributes to East Hertfordshire Health Authority's strategy for providing a localized service for the elderly mentally ill. It functions as an independent nursing home, providing 20 permanent residential places, four relief-care beds and day-care for up to 15 people each day over a seven-day week. A 'total-care' approach is employed, where nursing staff have a generic role and are involved in all aspects of direct and indirect client care and hotel tasks.

Resourcing the Three Schemes

All three schemes were highly resourced in terms of staff. In comparison with conventional hospital wards, there was a substitution of untrained for trained staff in respect of direct client-care at Highgove and Seward Lodge. The use of generic workers at Seward Lodge is probably cost-effective, but was not a popular option amongst staff.

Economic Aspects of the Homes

No direct relationship was found between dependency and the way staff resources were distributed amongst residents. This has implications for the way nursing homes are funded, as current mechanisms may not reflect the actual 'demandingness' of clients.

The extra resources available were largely channelled into routine care, such as residents' hygiene, dressing and feeding, and produced only a limited return in terms of 'positive' life-enhancing care.

The research showed that the use of activity organizers or occupational therapy aides did result in higher levels of positive care. For clients with dementia, a care model which includes a considerable amount of task assignment stands a greater chance of maximizing positive care than one which relies on personalized care alone.

Staffing issues

There is no evidence that the use of largely unqualified care staff to provide direct care resulted in any detriment to residents.

Both Highgrove and Seward Lodge devolved responsibility for individual client care to unqualified staff. There is no research evidence to suggest that clients were disadvantaged by this, but the practice emphasized the importance of management support, in-service training, quality assurance procedures and staff recruitment policy.

Although based on a social services model of care with no direct nursing input, Highgrove was able to cope with residents with behavioural problems who would normally have been admitted to long-stay psychiatric or nursing care.

The physical environment

All three homes provided a more domestic and home-like environment than is often found in residential care settings and long-stay hospital wards in particular. The homes offered high levels of private space and encouraged independent behaviour amongst residents.

However, residential accommodation based on communal living is invariably 'un-homelike'. Long corridors, offices and large communal lounges were features that are not found in truly domestic environments. With the exception of Highgrove, the care regimes were geared towards communal living.

Quality of life

- Measuring 'quality of life' is particularly difficult with this client-group because they are generally unable to conceptualize their needs or to express their feelings and attitudes. Existing concepts and measures of quality of life in residential and nursing-home settings reflect the needs of the physically frail rather than the mentally impaired.
- *Relatives* were interviewed as advocates of the residents: their response to the three homes was very positive. Relatives felt that the standard of care was high and that staff had a very caring attitude.
- The *pattern of daily life* in the three homes was relatively unstructured. Rather than making residents fit an institutional routine, the homes provided flexible regimes that accommodate the varying needs and wishes of individual residents.
- Admission to the three homes, and to long-term care in general, led to the *disengagement* of residents from their families and the wider society. In this sense, the three schemes are still very much in the traditional pattern of old people's homes.
- The research showed that beyond being able to feed themselves, residents were typically able to do very little in terms of *self-help*. Residents' abilities to do things for themselves is limited by their mental functioning. However, the effect of 'learned dependency', which is associated with institutional environments, was also a limiting factor.
- A lack of insight and understanding meant that residents were often unable to exercise *choice* in a conventional sense. The role of the key worker is crucial here.

- Although the experimental homes aimed to provide a better quality of life for residents, *positive aspects of lifestyle* – such as leisure and social interaction – were found to be no higher than in conventional long-stay psychiatric wards. The most common use of time by residents was 'doing nothing'.

Outcomes of Care

- Although the research data only allows tentative conclusions about survival, all three schemes had *low death rates*. The indications are that the protective and specialist residential environments afforded by the homes promote the longevity of residents.
- *Psychological well-being* is very difficult to define and measure for people who are cognitively disordered. However, some residents appeared to benefit or improve in terms of emotional well-being, agitation, aggression and cooperation. This suggests that those people who have psychological, behavioural or psychiatric disorders, as well as cognitive impairment, are likely to benefit most from the sort of care provided by the three homes.
- Overall, clients exhibited a pattern of *gradual deterioration* over time in respect to physical condition, cognitive functioning, and daily tasks of living. However, this general picture hides considerable individual differences.
- The benefits of the homes to *relatives* were: relief from constant worry; relief from the task of continuous caring; knowledge that the relative is well cared for. This last point is important in reducing the burden of guilt which often arises when a relative is admitted to care.

Researchers

Professor John Copeland, Dr Charles Crosby, Dr Andrew Sixsmith and Professor John Stilwell

Institute of Human Ageing, University of Liverpool, PO Box 147, Liverpool L69 3BX. (051 794 5074/5081; FAX 051 794 5077)

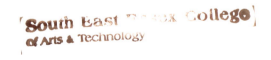

The Disabilities and Circumstances of Patients with Chronic Schizophrenia

This project was devised against the background of developing community care policies for psychiatric patients. Policies of closure of the mental hospitals and transfer to community services have been advocated for some time and have been in partial operation in Harrow. As elsewhere, the attempt to turn the pattern of treatment away from continuing in-patient care has been made without the organized development of appropriate alternatives. While the policy of community care has much to commend it, many difficulties have been encountered in relation to such policies and a good deal of controversy has been engendered. Much of this difficulty related to a lack of information about the long-term course and outcome of psychiatric illness managed in various ways. Studies have, however, been conducted on schizophrenic patients from the Harrow area (Johnstone, et al., 1981[12], Johnstone, et al., 1984[13]) and in the North West Thames Region (Macmillan, et al., 1986[14]) and they have indicated that the disabilities of these patients may be severe and persistent. Nonetheless, despite services which left a good deal to be desired, neither patients nor relatives wished a return to in-patient care. These views lend support to the concept of community care, but the findings of the studies emphasize the seriousness of the problems associated with schizophrenia.

The purpose of this study was to identify and trace all schizophrenic patients discharged from in-patient or day-patient Harrow psychiatric services between 1 January 1976 and 1 January 1985, and to examine them in terms of mental state, cognitive functioning, extrapyramidal function and social disability, and to relate these assessments to demographic, historical and treatment variables. This would provide firm information about the disabilities and unmet needs of this group of patients. Details of the method are described in the full report.

FINDINGS

During the relevant period, 532 patients who fulfilled stringent standardized criteria for schizophrenia were discharged from the psychiatric unit of Northwick Park Hospital and from the beds of Shenley Hospital to which Harrow patients are admitted.

Since 93.6 per cent of the sample was traced and 6.4 per cent untraced, the findings are truly representative of the sample: 12.5 per cent were dead, 7 per cent were abroad, and in 9.5 per cent either the patient, a relative, the GP or a legal representative refused. But 328 (61.7 per cent) of patients were interviewed and, where applicable and possible, a relative and/or a professional informant was

---

[12] Johnstone, E. C., Owens, D. G. C., Gold, A., Crow, T. J., and Macmillan, J. F. (1981) 'Institutionalisation and the defects of schizophrenia', *British Journal of Psychiatry*, **139**: 195–203.

[13] Johnstone, E. C., Owens, D. G. C., Gold, A., Crow, T. J., and Macmillan, J. F. (1984) 'Schizophrenic patients discharged from hospital – a follow-up study', *British Journal of Psychiatry*, **145**: 586–590.

[14] Macmillan, J. F., Crow, T. J., Johnson, A. L., and Johnstone, E. C. (1986) 'The Northwick Park study of first episodes of schizophrenia. III. Short-term outcome in trial entrants and trial eligibles', *British Journal of Psychiatry*, **148**: 128–133.

interviewed. Of the 69 deaths, 24 were clearly unnatural and it is probable that these patients killed themselves. This is greatly in excess of the rate of suicide in the general population. The total sample consisted of 291 males and 241 females. The mean ages in 1990 of those patients who were alive were 42 years for males, and 48 years for females. 75.7 per cent of patients were white Europeans, 6.4 per cent Afro-Caribbeans, 15.5 per cent Asian, 0.6 per cent White/Afro-Caribbeans and 1.7 per cent White/Asians. Few of the patients were entirely well and 50 per cent had a morbid rating on psychotic symptoms when seen. 24 per cent of patients lived alone and 59 per cent with relatives, most commonly parents. Only 5.3 per cent of families lived in hostels. Sixty-eight per cent of patients were satisfied with their accommodation and only two of them sought a return to hospital. Seventy per cent of relevant respondents were satisfied with the arrangement of the patient living with them and, although the remainder thought that this was difficult, only one person thought the patient would be better off in hospital.

At their best, these patients had performed well: 26 per cent had GCSE/CSEs or O-levels, a further 10.4 per cent had attended university or equivalent place of education and a further 5.3 per cent had obtained a degree. Over 60 per cent had a best occupational-level in work classed as 1, 2 or 3 according to the Registrar General's classification. This had shown a marked decline by the time of the index admission in 1975 and 1985 and when seen for the survey, 19.7 per cent of the sample worked full-time in some capacity and 11.8 per cent did part-time work, but 63.8 per cent were unemployed. Patients led impoverished lives, with 38 per cent going to no place of entertainment, even a cafe, club or public house, in the month prior to interview, 50 per cent showing a lack of interest in current affairs and 60 per cent having no strong interest or hobby.

Some of the assessments used in this survey were the same as those used in the earlier survey of all patients fulfilling the same criteria for schizophrenia dis-charged from Harrow beds between 1 January 1970 and 1 January 1975 and it is possible to compare the two studies. One hundred and twenty patients were discharged between 1970 and 1975, and 532 between 1975 and 1985. This much larger number may reflect more active discharge policies but it is likely also to be due to the fact that Northwick Park Hospital, a district general hospital with 12 national beds catering for psychiatric, largely schizophrenic patients, opened in 1975. The two samples are closely similar in age and sex distribution. A particular cause for concern in the earlier study was the lack of contact with any medical, social or psychiatric services of substantial numbers of patients. A comparison of the contact with services of the present sample with the earlier sample is shown in table 4.1, and it is clear that is has been possible to effect major improvements.

Table 4.1: *Contact with Services*

	1975–85 (present sample % of cases)	1970–75 (previous sample % of cases)	Significance of difference between samples
No medical or social support	5.8	27.2	p < 0.001
Contact only with CPN	2.7	13.6	p < 0.001
Contact only with GP	13.4	23.0	ns
Attending psychiatric clinic + other agencies	45.4	16.6	p < 0.001
Attending > one agency but not psychiatric clinic	11.5	20.0	ns

In spite of this greater degree of care, there were no significant differences between the two samples with regard to the morbid features of the mental state. The living circumstances of the patients did not show much change and it is clear that relatives continue to provide a great deal of care for these patients. There have, however, been significant reductions in the burden of care that the relatives experience (table 4.2). It seems reasonable to suggest that this lesser degree of burden, in particular the striking reduction in the anxiety about what will happen to the patient when the relatives die, may be due to the greater degree of contact with the services – especially the specialist services.

Table 4.2: *Burden of Care on Relatives of Patients*

	1975–1985 (present) sample % of cases	1970–1975 (previous) sample % of cases	
a) *Specific Questions*			
Time off work to look after patients	6.7	16	ns
Stopped work to look after patients	2.5	16	$p < 0.001$
Emotional illness in family	16.8	13	ns
Physical illness in family	9.2	6	ns
Social restrictions for family	30.8	48	ns
Disruption of family	16.7	35	$p < 0.005$
Financial difficulties	10.8	19	ns
b) *Additional Items of Concern*			
No further worries	47.3	20	$p < 0.01$
Concern over future, particularly when relatives die	3.6	38	$p < 0.0001$
Distress over patient's evident suffering	0	10	
Patient's independence	7.6	13	
Patient's loneliness	9.2	13	
Patient's apathy/slowness	8.4	5	
Fear of relapse	4.2	5	

Note:

Considerable additional detail on the treatment and care of these patients and their psychiatric, psychological, neurological and social disabilities is available, including details of physical illnesses and medical contacts.

Researchers

Professor Eve C. Johnstone, J. Leary, C. D. Frich, D. G. C. Owens, S. Wilkins

North West Thames Regional Health Authority, Harrow Health Authority, Northwick Park Hospital, Watford Road, Harrow, Middlesex HA1 3UJ. (081 864 3232)

Present address:

Professor Johnstone, Department of Psychiatry, The University of Edinburgh, Kennedy Tower, Royal Edinburgh Hospital, Morningside Park, Edinburgh EH10 5HF. (031 447 2011)

Publications

Johnstone, E. C. (ed.), 'Disabilities and Circumstances of Schizophrenic Patients – A Follow-Up Study', *British Journal of Psychiatry*, **159**, supplement 13.

The Buckingham Project – Preliminary Analysis

BACKGROUND

The Buckingham Project began in 1984, when a comprehensive mental health service was established in the northern region of the Aylesbury Vale Health District. This service aimed to provide all mental health care in a manner that integrated primary, secondary and tertiary mental health care. Assessment and treatment was conducted within a general practitioner setting, emphasizing early detection, home-based crisis management, and community-based, long-term rehabilitation. A multi-disciplinary team of mental health professionals, similar to that allocated to a hospital service, was trained in the latest biomedical and psychosocial management strategies, and was integrated with all four primary care teams in the area. Hospital and other specialized resources were contracted when needed to supplement the service. The goals of the service were to enhance:

Accessibility: making services readily available to all members of the community in need of them at all times.

Acceptability: providing services that were welcomed by the client-group, who complied readily with recommended clinical management.

Accountability: strategies for continuous assessment of the quality of the service provided in terms of its benefits and costs were devised.

Adaptability: the service was expected to be able to adapt to the varied needs of specific clients as well as the changing needs of the community as a whole.

A series of projects was established in order to evaluate the success of the project in achieving these goals. Four projects are summarized here:

(1) Assessment of the Benefits and Costs of Integrated Mental Health Care;

(2) Early Detection and Intervention for Schizophrenia;

(3) The Benefits and Costs of Long-Term Mental Health Care in the Community;

(4) The Stress of Caring for People with Long-Term Disabilities in the Community.

1. ASSESSMENT OF THE BENEFITS AND COSTS OF INTEGRATED MENTAL HEALTH CARE

A review of all cases assessed by the service during a 12-month period was conducted. This revealed a considerably higher rate of consultation than had previously been observed with a hospital-based community service. Approximately 1,100 people per 100,000 were assessed annually. Two-thirds were people who had not had previous contact with specialist mental health services. Almost half had no evidence of mental disorders, consisting primarily of psychosocial problems associated with family, marital or work stress; and 12 per cent had no significant disorders. Of those considered to have primary mental disorders, 80 per cent were suffering from either anxiety disorders, adjustment disorders or somatization. Functional psychoses formed only 5 per cent of the cases of mental disorders which were assessed.

It was clear that mental health care could be delivered in this community-based manner, and that supplementary hospital and social services were seldom required. In-patient care was used at a rate of less than 5 beds per 100,000.

Acceptability of the integrated approach seemed to be high, with 90 per cent of cases of mental disorders completing the recommended clinical management plan. Treatment was complete within three months for 70 per cent, while 3 per cent were considered to need continued clinical management after 12 months. The average number of clinical sessions per case was 7.5 by mental health clinicians and 2 from the primary care professionals.

A straightforward method of measuring the benefits of clinical management in terms of reductions in ratings of clinical, social and carer morbidity was piloted successfully. Clinicians were trained to make reliable ratings which were monitored by a quality assurance team. Benefits were most readily achieved with reductions in clinical morbidity, but worthwhile improvements in disability and carer stresses were measured. However, the benefits achieved from involvement with people suffering from mental disorders was three times greater than that achieved when psychosocial problems were the primary target of intervention.

An economic analysis showed that the major cost of the service was the clinical personnel, who spent 48 per cent of their time at work in direct patient-contact. This time was evenly divided between early intervention, crisis management and long-term care. The comprehensive cost (including all overheads) of one hour of face-to-face clinical contact with a mental health professional was £29. When these costs were compared with the benefits achieved on the clinicians' ratings, the cost to the community of achieving a unit of benefit was approximately £90, of which £60 was associated with the mental health budget. The cost of achieving one unit of benefit for those people suffering primary psychosocial problems was around £150.

A similar analysis of people who continued with the scheme after 12 months showed that benefits continued to accrue, although at a slower rate and a consequently higher cost. The mean cost per additional unit of benefit was £1,500, which took around one year of long-term care to achieve. The integrated service employed minimal specialized rehabilitation or supplementary social services to achieve these benefits. Evidence that the home-based approach did not appear to add to the burdens of informal carers was investigated in a study that is presented later in this report.

Surveys of the consumers, GPs and mental health clinicians indicated a high level of satisfaction with the integrated approach. Criticisms related to the lack of adequate resources for managing serious crises, and the concern that the team approach reduced the choice of therapist; a few carers felt they would like to become even more involved in the clinical management of their relatives than they had been. Staff concerns focused mainly on administrative arrangements at district level.

The study shows that the integration of mental health services with primary care teams is a highly effective means of delivering comprehensive mental health care to communities. Moreover, it is clear that this approach has considerable economic advantages as the need for hospital-based crisis care and specialized rehabilitation resources is reduced. The success of this project was generally attributed to *extensive training of the multi-disciplinary staff* in the assessment and treatment of mental disorders and their associated disabilities, including the training of primary care professionals and informal carers. A training project has therefore been developed to disseminate these strategies throughout the NHS, and is currently operating in more than 20 districts.

2. EARLY DETECTION AND INTERVENTION FOR SCHIZOPHRENIA

Training
Family observation
Self-report

Close collaboration with primary care services offered the potential for enhanced screening of people who might be experiencing the preliminary stages of major mental disorders, such as schizophrenia, and to enable effective treatment to begin earlier than with hospital-based services. The Buckingham Project aimed to train all professional staff, including GPs and community nurses (health visitors, district nurses and midwives), to recognize the early signs of the functional psychoses, and to enhance their clinical interviewing skills. All mental health professionals were trained to research reliability in the use of diagnostic scales, as well as employing a standardized medical history that screened for risk factors for mental disorders. Primary care staff received less formal training in screening procedures, mainly through personalized case consultation.

Clearly-defined procedures were followed whenever early signs of a functional psychosis were suspected. These included immediate consultation with a psychiatrist to confirm the nature of the emerging disorder, and the immediate initiation of a clinical-management plan. This involved educational, psychosocial and biomedical strategies targeted to the specific problems experienced by the patient and his/her informal carers. It also usually involved intensive stress management, educating patient and carers about the disorder that was thought to be emerging, and drug therapy to counter any specific symptoms. The intervention was continued until the features of the disorder had all resolved and all reversible risk factors (such as life events, major stressors, substance abuse, hormonal disturbances and so on) had been minimized. Monitoring then continued for a further 24 months to ensure that any further early signs were tackled without delay.

Low incidence rates of schizophrenic and major affective disorders were observed. But many cases with *symptoms* of these disorders were treated and almost all experienced full and lasting recovery after intensive clinical management. **This suggested that one of the benefits of integrated care may be the ability to detect cases at an earlier stage than hospital-based services.** Improved assessment training of all primary care as well as mental health professionals seems to be crucial, so that responses can be distinguished efficiently, and resources channelled to those most likely to benefit. Concern that diagnosing people at an early stage might be harmful has proved unfounded. But the reason for this lies in the way in which staff were trained to educate patients and their carers about the nature of mental disorders, and the factors contributing to their development and to their effective resolution.

The encouraging results of this study require validation in extensive, controlled clinical trials before they can be recommended for clinical practice.

3. THE BENEFITS AND COSTS OF LONG-TERM CARE IN THE COMMUNITY

Burden of care
Quality of life

A further project (mainly funded by the Mental Health Foundation) examined the effects of integrated care on a cohort of 41 long-term cases. All cases had received at least one year of continuous treatment from the service before they entered this project. A three-monthly review of clinical, social and carer morbidity was conducted for an additional 24 months. Significant reductions in clinical morbidity and social disability were achieved during this period, as a result of continued biomedical psychosocial interventions aimed at enhancing the quality of life of both patients and their informal carers. The burden of caring was low in 83 per cent of cases and, despite a trend for reductions in the six cases where carers experienced moderate or high levels, this was insufficient to establish a statistically-significant result overall. Clinical symptoms became worse in 17 per cent of cases during the first year and 9 per cent in the second year: two other cases remained severely mentally ill throughout the two-year period. Two cases required periods of in-patient care to supplement home-based crisis management during the first year, and one during the second year. **More than two-thirds of all clinical crises were successfully managed by intensive care in the community.**

An economic analysis, based upon the concept of additional years of healthy life that result from therapeutic intervention (QALYS), was undertaken. The cost to achieve one additional year of healthy life, free from disability and distress, was estimated at £10,934 for cases suffering from schizophrenia. The alternative method of assessing the efficiency of clinical interventions, described earlier, showed that units of benefit during the first 12 months averaged almost one unit per case, each unit of benefit costing around £1,500.

It is clear that the integrated-care approach to long-term rehabilitation was able to achieve continuing added benefits, both in terms of clinical and social recovery. This was achieved with low use of specialized resources and hospital care. There was no evidence of additional burdens being placed upon informal carers. Problems in assessing the economics of rehabilitative care were highlighted, and further research is needed to establish measures which will allow valid comparisons between different approaches and different health problems.

4. THE STRESS OF CARING FOR PEOPLE WITH LONG-TERM DISABILITIES IN THE COMMUNITY

Coping

This study examined the stresses of caring for people with disabilities in the community, and their association with subjective distress and health problems for the carers. A cohort of 48 people receiving long-term mental health care for functional psychoses and anxiety disorders were matched with 48 people receiving long-term physical health care in terms of disability levels, age, sex and marital status. Their key informal carers were assessed in terms of the stresses currently experienced in all aspects of their lives, including those which they attributed to the care-giving role. The effectiveness of the coping skills they applied to each stress factor was assessed, as well as their overall subjective distress and the burden associated with being a carer. An index of health status was devised.

Almost half of the key carers of people suffering from long-term health problems were found to be burdened by their care-giving roles, and a similar proportion suffered from health problems themselves: 1 in 4 suffered from major disorders. Environmental stress factors, of which the stress of care-giving comprised more than half, and the ability to cope effectively with them were closely associated with perceived burden. Almost three-quarters of carers expressed positive attitudes about their care-giving role, and very few expressed any desire to give up. However, many emphasized how important it was to have effective and flexible community services which could deal with all their needs.

There were few differences between the carers of people with long-term mental and physical disorders. Carers of people with physical illnesses thought that the overall expenses and lost earning-capacity of their households were double that of households with people suffering mental disorders.

The most striking findings of this study were found in the comparisons between the two major categories of mental disorders. Carers of people suffering from long-term anxiety experienced higher levels of burden and distress than those caring for people with functional psychoses, despite a lack of any differences in the levels of disability of patients in the two groups. The *anxiety cases* tended to be younger, had experienced the disorder, informal and professional care for a much shorter time, and two-thirds were working: only a third of people receiving long-term care for *functional psychoses* were employed.

Almost all the carers of anxiety disorders were themselves working, and almost 10 years younger than carers of the functional cases. It was clear that many carers of people suffering from mental disorders had difficulties in continuing to lead the lives that they had expected; and that persisting anxiety disorders tended to interfere with the carer's life on an everyday basis. People with functional disorders, on the other hand, tended to have quiescent periods between episodes of disturbance.

This study showed that the integrated community care of people with long-term mental disorders – particularly those with functional psychoses – compared favourably with that for people with long-term physical disorders. However, it highlighted the problems associated with the long-term care of people with persisting anxiety disorders, who showed levels of disability similar to those of people with functional disorders, and were associated with greater burdens for carers. These cases require very skilled management from a well-trained multi-disciplinary team, and present a strong argument for the provision of extensive community-based services.

Researcher

Dr Ian R. H. Falloon

Buckingham Mental Health Services, 22 High Street, Buckingham MK18 1NU. (0280 812925)

Present address:
COMMEND Project, The Coach House, Finmere, Nr Buckingham, MK18 4AR. (0280 848698)

Publications

Andrews, G. (1990) 'England: An innovative community psychiatric service', *Lancet*, **335**: 1087–1088.

Andrews, G. (1991) 'The Tolkien Report: a description of a model mental health service', Darlinghurst, Australia, Health Services Research Group.

Falloon, I. R. H. (1986) 'Family Stress and Schizophrenia: Theory and Practice', *Psychiatric Clinics of North America*, **9**: 165–182.

Falloon, I. R. H. (1987) 'Informing the consumer: Developments in patient and family education', Proceedings, International Conference on Mental Health Education, Dublin.

Falloon, I. R. H. (1988) 'Behavioural family therapy and the management of schizophrenia', in P. Williams, G. Wilkinson, and K. Rawnsley (eds), *Scientific Approaches in Epidemiological and Social Psychiatry*, London, Tavistock.

Falloon, I. R. H. (1988) 'Behavioural family therapy in the prevention of morbidity of schizophrenia', in I. R. H. Falloon (ed.), *Handbook of Behavioural Family Therapy*, New York, Guildford Press.

Falloon, I. R. H. (1988) 'Social skills training for schizophrenia', in F. Flach (ed.), *The schizophrenias*, New York, W. W. Norton.

Falloon, I. R. H. (1989) 'Family management of Schizophrenia', in M. Weller (ed.), *Innovations in the Treatment of Schizophrenia*, London, Tavistock Press.

Falloon, I. R. H. (1990) 'Behavioural family therapy for schizophrenic disorders', in M. Herz, S. Keith, and J. Docherty, *Handbook of Schizophrenia: Psychosocial Treatment for Schizophrenia*, New York, Elsevier.

Falloon, I. R. H. (1990) 'Integrated family, general practice and mental health care in the management of schizophrenia', *British Journal of Hospital Medicine*, **83**: 225–228.

Falloon, I. R. H. (1991) 'An asylum in the community – a future view of psychiatric care', *Linc-Up*, **1**: 8–9.

Falloon, I. R. H. (1991) 'Family stress management approaches and schizophrenia', in H. Stierlin, *et al.* (eds), *Treatment of psychotic behaviour*, Berlin, Springer-Verlag.

Falloon, I. R. H. (1992) 'Early intervention for first episodes of schizophrenia: a preliminary exploration', *Psychiatry*, **55**: 1–12.

Falloon, I. R. H. (in press) 'Family therapy for schizophrenia and affective disorders', in M. Herson and A. Bellack (eds), *Handbook of behavior therapy in the psychiatric setting*, New York, Plenum.

Falloon, I. R. H. (in press) 'Prevention of major depressive episodes: Early intervention with family-based stress management', *Journal of Mental Health*.

Falloon, I. R. H., and Fadden, G. (in press) *Integrated Mental Health Care*, Cambridge, Cambridge University Press.

Falloon, I. R. H., Harpin, R. E., and Pembleton, T. (1988) 'Behavioural family therapy in primary health care settings', in I. R. H. Falloon (ed.), *Handbook of Behavioural Family Therapy*, New York, Guildford Press.

Falloon, I. R. H., and Hole, V. (1990) 'Family care as an alternative to the mental hospital', in P. Hall, and I. Brockington (eds), *Closure of mental hospitals*, London, Royal College of Psychiatrists.

Falloon, I. R. H., Hole, V., Mulroy, L., Norris, L. J., and Pembleton, T. (1988) 'Behavioural family therapy', in J. F. Clarkin, *et al.* (eds), *Affective Disorders and the Family*, New York, Guildford Press, 117–133.

Falloon, I. R. H., Hole, V., Shanahan, W. J., Laporta, M., and Krekorian, H. (1989) 'Developing family based care for schizophrenia: A training project', *Bulletin of the Royal College of Psychiatrists*, 675–676.

Falloon, I. R. H., Krekorian, H., Shanahan, W. J., Laporta, M., and McLees, S. (1990) 'The Buckingham Project: a comprehensive mental health service based upon behavioural psychotherapy', *Behaviour Change*, **7**: 51–57.

Falloon, I. R. H., and Laporta, M. (1991) 'Prevention strategies in schizophrenia', in D. Kavanagh (ed.), *Schizophrenia: an overview and practical handbook*, London, Chapman Hall.

Falloon, I. R. H., and Laporta, M. (in press) *Managing stress in families*, London, Routledge.

Falloon, I. R. H., Laporta, M., and Shanahan, W. J. (1991) 'Behavioural psychotherapy', in J. Holmes (ed.), *Psychotherapy in psychiatric practice*, London, Churchill-Livingstone.

Falloon, I. R. H., and Lillie, F. J. (1988) 'Service in the community', *Health Service Journal*, 7 April, 392.

Falloon, I. R. H., Mueser, K., Gingerich, S., Rappaprot, S., McGill, C. W., and Hole, V. (1988) *Behavioural Family Therapy: A Workbook*, Buckingham Mental Health Service, England, (translated into Italian, Greek, Spanish, German).

Falloon, I. R. H., and Shanahan, W. J. (1990) 'Community management of schizophrenia', *British Journal of Hospital Medicine*, **43**: 62–66.

Falloon, I. R. H., Wilkinson, G., and Burgess, J. M. (1989) 'The Buckingham Project: An integrated mental health service with primary care', *Communication and Handicaps*, Paris, Conservatoire national des Arts et Métiers, 79–81.

Falloon, I. R. H., Wilkinson, G., Burgess, J., and McLees, S. (1987) 'Evaluation in psychiatry: Planning, developing and evaluating community-based mental health services for adults', in D. Milne, (ed.), *Evaluating Mental Health Practice*, London, Croom Helm.

King's Fund Centre (1991–2) 'Alternatives to Acute Hospital Admission', *Bulletins 1–5, Keyhole Group*, (R. Echlin, Convenor; I. Falloon and V. Graham-Hole, Members).

Shanahan, W., Laporta, M., and Falloon, I. R. H. (1990) 'The Buckingham Project – A home-based mental health service', *Irish Journal of Psychological Medicine*, **7**: 151–153.

National Institute of Mental Health (1991) 'The Prevention of Mental Disorders: Progress, Problems and Prospects', Preliminary Report of the National Conference on Prevention Research, Rockville, MD, (I. Falloon, Member).

WHO Scientific Group (Falloon, I. R. H., Member) (1991) 'Evaluation of methods for the treatment of mental disorders', *WHO Technical Report Series*, 812, Geneva.

Wilkinson, G., Croft-Jeffreys, C., Krekorian, H., McLees, S., and Falloon, I. R. H. (1990) 'QALYS in psychiatric care?', *Psychiatric Bulletin*, **14**: 582–585.

Wilkinson, G., Falloon, I. R. H., and Sen, B. (1985) 'Chronic mental disorders in general practice', *British Medical Journal*, **291**, 1302–1304.

Wilkinson, G., William, B., Krekorian, H., McLees, S., and Falloon, I. (in press) 'QALYS in mental health: A case study', *Psychological Medicine*.

Community Versus Standard Psychiatric Care

INTRODUCTION

Psychiatric-bed numbers in Britain have fallen by over two-thirds since their peak in the mid-1950s – a pattern which has been observed in many countries. Despite this, spending on mental health services has increased from 0.2 per cent of GNP in 1954 to 0.3 per cent in 1988. Consultant provision has increased by 3.5 per cent and nurse provision by 22 per cent between 1976–86. In-patient services dominate nurse employment, with only 5,000 Community Psychiatric Nurses (CPNs) out of a total establishment of 58,000 in 1990. Hospital care continues to absorb around 80 per cent of NHS mental health expenditure.

Well-publicized studies of alternatives to hospital treatment have had only a modest impact on psychiatric practice. Common reservations expressed are that the patients are too selected, the experimental teams are too highly resourced and/or motivated, and that the working practices of these experimental teams could not be sustained over time

THE STUDY

This study contrasted an existing home-based model (HB) against standard care (SC) with no clinical exclusion and no extra resources. The teams were asked to offer all referred patients an assessment in their own homes, within two weeks of referral. The assessment was to be by two team members – one medical and one a trained CPN, social worker or psychologist. Where possible, treatment was also based at home, and the teams operated without waiting-lists. No other restrictions on clinical practice were specified.

Three South London sectors were studied: each was served by two consultant-led teams, one of which acted as the experimental team (HB) and the other as control (SC).

METHODS

All referred patients, including emergency admissions, aged between 18 and 74 who had not been in contact with local psychiatric services within the preceding 12 months were randomly allocated to the two services. Patients were assessed by independent researchers at intake, at 6 weeks, 6 months and 12 months. These research interviews contained a battery of measures of symptoms (Present State Examination, Clinical Interview, the Brief Psychiatric Rating Scale), social functioning and consumer satisfaction, as well as collecting basic demographic data. Where informants were available, their assessments of the patient's progress plus family and economic burden were obtained.

One hundred and seventy-two patients (78 SC and 94 HB) entered the study and were followed up for one year.

RESULTS

Just over 30 per cent of patients were suffering from a psychotic disorder at intake, the remainder mainly adjustment and neurotic disorders. Just over half had a previous psychiatric history.

> Both groups showed significant improvements in clinical and social functioning with no significant differences between them. Similarly, no significant differences were observed in consumer satisfaction or family burden.

Half of patients in both groups were seen within one week and this included all the psychotic patients. Of those not seen within one week, there was a greater delay for those receiving standard care. The improved access to care demonstrated in HB was clearly related to long waiting-times for routine out-patient appointments in SC. Of the four suicides in the study, three were in the SC group.

The number of out-patient contacts were similar in both groups (5.5 per patient). On average, HB appointments were 10 minutes longer (plus 10 minutes travel), so each HB patient received an average of *one hour extra therapeutic contact*.

There was a marked shift to *more multi-disciplinary working* in HB. Non-medical staff accounted for 50 per cent of all patient contacts in HB, compared with only 25 per cent in SC. The role of the CPNs, in particular, was enhanced, and there was clear evidence that they began to adopt a key-worker role. An analysis of the content of these contacts demonstrated an increase in psychotherapeutic work – behavioural work and counselling. The proportion of patients treated *totally drug free* was 41 per cent in HB and 20 per cent in SC.

The proportion of *patients admitted* was substantially reduced from 33 per cent to 19 per cent in HB. These HB admissions were on average shorter (35 days compared with 41 days) and there were fewer patients readmitted (4 per cent compared to 13 per cent). The overall bed usage was significantly lower in HB when averaged out across the whole patient population.

Day hospital care was surprisingly under-used in this study in both groups. *GP and local authority social service usage* was essentially similar in both groups.

Detailed costing was undertaken which shows significant *cost advantage to HB* – on average, SC costs 40 per cent more. The addition of capital charging will widen this difference, since the cost differences derived almost entirely from differences in in-patient care.

Schizophrenic patients were not the most expensive over the course of the one-year follow-up. Brain-damaged patients and those with severe affective disorders accounted for the highest costs.

Specialist care accounted for a large increase in treatment costs in non-psychotic patients. This may be due to the special nature of the treatment setting. But, even including these costs, the advantage to HB is maintained.

CONCLUSIONS

The kind of multi-disciplinary assessment of all psychiatric referrals which was used in this study encourages effective key-worker management and substantially reduces hospital admissions.

It appears to achieve this by promoting multi-disciplinary working and an increase in 'psychosocial' rather than medical interventions – twice as many patients in HB were treated wholly without prescription. The failure to improve consumer satisfaction may reflect the fact that there was no change in practice, within an individual patient's treatment in the research design. The study raises some doubts about the improved consumer satisfaction reported in previous studies.

There was no evidence that improved access attracted the referral of less ill patients; nor was there any evidence of burden-shifting. The modest alterations to the teams' approach required by the study involved no new skills or resources and yet achieved the same clinical results for less cost, with a corresponding increase in cost-effectiveness.

Researcher

Dr Tom Burns

West Wimbledon Community Mental Health Team, Nelson Hospital, Kingston Road, Merton, London SW20 8DB. (081 544 1499)

Publications

Burns, T. (1990) 'The Evaluation of a Home Based Treatment Approach in Acute Psychiatry', in D. Goldberg, and D. Tantam (eds), *Public Health and Social Psychiatry*, Hogrefe and Huber.

Burns, T., and Raftery, J. (1991) 'Cost of Schizophrenia in a Randomised Trial of Home Based Treatment'. *Schizophrenia Bulletin*, **17**, 3: 407–410.

Evaluation of Community Mental Health Centres

THE PURPOSE OF THIS STUDY

CPNs

Social support

Key workers

Community Mental Health Centres (CMHCs) multiplied dramatically in Britain during the 1980s. They were doubling every two years up to 1988, the last year for which figures are available, according to surveys by Research and Development in Psychiatry. By 1990 there were probably 160 CMHCs nationally.

'Comprehensive' CMHCs were intended as a major vehicle for community services for sufferers from serious mental illness. At the same time, they often clearly embraced the long-standing CMHC commitment to making psycho-therapies accessible to people with relatively minor mental health problems. Can CMHCs serve both the 'traditional' psychiatric clientele and the new clientele of unserved mental health needs among a much broader public? This is a crucial question if CMHCs are to become a key component of the new localized psychi-atric services. In 1986, the Department of Health gave start-up funding to some new mental health projects. These included ten CMHCs, of which six aimed to provide a comprehensive catchment service. When Good Practices in Mental Health (GPMH) was commissioned to research these projects, we focused on the viability of these six comprehensive CMHCs. In particular, we concentrated on what service to sufferers from serious mental illness could be provided within this model.

There were three main questions which our study set out to answer:

- How far was the traditional psychiatric clientele being served through comprehensive CMHCs – and how far were their resources going to a different group of people instead?
- Do CMHCs provide a genuinely comprehensive service to people with a psychotic diagnosis?
- What are the advantages and disadvantages of serving a widely-varied clientele from a single, comprehensive CMHC?

KEY FINDINGS

Large variations emerged in the extent to which comprehensive-catchment CMHCs served sufferers from serious mental illness. Whatever measures were used for the presence of people with more serious problems, the same large differences between CMHCs were evident. These six Centres then do demonstrate how this type of service can sometimes concentrate on people other than the traditional priority clientele of psychiatric services. Some simple factors influenced this process.

A key factor is whether a CMHC incorporates the existing long-term service for its catchment very early on. Early incorporation of existing long-term Community Psychiatric Nurse (CPN) and day-unit caseloads characterized the Centres which reached most sufferers from serious mental illness. Without wholesale caseload transfer, known long-term clients were unlikely to benefit from the CMHC, owing to tensions concerning their respective roles between the new CMHC and the established services outside it. The presence of an established long-term service parallel to a new CMHC could likewise divert new referrals of people with more serious problems away from the CMHC.

At all comprehensive Centres where planners had not initially incorporated existing CPN caseloads, eventually such posts were either incorporated or withdrawn by their managers – sometimes shortly after our research. The CMHC was then told to take over their work. But by then, many CMHC staff had acquired sizeable personal caseloads of previously unserved people with minor mental health problems. They had little space to work with transferred CPN caseloads, which could be very large. Sometimes, even, late-transferred CPN clients were discharged by the CMHC to receive medication from GPs instead.

Delaying incorporation of these long-term caseloads could mean a one-to-three-year false start for a 'comprehensive' CMHC. During this time it would consolidate its workload, staff skills and referrer expectations around people with minor mental health problems. The timing of the incorporation of existing long-term caseloads is as important as ensuring that it occurs.

Centres which offered services particularly relevant to people with serious mental illness were more successful in reaching them. Some planners equipped their CMHC with resources often used by this group. There were four teams in the whole 12-project series where clearly relevant resources brought ample referrals of long-term clients despite possible barriers – such as no formal links with a Consultant Psychiatrist.

Centres rarely employed any 'gate-keeping' system. Selection of referrals was often devolved to individual team members, with little clear team policy or supervision: they accepted indiscriminately clients without histories of in-patient care or psychotic diagnosis. New clientele were predominantly women, by ratios between 2:1 and 4:1. They often had diagnoses of anxiety or depression. Life events, like bereavement and the breakdown of marital relationships, figured substantially among a small sample studied in detail; but they do include a proportion who are seriously incapacitated by their problems. Clients without histories of in-patient care or psychotic diagnosis came overwhelmingly from GP referrers.

There was often no means of assessing whether a CMHC was adequately reaching people with serious mental illness. There were no target caseload figures nor any opportunity for comparison with other services. Often no one knew either what the caseload should comprise or what it actually comprised. Difficulties of access were the main CMHC shortcoming for sufferers from serious mental illness: once on the caseload, the quality of Centre services could be good.

Attachment of small day-centres to some Centres had a major effect. These enabled substantial regular social support to more disabled clients, which would have been difficult, in terms of staff time, to provide in any other way. Day-centres brought clients into contact with staff other than their key-worker. Such wider relationships enabled continuity of service if key-workers were absent or changed jobs.

Centres often treated clients as the responsibility of individual key-workers rather than of the team. Cover-and-review systems, which depend on team members knowing each other's clients, could suffer accordingly. But a day-centre attached to the CMHC could readily involve other workers and counter this aspect of keyworker-centred models.

A keyworker-centred model often meant key-workers were expected to secure for their clients all necessary therapeutic and practical services without assistance from colleagues. In practice, clients risked missing types of practical help with which their key-worker was unfamiliar. A particular problem occurred if clients with psychotic diagnosis, who are more likely to need practical assistance, were concentrated on one or two over-burdened key-workers.

There was often little managerial knowledge or supervision concerning how key-workers were managing their caseloads. Yet many key-workers were new to community mental health work. Within the same CMHC they often varied widely in their policies – for instance on length of service to clients. They might have benefited from greater induction, supervision and training.

A contrasting model of care was offered by two high-care support teams which were also studied. These served very small caseloads of particularly vulnerable people. They demonstrated procedures for systematic teamworking around each client. They illustrated conditions and resources necessary for such teamworking.

Researchers

Charles Patmore and Tim Weaver

Good Practices in Mental Health, 380–384 Harrow Road, London W9 2HU. (071 289 2034)

Now at:

Charles Patmore

20 Talbot Road, Wembley, Middlesex HA0 4UE.

Tim Weaver

Health Care Development Unit, (St Mary's Hospital Medical School), c/o The Bungalow, Central Middlesex NHS Hospital Trust, Acton Lane, London NW10.

Publications

From 1987 to 1990 the Department of Health funded a research project on 12 new Community Mental Health Teams. This was written up in detail in:

Patmore, C., and Weaver, T. (1991) 'Community Mental Health Teams: Lessons for Planners and Managers', GPMH Publications. (This can be obtained from GPMH at the above address. Price £15 plus £1.35 postage.)

The following articles also feature aspects of this research:

Patmore, C. (1990) 'How Can Community Mental Health Centres Give Good Service to Sufferers from Serious Mental Illness?', 2,700-word paper at RDP seminar on CMHCs, April 30, 1990.

Patmore, C. (1991) 'New research on community care', *NSF News*, November 1991.

Patmore, C., and Weaver, T. (1991) 'Care liaison vital', *Hospital Doctor*, September 19.

Patmore, C., and Weaver, T. (1991) 'Falling Through Holes in Community Care Net', *Guardian*, Summer 1991.

Patmore, C., and Weaver, T. (1992) 'Improving community services for serious mental disorders', *Journal of Mental Health*, June.

Patmore, C., and Weaver, T. (1989) 'Measures of Care', *Health Service Journal*, March 16, **99**, 5142: 330–331.

Patmore, C., and Weaver, T. (1991) 'Missing the CMHC Bus', *Nursing Times*, April 24.

Patmore, C., and Weaver, T. (1990) 'Mixed blessings in mental health care units', *Doctor*, April 18.

Patmore, C., and Weaver, T. (1991) 'Unnatural Selection', *Health Service Journal*, October 10.

Patmore, C., and Weaver, T. (1990) 'Rafts on an Open Sea', *Health Service Journal*, October 11, **100**, 5222: 1510–1512.

Patmore, C., and Weaver, T. (1991) 'Strength in Numbers', *Health Service Journal*, October 17.

Patmore, C., and Weaver, T. (1990) 'Working with a New Clientele', *Nursing Times*, December 19, **86**, 51: 67–68.

Weaver, T., and Patmore, C. (1990) 'United Fronts', *Health Service Journal*, October 18, **100**, 5223: 1554–1555.

Community Mental Health Centres – Literature Review

INTRODUCTION

Access
Account-
ability
Evaluation

This review of American and British literature relating to the Community Mental Health Centres (CMHCs) involved the creation of a framework for the analysis of existing services, and their aims and outcomes.

The framework we have developed describes the fundamental goals of Community Mental Health Centres and community mental health services. It describes underlying principles of service delivery, in terms of ultimate aims. At the same time, the elements of the model can produce operational standards of service delivery against which performance can be judged.

Service planners and providers are striving to offer mental health services which achieve certain fundamental goals. These goals, (and the elements of our framework) are that services should be: comprehensive; coordinated; accessible; acceptable; efficient; effective; and accountable.

The main findings of our study are organized in relation to these goals.

An important lesson from the literature is that it is dangerous to think of CMHCs as providing only one model of care. It is clear that no single physical location can hope to provide all the care which is required. The 'mental health centre' describes a network of resources, based on common principles, but expressed in a variety of forms. United Kingdom services should strive to emulate the goals of community mental health services, but should not become tied to one service-delivery strategy. The greatest danger is that the community or social-service model comes to be seen as separate from the health service, or institutional model. A genuine multi-site 'Centre' should include all relevant forms of service which the client and his/her family need.

FINDINGS

Comprehensiveness and Coordination

Comprehensiveness and coordination are very widely accepted service objectives: they are regarded as essential to the efficiency and effectiveness of services.

The term comprehensive, when used in relation to CMHCs, usually means the provision of the five essential services. These are in-patient care, out-patient services, emergency services, partial hospitalization, and consultation and education.

Coordination usually refers to continuity of individual care. The most common problem in the achievement of coordinated services is client 'drop-out'. The reasons for client drop-out could include successful treatment, inappropriate services or their own dissatisfaction.

Among the CMHC services features which have been introduced deliberately to improve coordination and/or extend service coverage are: multi-disciplinary teams; key-workers; joint planning; consultation and education; targeting; catchments and sectorization; needs assessment; the use of volunteers; self-help groups; service guides; community involvement in planning; and private care. There is little evidence that any of these have actually resulted in more comprehensive or better-coordinated care, nor that they have improved outcome for clients; but clear definitions of sectors or specific catchment areas *do* seem to improve the coordination of care.

Accessibility and Acceptability

We located the following meanings of accessibility and acceptability in the literature: geographic accessibility, or proximity; cognitive (do people know where the service is, what it is for, who is eligible, and how to access it?); bureaucratic (is there a referral system, is there a waiting-list, etc.?) and psychological. The last of these is synonymous with acceptability (is it the sort of service which the person wants, likes and is satisfied with?).

There are several reasons why a simple judgement about the accessibility of CMHC services cannot be made. The main one is the great variability between centres. The proportion of the service used by known priority groups varies from *none*, in some cases, to *all* in others.

The CMHC movement hoped to overcome unnecessary barriers to care by removing the bureaucratic and cumbersome procedures often encountered by those in need of mental health care. CMHCs appear to have made self-referral easier to some extent, in comparison with other sources of care such as public mental hospital, private mental hospital, and general hospital.

Ethnic minorities failed to make use of services once referred to them. The failure to show up for the first appointment, the reluctance to attend for more than one appointment, and the early drop-out from treatment could all be indicators of an unacceptable service.

Efficiency

Cost-benefit studies have been conducted in CMHCs, but these display several methodological problems, such as the use of dubious methods in assigning monetary values to patient improvement, the use of a narrow definition of costs, the failure to specify whether average or marginal costs are being reported. Cost-effectiveness studies suffer from similar methodological shortcomings.

Some tentative conclusions can be drawn. These are that the costs of maintaining more-severely-disabled patients tend to be higher; a substantial proportion of the cost savings in community services is due to savings on hospitalization, and a large proportion of the costs incurred in community services is due to patient hospitalization. Day services appear to be as effective as district general hospital services, without being more costly, for certain categories of patient.

Effectiveness

The use of readmission rates as outcome measures is highly dubious. In many studies, hospitalization is treated as a homogenous entity: periods of 'wellness' in hospital are not reported, nor are renewed episodes of ill-health.

Successful services work out the proper place for hospital treatment in the spectrum of services. Adequate after-care is essential to a successful service, but most standard after-care provides very little contact. Almost half of discharged patients receive no after-care at all, and those who do receive it infrequently.

There are hardly any well-designed and controlled studies of the effectiveness of residential services. There have been no serious attempts to demonstrate the effectiveness of preventive effort, even with high-risk groups.

Accountability

The main stakeholders involved in the delivery of mental health services appear to be: the employees' managing agency; the professional body (or bodies) of which the employee is a member; the workers who share responsibility with an individual employee for the delivery of services; the people using services and their carers (usually families); the communities (or their representative) within which services are delivered.

The growth of the 'consumer movement' in mental health mirrored the general impact of consumerism in the United States during the 1960s and 1970s. Health care consumption is a very different form of consumerism from that of cash exchange for an industrially-manufactured product. Client satisfaction scales were developed during the late 1970s and early 1980s, but these have some serious drawbacks.

Other research argues that client representation can be obtained, but requires the active recruitment, orientation and training of clients with regard to the mental health and social-service delivery systems to ensure informed participation as well as the training of clients to serve as advocates, self-advocates and members of boards.

Evaluation

An entrepreneurial evaluation 'industry' grew up in the US and a great deal of service development takes place without regard to the existing evidence about effectiveness and efficiency. 'Advocacy research' tends to exaggerate and overstate its case: 'management review'-type research tends to avoid controversial findings. Needs assessment approaches seem to be of potential value but none of the US Department of Health and Welfare publications which used the term ever defined it.

It is important to establish the purpose of evaluation and its likely use, before the evaluation begins. Use of information in policy-making is more likely to occur where the service provider funds the evaluation.

Many of the problems of the CMHC programme in the US were due to the wrong evaluation mandate. A major mistake was to require self-evaluation: routine monitoring by the service is essential, but formal evaluation should be conducted by an outside evaluator.

Client outcome (from the client's and an independent perspective) is the most important target for evaluation effort.

Researcher

Professor Peter Huxley

Mental Health Social Work Unit, University of Manchester, Department of Psychiatry, Mathematics Tower, Oxford Road, Manchester M13 9PL. (061 275 2000; FAX 061 275 3924)

Publications

Huxley, P. (1990) *Effective Community Mental Health Services*, Gower.

A Comparison of Day- and In-Patient Treatment for Psychiatric Illness

1. Completed Studies

Costs
Benefits
Staffing

The treatment of patients in a day hospital rather than an in-patient unit means firstly, that patients are not removed from their homes and secondly, that it is cheaper for the hospital service, since patients do not stay overnight. Day-hospital treatment may also carry less stigma than in-patient treatment, but may, on the other hand, cause additional burden on relatives. The aim of this study was to discover what proportion of all patients admitted to a psychiatric unit could be treated in a well-staffed day hospital and to discover if the effects of treatment are different in the two settings.

Our psychiatric service serves an inner-city population with high psychiatric morbidity. In 1983, a new 50-place psychiatric day hospital on a main hospital site was opened. The district had a relatively small number of in-patient beds seven miles away. This meant that acutely ill patients were admitted directly from the community to the day hospital. Our preliminary study demonsrated that we were able to treat acutely ill patients (including those with suicidal ideas or psychotic illness) in the day hospital.

In order to compare the effects of day hospital and in-patient treatment, we used a random allocation procedure. The patients admitted under the Mental Health Act, and others who were seriously disturbed, had to be excluded. We found that approximately 40 per cent of all patients presenting to our service could be treated in the day hospital.

Reduction of psychiatric symptoms was similar in the two groups, (see figure 4.1): Improvement in social role performance was also similar, (see figure 4.2).

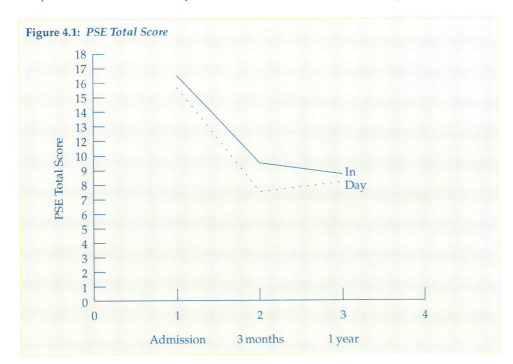

Figure 4.1: *PSE Total Score*

Figure 4.2: *Social Role Performance*

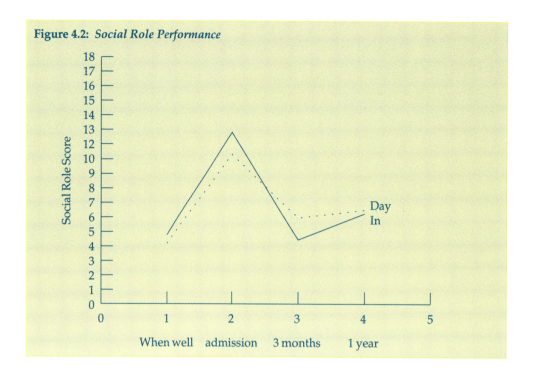

In the short term, it appeared that in-patient treatment had two advantages. Two-thirds of the in-patients had been discharged from hospital by three months, whereas 56 per cent of the day-hospital patients were still attending the day hospital. In-patients also appeared to improve in social functioning more rapidly than day-patients.

On the other hand, at the end of one year, ten of the 48 in-patients (21 per cent) had been readmitted to hospital compared to only two (5 per cent) of the day-patients – the remaining day-patients were living in the community. This raises the possibility that day hospital treatment helps the person to stay out of hospital in the months or years following treatment.

We performed an identical study in a neighbouring district, which had a less well-staffed day hospital. They were unable to treat acutely ill patients to the same extent: only 16 per cent of the admissions in that district could successfully be treated in the day hospital. The results showed that any patients with disturbed behaviour could not be tolerated in the day hospital and had to be transferred to the in-patient unit.

CONCLUSION

These studies have shown that it is possible to treat nearly half of all new admissions in a psychiatric day hospital, but only if there are adequate staff. The outcome is similar to in-patient treatment, although the return to normal social functioning may be slower. The additional staff, coupled with this longer initial period of treatment, make day treatment more expensive than in-patient treatment in the short term. However, if day hospital treatment really does reduce the chance of further rehospitalization, it might prove to be both preferable and cheaper in the long term. We are now engaged in a longer follow-up study and a cost-benefit study to examine these possibilities.

2. Modified cost-benefit analysis comparing day- and in-patient treatment for acute psychiatric illness

This study is still under way. We are using the same method of randomly allocating patients to day- and in-patient treatment as described in the previous project. Since we have demonstrated that the outcome of treatment is similar, this study is measuring the costs involved in treatment, and the burden on relatives.

The costs of treatment include the direct costs to the hospital. These are inevitably cheaper for day-patients, who do not require 24-hour nursing care. However, patients appear to improve more slowly in the day hospital, which means that the period of admission is longer. This increases the cost of day hospital treatment, even though it is cheaper per day.

There are numerous indirect costs to be considered. Day hospital treatment may be accompanied by excessive demands on GPs, community psychiatric nurses and social workers. These contacts are being measured in the present study. Acutely ill patients in the day hospital might be more of a burden to relatives when they are at home at night and at the weekends. However, the relatives of our in-patients report that visiting their relatives in hospital is worrying and time-consuming.

Psychiatric illness may impair the performance of tasks around the home, interfere with close relationships and lead to disturbed behaviours. Although in-patient treatment leads to rapid suppression of psychiatric symptoms, the disruptive effect of removal from the community and equally abrupt return after treatment may impair family relationships, and confidence with tasks at home. For this reason, we are measuring the degree of stress associated with each form of treatment, as one of the hidden 'costs'.

If these two treatments are demonstrated to have similar outcomes, our analysis of costs will be crucial to determining which pattern of treatment should be recommended in the future.

Researcher

Professor Francis Creed

Department of Psychiatry, University of Manchester, Rawnsley Building, Manchester Royal Infirmary, Oxford Road, Manchester M13 9WL. (061 276 5331/5397)

Publications

Anthony, P., Black, D., and Creed, F. (submitted) 'Barriers to the successful utilisation of day hospital treatment'.

Anthony, P., Creed, F. H., and Lancashire, S. (1991) 'Side effects of psychiatric treatment. A qualitative study of issues associated with a random allocation research study', *Sociology of Health and Illness*, **13**: 131–137.

Creed, F. H. (1989) 'Comparison of Day and in-patient treatment for acute psychiatric illness'. *DH Yearbook of Research and Development*, London, HMSO, 17–26.

Creed, F. H., Anthony, P., and Black, D. (1989) 'Day hospital and community treatment for acute psychiatric illness: A critical appraisal', *British Journal of Psychiatry*, **154**: 300–310.

Creed, F. H., Anthony, P., Godbert, K., and Huxley, P. (1989) 'Treatment of severe psychiatric illness in a day hospital', *British Journal of Psychiatry*, **154**: 341–347.

Creed, F. H., Anthony, P., and Tomenson, B. (submitted) 'Predicting length of stay in psychiatry'.

Creed, F. H., Black, D., Anthony, P., Osborn, M., Thomas, P., Franks, D., Polley, R., Lancashire, S., Saleem, P., and Tomenson, B. (1991) 'Randomised controlled trial of day and in-patient psychiatric treatment: II Comparison of two day hospitals', *British Journal of Psychiatry*, **158**: 183–189.

Creed, F. H., Black, D., Anthony, P., Osborn, M., Thomas, P., and Tomenson, B. (1990) 'Randomised controlled trial of day patient versus psychiatric treatment', *British Medical Journal*, **300**: 1033–1037.

Compulsory Treatment of Psychiatric Patients in the Community: Who is likely to be Recommended, and with what Effects?

In the past, some patients – admitted for in-patient psychiatric treatment under Section 3 of the Mental Health Act (1983) – have remained on Section after discharge. This practice of treating patients on 'extended leave' from hospital was judged illegal by the High Court in 1985. Patients treated in this way would probably have been placed on a community treatment order, if such a thing existed. This project, therefore, was designed to investigate the feasibility and utility of compulsory community treatment, by a study of the characteristics of extended-leave patients.

A representative sample was identified of patients treated with extended leave (comprising 35 patients, and a total of 42 episodes of extended leave). This 'Extended Leave' group was compared with two other patient samples, matched for age, sex and psychiatric diagnosis. The 'Nominated' group comprised 29 patients whom consultant psychiatrists would recommend for a community treatment order, if it were available. The 'Control' group, selected by the same consultant psychiatrists, included 49 patients considered by the consultants as not requiring compulsory community treatment. The three groups were compared using data from medical records and other available sources.

'Extended leave' Medication Follow-up

FINDINGS

Overall, the use of extended leave was found to be uncommon. Of 26 psychiatric units contacted directly, 19 had not used extended leave.

All those patients treated with extended leave had a diagnosis of functional psychosis, predominantly schizophrenia or schizo-affective disorder. The mean duration of extended leave in the sample was 113 weeks, with 40 per cent of the episodes lasting one year or less, and 69 per cent less than two years. Use of extended leave in most instances followed a long history of psychiatric disorder, with multiple previous admissions. Sixty-seven per cent of episodes of extended leave followed four or more psychiatric in-patient admissions, including one or more Mental Health Act admissions in most cases.

Contrary to expectations, the Extended Leave group was not conspicuously socially deprived. Forty per cent had attained an educational level beyond O-Level or its equivalent. Half were living with partners or families, and 62 per cent had lived at their current address for at least one year. The majority were registered with a GP. However, most of this group were unemployed: 48 per cent had been unemployed for at least three years. In all these characteristics, the Extended Leave group closely resembled the Control group. The Nominated patients differed from the Extended Leave group in that they were more likely to be single, living alone, and to have changed their address at least once in the preceding three years.

A lifetime's history of being seriously dangerous was common in all groups, including the Controls. The three groups differed very little in their histories of in-patient admissions, except that patients in both the Extended Leave and Nominated groups were significantly more likely than the Control patients to have been admitted under the Mental Health Act in the 12 months before being recommended for compulsory community treatment. Over the same time-period, the Nominated and Extended Leave groups were significantly more likely than the Control patients to have shown at least one episode of serious dangerousness. Compared with the Control patients, those in the Nominated and Extended Leave groups showed significantly poorer compliance with their out-patient appointments and medications, and were much more likely to be lost to follow-up. Only one patient (2 per cent) in the Control group was lost to follow-up for three months or more, compared with 40 per cent of the Extended Leave group and 31 per cent of the Nominated group.

The clinical course of patients in the Extended Leave group was compared for equal time-periods before, during and after their episodes of extended leave. Use of extended leave led to a significant reduction in the frequency of in-patient admissions and in the total time spent in hospital. Recorded episodes of serious dangerousness towards self or others were significantly reduced while patients were on extended leave. Full attendance at out-patient appointments rose for 17 per cent to 55 per cent while on extended leave, and compliance with medication improved in 43 per cent of instances. A small sub-sample of 13 patients was identified, whose extended leave had been discontinued not on clinical grounds, but as a result of the 1985 judgements which determined the practice of extended leave to be illegal. Overall, this sub-group fared poorly. Two committed suicide, and six had subsequent Mental Health Act admissions – in one case, within weeks of extended leave being ended. A further three were lost to psychiatric follow-up. Compared with the remainder of the Extended Leave group, those whose extended leave had been discontinued on legal grounds were significantly less likely to attend out-patient follow-up, and showed a tendency towards poorer compliance with their medications.

CONCLUSIONS

These results indicate that if a community treatment order were available, consultant psychiatrists would be capable of recommending its use consistently for a selected group of patients. These patients are likely to have a history of previous in-patient admissions for functional psychosis, but are particularly characterized by a recent history combining episodes of serious dangerousness and poor compliance with medications and/or out-patient follow-up. There is a fear among some professionals and others that a community treatment order would be used primarily to coerce patients to accept treatment in their own homes; but no recorded instances of such practice were found in the Extended Leave group. Use of extended leave significantly improved patients' compliance with their out-patient psychiatric follow-up, and more regular contact with patients offers greater opportunities to work towards better compliance with medications. The psychiatrists who participated in this study generally viewed the community treatment order as offering the power to recall patients into hospital when necessary, rather than as a means of *imposing* treatment in the community.

Judging by the impact of extended leave when this was still in use, compulsory community treatment can lead to significant reductions in in-patient admission and in serious dangerousness. It is likely to benefit a small percentage of patients suffering from serious mental disorders, mainly schizophrenia. Without the possibility of compulsory community treatment, this small group of patients is particularly likely to fare poorly, especially in terms of remaining in the community.

Researchers

Tom Sensky, Timothy Hughes, Steven Hirsch

Department of Psychiatry, Charing Cross and Westminster Medical School, West Middlesex University Hospital, Isleworth, Middlesex TW7 6AF. (081 565 5179; FAX 081 565 5315)

Publications

Sensky, T., Hughes, T., and Hirsch, S. (1991) 'Compulsory psychiatric treatment in the community: I. A controlled study of treatment with 'extended leave' under the Mental Health Act: special characteristics of patients and impact of treatment', *British Journal of Psychiatry*, **158**: 792–799.

Sensky, T., Hughes, T., and Hirsch, S. (1991) 'Compulsory psychiatric treatment in the community: II. A controlled study of patients whom psychiatrists would recommend for compulsory treatment in the community', *British Journal of Psychiatry*, **158**: 799–804.

This study was concerned with the problems of elderly mentally ill people, over 75 years of age, registered with the Worcester Development Project. Our objectives were to diagnose mental illness, both organic and functional, to identify the needs imposed by it, to determine on whom the burden fell, and to find out to what extent the needs were being met. From the original sample of 759 subjects, we excluded 38 who had died before it was drawn and one who was under the age of 75, leaving 720 for interview. Sixteen were lost altogether, 69 died between sampling and approach, and 210 refused the interview; every attempt was made to obtain information on those who had died or refused interview. In the end, we interviewed 413 and had some information on 642.

Elderly people
Services
Private sector

We used a screening interview which was designed to cover mental and physical health, social support, and the circumstances of daily living. Our definition of functional mental illness required subjective or objective evidence of anxiety or depression lasting at least a month; and that the subject had sought treatment, wished to die, or had a functional deficit resulting from those symptoms.

RESULTS

- *Severe forgetfulness.* This was defined by evidence of a failure to learn on memory testing and a small number of errors on the cognitive testing, without any functional deficit due to brain failure. This was very common: 10 per cent of the sample interviewed suffered from it; and we could detect minor but definite degrees of memory failure in a considerably larger number – perhaps 25–30 per cent of those aged over 75. It was more common in women: 33 per cent of women of extreme age (90 or above) had severe forgetfulness.
- *Dementia.* We found 67 subjects with dementia. Many had died between sampling and approach, and it seems important in this kind of research to conduct a 'rolling survey', because of the high death-rate among demented people. It is essentially a problem of the over-85s, especially in women. If dementia and severe forgetfulness are combined, then 80 per cent of women in extreme old age had mental impairment.

How Are These People Supported and Cared For?

There were 78 subjects in the whole sample in residential care: 41 in private residential care, 10 in voluntary-aided care, 21 in Part-III accommodation, 2 in a geriatric ward, and only 4 in a psychiatric ward. Of the subjects with dementia, 40 out of 67 were in residential care: 17 of those were in private nursing homes, 7 in private rest-homes, only one in voluntary-aided home, 10 in Part-III accommodation, 2 in a geriatric ward, and 3 in a psychiatric ward.

We found no evidence that the more severe cases were in hospital, rather than in social-services homes or private homes; in fact, the opposite was true. It was possible to determine which patients had severe physical disorder as well as dementia, and we found that 17 of 32 people in private homes and only 7 of 23 in the social-services homes or the hospitals had this combination. In other words, it appeared that the *more severely ill people were in private homes*. We also noted that there were five people with extreme incapacity – three of whom were in private homes, one in a social-services home, and one in a hospital.

The costs of the private nursing homes were between £125 and £250 per week. Part-III accommodation cost £161 per week, which is quite moderate in comparison, but it was difficult to obtain comparable data for hospitals. The estimated cost of private residential care in Worcester and Kidderminster health districts is £10 million a year, whilst the total budgets of the National Health Service mental health units are somewhat higher than that. Families provided some of the 'residential care'.

It seemed clear that the majority of people who were taken into residential care had never had any assessment by psychiatrists or by social workers.

Of the demented subjects who were not in residential care, six were living alone, some of them having physical illness as well; one was in day-care for two days a week. Two were largely supported by wardens, and another two had much support from home-helps. Fifteen other subjects were living out of residential care, with family members or with their spouses; some of them had a major physical illness as well as dementia. Of these 15 living with families or their spouses, two were in day-hospital care for 5 days a week and one was in day-hospital care for 2 days a week, so that there was an underprovision of day-care. Two of them had daily visits from a nurse, one had twice-weekly visits and one had once-weekly visits. There appeared to be unmet need in eight subjects.

It was surprising how little functional mental illness was found: there were only 5 definite 'cases'. It was also remarkable what a good state of morale most elderly people had, and how happy they were, how well adjusted, and what a very small number were severely depressed. Even so, it was disturbing that well over half of those who *were* depressed were not in treatment, perhaps because elderly depressed people do not refer themselves for treatment.

Who is Supporting the Elderly?

We counted the number of visits (made at least once a week) by different people – 1,194 visits to 366 subjects not in residential care. On average, two visits per week were made by family members and two-thirds of all visits were made by them. The average number of visits was low if a person had already been taken into the home of a relative, and it was relatively low for fit subjects. The highest number of visits (over three a week) was made to those who were housebound by physical illness.

Another important source of support is neighbours and friends: we found that the amount of support offered by them was about the same as the statutory support – a total of about 150 visits per week in all. On the other hand, the private sector, which is making a major contribution to residential care, makes only a very small contribution to domiciliary care. As for statutory care, wardens are an important source of support for the elderly: they are financed partly by social services and partly by housing organizations. We found that just over one-fifth of all subjects were in warden-assisted accommodation, and to some extent this was given preferentially to the mentally ill (54 per cent); however, there was only one demented person on our list who was in warden-assisted accommodation. Apart from wardens, the main source of statutory help was the home-helps, provided by social services.

CONCLUSION

There was evidence from this study that a great deal is being done to help the aged in the Worcester Development Project area and that it is being done by a wide variety of people. Worcester and Kidderminster are well supplied with psycho-geriatric services – more so than most districts. Even so, these services are seriously overstretched: they have too many people to see, and yet the psychogeriatric services are making a very small contribution to the total picture of care. There is clearly a major problem in setting up services to deal with the challenge of mental illness in the elderly.

Researchers

Ian Brockington, Wendy Morris and Eric Jones

Department of Psychiatry, University of Birmingham, Queen Elizabeth Psychiatric Hospital, Mindelsohn Way, Birmingham B15 2QZ. (021 627 2835; FAX 021 627 2832)

Publications

Brockington, I., *et al.* (1987) *A Survey of the Mentally Ill in Kidderminster*.

Brockington, I., *et al.* 'Senile Dementia: Prevalence and Support'.

Brockington, I., Morris, W., and Jones, E. (1991) 'The needs and burdens of the elderly mentally ill', in *The Closure of Mental Hospitals*, Royal College of Psychiatrists, **13**: 86–91.

Hassall, C. (1988) *The Elderly in the Psychiatric Services Worcester Development Project*.

Jones, E., Morris, W., Cooper, P., and Brockington, I. (1988) *Needs and Burdens of the Elderly Mentally Ill*.

Cost of Care for the Elderly Mentally Ill in Worcester and Wyre Forest

THE STUDY

This study investigated the productivity of six institutions offering residential care to the elderly mentally ill, by means of an activity analysis and a study of engagement patterns among residents. The study was complementary with elements of the project *Three experimental homes for the Elderly Mentally Ill*, directed by Professor J. R. M. Copeland[15], Department of Psychiatry, University of Liverpool. The report which follows is based upon observations in three homes from the Copeland study, the control being provided by the Worcester study. The conclusions of this report are reinforced by analysis of the other homes in Worcester.

Data were collected for a complete week in each home and a comparison unit, in order to find out what tasks were performed, by whom, and with which clients. This information could then be interpreted in the light of each home's objectives, and be used to see how evenly, or unevenly, the care was distributed between staff and among all the clients, and whether any particular type of client laid an especially heavy burden upon staff. It could also be combined with information from observational studies, and some ethnographic work, in order to throw light on areas of importance to health facility planners.

Productivity
'Positive care'
Staffing

RESULTS

Table 4.3 shows the total number of observations for the three units, and the percentage split between time spent 'with' or 'not with' clients.

Table 4.4 shows the percentage of time each staff-group spent 'with clients', indicating that home A's trained staff spend the lowest proportion of time with

Table 4.3: *Summary of Observations*

Home	No. of observations	Observations	
		With clients (%)	Not with clients (%)
A	3795	2010 (53)	1785 (47)
B	3337	2123 (64)	1214 (36)
C			
Day	941	533 (57)	408 (43)
Residential	3009	1687 (56)	1322 (44)
Control	2288	1399 (61)	889 (39)

---

[15] See p 198.

Table 4.4: Percentage of Time Spent with Clients, by Staff Group

Home	Trained	Untrained	Night	Other
A	38	71	—	40
B	62	71	55	85
C	49	59	56	—
Control	59	63	61	—

residents. B has the highest proportions of staff with clients for all except night staff. Table 4.4 also reveals a very large difference between the ratios for Other staff at A and B.

We divided not-with-clients records into four categories: administration, task, break and observation at night. The main category of staff activity not undertaken with clients is the classification 'task'. Tasks can be subdivided into housekeeping and professional/clerical, such as report writing.

It is immediately clear that A stands on its own, with a heavy professional/clerical load, equivalent to about eight full person-days. C has far more housekeeping than the others. This is because the staff at C also perform the jobs done in the other homes by domestic staff. There are low domestic loads at B and the Control, and a low overall figure at the Control.

Table 4.5: Breakdown of Time Spent not with Clients

	A	B	C	Control
Total not-with-clients	1785	1214	1730	889
Administration	195	128	208	112
Tasks				
(a) Professional/clerical				
Supervision	67	14	0	3
Handover	252	140	130	224
Report writing	214	188	25	3
Other writing	56	19	33	3
Discussion	192	36	7	66
Meeting	105	19	70	17
Sub-total	1081 (61)	544 (45)	473 (27)	428 (48)
(b) Housekeeping				
Tidying	53	9	11	23
Washing/laundry	74	14	237	28
Cleaning	17	8	90	12
Ironing	0	0	26	0
General domestic	2	0	68	0
Sub-total	146 (8)	31 (3)	432 (25)	63 (7)
(c) Residual	320 (18)	220 (18)	404 (23)	269 (30)
Break	238 (13)	274 (23)	363 (21)	109 (12)
Observation	0 (0)	145 (12)	58 (3)	20 (2)

As regards time spent with clients, we wanted to investigate two questions: firstly, did *positive* (as opposed to what we defined as 'routine' or 'demanding') care increase with staff numbers; and secondly, as total staff increased, did positive care increase at an increasing rate. We considered both comparisons between units and within each unit, since there were different staffing levels at different times.

CONCLUSIONS

The basic question which the study aimed to answer focused on the productivity of the extra labour at the three experimental homes.

There were an average of nine staff on daytime duty at A, compared with 4.8 at the Control. But of these additional 4.2 staff at A, 3.2 were engaged in extra routine care and only 1 in extra positive care. Yet we have no reason to believe that the standard of routine care at the Control was in any way unsatisfactory. No short cuts to hygiene care were adopted; all residents received appropriate nutritional care; there was a constant supply of tea, coffee and biscuits. Physical needs were monitored and attended to. So even if we assume a very considerable sampling error, we are still left with the conclusion that we could have expected far more extra, specialist, positive care than was actually delivered. Daytime resources were almost doubled, but this resulted in only a 25 per cent increase in positive care.

Is the failure of an increase in staffing levels to deliver relatively more positive care due to the lack of training of the staff, or the way in which care was organized, or the very nature of the job?

Primary nursing, which is part of the professional model, was in place at all units; the qualified staff were perfectly aware of up-to-date thinking in their professions. Yet the qualified staff, apart from the nurses or officers in charge, were just as likely to take part in manual, not-with-clients activities as the unqualified staff. **There was no obvious evidence that a professional training would make a member of staff more likely to deliver additional 'positive' care.**

Moreover, although most staff spent less than a quarter of their time on positive care, there were two categories of staff who spent about three-quarters of their time on positive care. These were the staff at B and C who were employed as activity organizers, or Occupational Therapy Aides (OTAs). There was a corresponding member of staff at the Control, who was the OTA in the day hospital which two residents attended occasionally.

These five part-time staff were unqualified but highly motivated and many activities revolved around them, although they accounted for only a small part of the Homes' budget. Their job descriptions concentrated on the specific positive activities of Reality Orientation, Occupational and Diversional Therapy, and excluded help with physical caring activities.

All the homes subscribed to the philosophy that the care of persons with dementia-like illnesses is a skill which can be taught in the manner of an apprenticeship, with emphasis on practical aspects, but without ignoring the necessary intellectual – and the moral – content. Yet this was in conflict with their equal acknowledgement of the professional content of nursing and residential social work. The conclusions to be drawn from our observations are that when individual nurses were wholly responsible for the nursing care of small groups of patients suffering from dementia, a care model that includes a considerable element of task assignment appeared more likely to maximize positive care than a model that relies on personalized care alone.

Researcher

Professor J. A. Stilwell

Health Services Research Unit, University of Warwick, Coventry CV4 7AL. (0203 523523)

The Interface between Primary Care and Specialist Mental Health Services in the Community

Introduction

This was a prospective study comparing a group of patients and doctors with access to a new community team – the Pathways team – with a group who continued to use the established services only. The new team liaised closely with 11 General Practitioners (the 'index GPs') and patients registered with these GPs (the 'index patients') had access to their services. A control group of patients registered with 11 control GPs were defined: these patients and doctors had no access to the team but continued to use the established services as before. There were 19,345 patients in the index group and 20,934 in the control. The two groups were matched for socio-demographic characteristics, and prior use of services.

Summary of findings

The new service succeeded in greatly increasing the availability of specialist mental health care to patients: the rate of introduction to psychiatric care was increased almost three times, leading to a doubling in the treated prevalence of psychiatric disorder. This was achieved by making new resources available, the savings in hospital resources did not offset the cost of the new team. The treatment of patients with neurotic disorder by the team was of higher quality in several important respects and the NHS costs of treatment were less. Patients treated by the new team were more satisfied, waiting-times were shorter and continuity of care improved. The new team also offered a better quality service to patients with chronic schizophrenia: more of the patients' needs were met and patient satifaction was higher. However, this was achieved at the expense of higher NHS costs. The GPs with access to the new team were more satisfied with the psychiatric services available to their patients.

Detailed Findings

(1) Impact of the New Team on Service Use

The new team greatly increased the availability of specialist mental health care. The rate of inception to care from the index population in 1990 was 16.9 per thousand, which was almost three times that in the control. This gave rise to a treated prevalence rate in the index group of 30.2 per thousand, more than twice that in the control.

Anxiety disorders and adjustment disorders showed the greatest rise in treated prevalence, being five times higher in the index group. However, the rate of treated depressive illness was increased three times, and substance abuse 1.5 times.

Index patients were more likely to be women, indicating that the presence of the team had reduced the barrier to care for distressed women normally seen in traditional services. Overall, a lower proportion of the index patients had a past psychiatric history; a higher proportion of index patients were married and fewer unemployed.

Consumer views
Specialist services
Costs

The index group incurred higher NHS costs than the control as the cost of the new team was not offset by savings in hospital resources. The numbers of patients using the hospital-based psychiatric services was reduced but the reductions were in the less costly areas, and were outweighed by the lack of any reduction in the use of in-patient beds.

The average cost to the NHS per control patient in 1990 was £1,039, the average marginal NHS costs per extra patient treated in the index group was £606. The new patients treated by the team cost less per patient than those seen by the traditional service, but many of the additional patients treated were suffering from less severe illnesses.

(2) Care of Patients with New Episodes of Neurotic Illness

Two well-matched samples of 30 patients with new episodes of neurotic illness from each study group were interviewed. Psychiatric and social outcomes at six months were similar in the two groups. Mean waiting-time for non-urgent referrals were 13.5 days for index patients and 47.5 days for controls. Control patients were found to be more likely to have seen excessive numbers of staff and to be dissatisfied with the continuity of care.

The quality of the notes was rated. There was no difference in the amount of missed information in the notes, but the community notes were more likely to have an inadequate assessment of mood and the hospital records an inadequate assessment of the patients' current social situation. The index group were more likely to have been offered a home visit, and their relatives to have received coping advice.

The index patients were more satisfied with the care they had received and the information they had been given. The health service costs of the index group were about half those of the control. The extra cost of the Pathways team was far outweighed by the savings in the other NHS services. The largest saving was in the use of in-patient resources, but other hospital and community costs and primary care costs were also reduced. The costs to the patients were also less in the index group.

(3) Quality of Care for Patients with Chronic Schizophrenia

All patients in the index and control groups with chronic schizophrenia were approached for interview. There were 108 eligible patients and 82 per cent agreed to participate.

The group with access to the new team had more met-needs and fewer unmet needs than the group cared for only by the established services. These differences were all highly significant for clinical problems, but less so in relation to social problems. There were no specific problem areas where the control group's needs were better met.

The main types of care identified as *underprovided* to the control group were psychotherapeutic interventions, and monitoring of symptoms and treatment. In both groups, about 50 per cent of social needs were met by the sheltered residence provided by relatives.

The patients with access to the new team reported overall satisfaction with the service they had received and expressed higher satisfaction on a number of specific issues.

The control relatives had more unmet needs. There was no difference in the numbers of problems reported by relatives in the two groups or in their views of the service.

The index group incurred higher health service costs in that the extra cost of the Pathways team was not offset by savings in hospital resources. They used less local-authority-funded residential care but more day-care. The cost of relatives' time was similar in both groups.

(4) The Satisfaction, Attitudes and Practices of Study GPs

The impact of the Pathways Team on the satisfaction, attitudes and practices of general practitioners was examined by comparing the ten index GPs with the ten control GPs who were practising throughout the study period.

There had been no impact on detection of psychiatric disorder, diagnosis or treatment practices. The index GPs expressed a greater level of satisfaction with the service for all five major diagnostic groups about which we enquired. They rated the service as more helpful in reducing the practice burden generated by acute and chronic neurotic patients and those with family problems.

They were more satisfied than controls with the service received from all five professional groups in the team. They gave higher priority than control GPs to community psychiatric nurses, social workers and occupational therapists, in a theoretical exercise asking them to allocate part of their practice budget to support psychiatric services.

Researchers

Professor Goldberg, Dr Gayle Jackson

Department of Psychiatry, University of Manchester, Withington Hospital, West Didsbury, Manchester M20 8LR. (061 445 8111)

Publications

Jackson, M. G., Gater, R. G., Goldberg, D. P., Tantam, D., Loftus, L., and Taylor, H. (in press) 'A New Community Mental Health Team Based in Primary Care i) A description of the service ii) Impact on service utilisation in the first year', *British Journal of Psychiatry*.

Tantam, D., Gater, R., Jackson, G., Percival, C., Purlackee, R., Stratton, M., and Amaee, S., (submitted) 'Auditing The Community Team', *Health Trends*.

The Prevalence and Outcome of Minor Psychiatric Disorders in Social Workers' Clients

Background

Social services departments in the UK are major providers of services for mentally ill people in the community. Until recently, the extent of psychiatric morbidity in the clients of social services was not acknowledged, and many cases remained undetected and without clinical help. The attachment of social workers to general practices usually involves social workers in considerably more work with clients with mental health problems, and promotes joint medical and social care. But this kind of arrangement is increasingly uncommon and unfashionable in the UK, and its potential benefits are being lost.

This study was designed to investigate the clinical and social outcome in two social services settings – local (area) teams and general practice attachments – and to examine whether the two organizational arrangements lead to differences in type of social work undertaken, in outcome, or in the benefit to clients.

The sample was acquired by taking a consecutive series of cases newly referred to two social services area offices and six general-practice-attached social workers.

FINDINGS

Prevalence

Of 158 clients referred to two area-offices and six general-practice-attached social workers, 141 were interviewed using standardized social and psychiatric research interviews. The General Health Questionnaire (GHQ) was completed by 138 clients. Their social worker completed a Case Review Form. Scores of 5 or more on the Present State Examination (PSE) Index of Definition (for the client) were used to indicate psychiatric 'caseness'. Using scores of 5 or more, 53 per cent of the sample were identified as cases. The GHQ (cut-off 4/5) identified 73 per cent of the clients as cases; and the GHQ (cut-off 10/11) identified 51 per cent as cases.

Morbidity was significantly greater in the general practice setting. Social workers' judgement (about the presence or absence of mental illness/emotional disorder) was not significantly better than chance in the identification of specific disorders, but was significant in relation to the whole sample.

Clinical Outcome

Out of 141 new referrals to a social services department, 101 were assessed at inception and 12-month follow-up using the PSE, the Social Maladjustment Schedule and the Case Review Form. Mental illness, financial and housing problems were the three problems most frequently identified by the social workers. At inception, 72 (51 per cent) of the subjects were PSE cases – 25 per cent at follow-up. The type of social work help offered to cases and non-cases did not differ.

Certain social factors are correlated with disorder at inception (housewife status and poverty) and other social factors are associated with case status at follow-up (housing and poor social functioning). Poor social functioning scores are also associated with limited clinical change. The social worker should be alerted to the possibility of the existence of clinical problems, and in the case of poor social functioning of the likelihood of long-term problems. A better outcome is suggested by acute long-term social crises, such as family break-up. The findings suggest that social workers could get valuable clues about long- and short-term clinical problems from the associated social difficulties.

The idea that people can be neatly divided into those who have clinical problems and present these to health services, and those who have social problems and present them to social services is clearly untenable. There is no way that Approved Social Workers or other specialist mental health social workers can be the only social workers in a social services department to deal with clients with mental health problems. There is every reason to suppose that substantial levels of clinical disturbance are present in the clients of other social workers, for example, probation officers, and in people presenting to other social welfare organizations, such as Citizens' Advice Bureaux, the NSPCC, and so on.

Social Outcome

Being a case at follow-up is clearly associated with poor social functioning or coping abilities identified at inception. This item is also the one which emerges as a predictor of clinical change over the year. At inception, the relationship between poor coping and case status is masked by more important acute disturbances in clinical and social circumstances. At follow-up, however, the cases with chronic management problems are those whose illnesses are long-lasting ones. Family break-up behaves in a different way, and is associated with non-case status and clinical improvement. This suggests that it reflects a social crisis which resolves over time. These two variables consistently identify different groups within the total sample.

CONCLUSION

From a social work point of view, it seems to us that the key to the provision of a successful social services contribution to the community care of people with mental health problems is the ability of all social workers – wherever they happen to be located – to have an understanding of the nature of psychiatric disability and to be able, in broad terms, to recognize it and to take account of it in their work with clients and their families.

A second, and perhaps equally important consideration is the extent to which the clients who present problems to their GPs can be integrated into, rather than separated from social services departments' work. What would have happened to the problems presented to the GP-attached social workers if there had been no attachments in the areas concerned? A complete answer to this question could be obtained by studying the same GP practices and area teams now that the social work attachment scheme is to be ended by the local authority. In the absence of such a study, some light might be thrown on to the question by comparing cases referred in non-inner-city areas where area teams do not have GP-attached social workers.

We have shown that – although there are common problems presented in both settings – the cases seen do differ. The nature of the work undertaken with the cases reflects these differences. The GP-attached workers see more people who have mental health problems and have a greater degree of success in helping to eliminate or ameliorate these over 12 months. The removal of a route to social workers through attachment or liaison schemes is likely to deprive a proportion of the population of the services of a social worker at the place and time they ask for help. In the absence of specific schemes such as attachment or liaison, it seems unlikely that close and profitable working relationships will develop between social workers and GPs. In this study, such contact as there was between area social workers and primary health care was predominantly with nurses, and this was in relation to child care rather than mental health issues.

Researchers

Peter Huxley, Hadi Mohamad, Jacky Korer, Caroline Jacob, Hitesh Raval and Phil Anthony

Mental Health Social Work Research Unit, Department of Psychiatry, University of Manchester, Mathematics Tower, Oxford Road, Manchester M13 9PL. (061 275 2000; FAX 061 275 3924)

Publications

Huxley, P. J., Korer, J., Raval, H., and Jacob, C. (1988) 'Psychiatric Morbidity in the Clients of Social Workers', *Journal of Psychiatric Research*, **22**, 1: 57–67.

Huxley, P. J., Korer, J., and Tolley, S. (1987) 'The Psychiatric 'Caseness' of Clients Referred to an Urban Social Services Department', *British Journal of Social Work*, **17**: 507–520.

Huxley, P. J., Mohamad, H., Korer, J., and Jacob, C. (in press) 'Psychiatric Morbidity in social workers caseloads: A comparison between an Inner City and a Suburban Area' *Social & Epidemiological Psychiatry*.

Huxley, P. J., Raval, H., Korer, J., and Jacob, C. (1989) 'Psychiatric Morbidity in Social Workers' Clients: Clinical Outcome', *Psychological Medicine*, **19**: 189–197.

Early Signs: Predicting Relapse in Schizophrenia

INTERIM REPORT

Assessment
Self-report
Family
observation

This project is concerned with the development and testing of instruments which could be used in a clinical setting to detect early signs of relapse in schizophrenia.

Recognition of the symptoms which precede and predict relapse offer the possibility of averting it, and avoiding the patient's readmission to hospital.

The clinical application of early drug-intervention once early signs are detected is constrained by the following factors:

1. the identification of 'early signs' by a clinician required intensive, regular monitoring of mental state which is rarely possible in clinical practice.
2. Some patients choose to conceal their symptoms as relapse approaches and insight declines.
3. Many schizophrenic patients experience persisting symptoms which may obscure the visibility of 'early signs'.
4. The predictive significance of **particular** early signs for an individual can only be detected by a clinician with close personal knowledge of the patient, of the kind which exists within the family; such close and continuous contact is not possible in clinical practice.

A continuous system of measurement, administered by patients and families themselves, might overcome these difficulties. The system could make use of behavioural observations by a family member (to compensate for under-reporting and declining insight in the individual) in addition to patient self-report. This would permit the identification of **changes** in symptoms, especially relevant if the individual is experiencing persisting psychiatric symptoms.

STUDY 1: DEVELOPMENT OF THE EARLY SIGNS SCALE (ESS)

Family informants from a sample of 42 schizophrenic patients were interviewed.

A structured interview, using open-ended questions, elicited precise details of changes in behaviour observed prior to the most recent period in hospital, and the interval between onset of symptoms and admission. The symptoms that relatives had noted were ordered into six time-periods prior to relapse and rank-ordered in terms of frequency of observation.

Results

Four separate groups of changes were distinguished: anxiety/agitation, depression/withdrawal, disinhibition and incipient psychosis. Table 4.6 shows the symptoms most commonly reported prior to relapse within each of these categories. The anxiety/agitation and depression/withdrawal categories revealed the highest frequency of prodromal signs.

Table 4.6: *Most Common Prodromal Symptoms Described by Relatives*

Subscale	Item	% of relatives reporting the symptom as present (N=42)
Anxiety/agitation	Irritable/quick-tempered	62
	Sleep problems	67
	Tense, afraid, anxious	62
Depression/ withdrawal	Depressed, low	57
	Quiet, withdrawn	60
	Loss of weight, poor appetite	48
Disinhibition	Restless	50
	Violent, aggressive	55
	Stubborn	36
Incipient/ psychosis	Behaves as if hearing voices	50
	Says he is being laughed at or talked about	36
	Odd behaviour	36

The results of this study were the basis of the 34 items included in the ESS scale, which measures changes in key symptoms in terms of the patient's own perceptions and those of an observer.

STUDY 2: PREDICTION OF RELAPSE USING THE ESS

A sample of 19 schizophrenic out-patients was recruited. Patients and informant – a relative or key-worker – were asked to complete the ESS fortnightly, either at their clinic appointment or through the post, rating the presence and severity of symptoms over the previous 14-day period. At monthly intervals, a clinician completed a well-validated mental-state assessment for each patient at their out-patient appointment. Patients were followed up for nine months or up to relapse, whichever was the sooner.

Results

Figure 4.3 illustrates the outcome for the total sample over the duration of the pilot study.

Discussion

The predictive validity of the ESS is supported by this pilot study. The external validity of the study is limited by the modest size and characteristics of the sample (predominantly young, generally compliant individuals). Nevertheless, the significant results suggest that the ESS system merits further research in view of its potential benefits.

Figure 4.3: *Early Signs and Relapse: Branching Diagram for Total Sample*

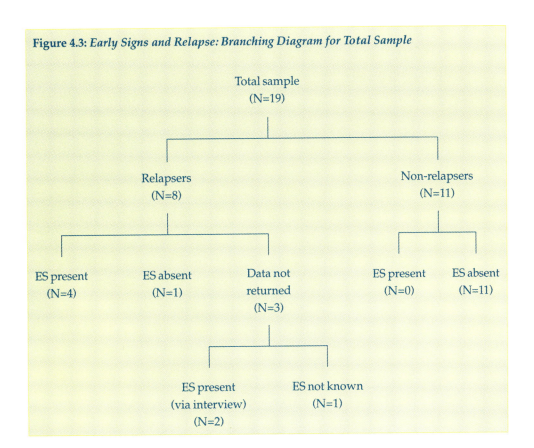

The ESS shows promise in its ability to detect prodromal symptoms which in turn might enable medical intervention to avert full relapse and readmission to hospital. This is supported by the two cases of incipient relapse in the pilot study. A replication and early-intervention study is now in preparation to explore fully the clinical implications of monitoring 'early signs', using a standardized monitoring system.

Researchers

Dr Max Birchwood, Dr J. F. Macmillan, Dr D. McGovern and Dr J. Smith

The Archer Centre, All Saints Hospital, Winson Green, Birmingham B18 5SD. (021 554 9000)

Publications

Birchwood, M. (1992) 'Early interventions in schizophrenia', *British Journal of Clinical Psychology*, **31**, 3: 257–278.

Birchwood, M., and Macmillan, J. (in press) 'Early interventions in schizophrenia', invited editorial, *Australian and New Zealand Journal of Psychiatry*.

Birchwood, M., Macmillan, J., and Smith, J. (1992) 'Ealry interventions', in M. Birchwood, and N. Tarrier (eds), *Innovations in the Psychological Management of Schizophrenia*, Chichester, Wiley.

Birchwood, M., Smith, J., and Macmillan, F. (1989) 'Predicting relapse in schizophrenia: An Early Signs Monitoring System, *Psychological Medicine*, **19**, 649–656.

Macmillan, J. F., Birchwood, M., and Smith, J. (1992) '"Early Signs" monitoring methodology', in D. J. Kavanagh (ed.), *Schizophrenia: An Overview and Practical Handbook*, London, Chapman and Hall.

Community Psychiatric Nurse Management of the Elderly Depressed in the Community – Interim Report

It was discovered by population screening in Gospel Oak ward in North London in 1987 that 18.5 per cent of the elderly residents in the community (including nursing homes) were suffering from depression of clinical severity. This finding was confirmed at re-screening in 1990, when a figure of 19.2 per cent was recorded. The research showed that depressed elderly people were likely to be female and living alone, and complain, primarily, of poor sleep and many physical symptoms. Depressed people visited their GP more frequently than others in this population, but prescription of anti-depressants appeared low – only 1 in 8 of the depressed people received such a prescription. It seemed, therefore, that a large-scale problem had been uncovered that needed further investigation and management.

Collaboration
Assessment
Service
planning

Aims of the study:

1. to obtain a diagnostic profile of the depressed subjects;
2. to draw up the ideal management plans; and
3. to investigate the success of a community psychiatric nurse (CPN) working closely with primary care staff in implementing these plans and the outcome for the depressed person.

Progress of the Study

One hundred and twelve subjects were identified in 1990 as suffering from probable clinical depression. Ninety-six (86 per cent) were included, assessed in detail by the research psychiatrist, and discussed with the local psychogeriatric team for management plans. Forty-nine were then randomly allocated to the GP for follow-up and 47 were allocated to the community nurse to implement the management plan in conjunction with the GP. Ninety out of the 96 were seen again, after three months, for standard assessment. At the same time, an independent research worker reapplied the screening questionnaire blind to the trial group. Management plans on the 49 control subjects were then fed back to the GP. Reassessment is now taking place six months later, to see, (a) how successful the GP has been in implementing the plans on his own, and (b) whether the changes that have been initiated during the three months' contact by the community nurse with the patient are still present.

PRELIMINARY RESULTS

Phase I

The initial screening cases were discovered by the psychiatrists to be clinically depressed. Thirty-eight per cent had declared their depression to the GP and 6 per cent were known to the psychiatric services.

The interventions requested by the management team were very broadly based. Increasing social network was considered necessary in 60 per cent of cases; introduction of anti-depressants in 44 per cent, and reviewing current anti-depressants in 28 per cent; specific behaviour therapy in 37 per cent, and counselling on current personal and social problems in 39 per cent.

Phase II

1. Three-month follow-up indicated that the CPN intervention had been successful in reducing levels of depression in that group compared with those followed up by the GP. Using the independent depression score, the mean fell from 8.6 to 7.1 amongst the control group, and from 8.5 to 5.8 amongst the intervened group. This was a significant difference; (the point on this scale indicating depression is 6–7). Similar changes occurred for those amongst the original sample who were diagnosed as suffering from a major depressive episode.

2. The CPN did encounter difficulties in certain of her interventions, particularly in the introduction of anti-depressants, largely because of patient refusal. In most cases, it was also difficult to increase the social network, particularly if this involved referral to a day hospital, as there was a long waiting-list. However, the CPN's personal counselling and behaviour therapy was always successfully introduced.

3. Checking with the control group, it was clear that the GP had not made any interventions or started any anti-depressants in the group allocated to him.

CONCLUSIONS

The analysis is still under way. The study so far confirms that clinical depression certainly exists in the community and that it remains out of the orbit of the mental health services, and often undeclared to GPs. The ideal management involves pharmacological, psychological and social elements. The CPN alone has some difficulties, but the contact with the nurse over three months made a significant difference in the level of depression.

Researchers

Investigator: Professor A. H. Mann

Research Workers: Dr M. Blanchard, Ms Anna Waterreus

Institute of Psychiatry, De Crespigny Park, Denmark Hill, London SE5 8AF. (071 703 5411)

Community Psychiatric Nurses and Psychosocial Intervention for Families Caring for a Relative with Schizophrenia:
Summary of Pilot Study Results

ABSTRACT

We were commissioned to examine whether or not Community Psychiatric Nurses (CPNs) could be trained to undertake psychosocial interventions with families caring for a member with schizophrenia. We also looked, in some detail, at the effect on families of these newly-acquired skills. Psychosocial intervention itself consisted of comprehensive assessments of all family members' needs, health education and the design of family stress-management programmes.

We employed a 'quasi-experimental' design and followed up a total of 54 families over a period of 12 months. The clients recruited to the study had to meet certain sample inclusion criteria which included: recent diagnosis of schizophrenia confirmed by a psychiatrist; aged 16–65 years; living with a relative (or in contact with a relative at least 10 hours a week or more); and apart from contact with a psychiatrist, the CPN had to be the principal professional involved. We observed a number of favourable improvements in 'experimental' families, but not in the controls.

Carers
Consumer
views

THE RESULTS

The Clients: We found that the 'negative' symptoms (namely depression, anxiety and retardation) of schizophrenia improved in the experimental group but not the controls. However, the frequency and severity of delusions improved equally well in both groups. In addition, we were able to show that the client's overall social adjustment improved in the group that received psychosocial intervention, but not in the control group. One further finding worth commenting on is that, somewhat contrary to our expectation, there was a trend for neuroleptic drug dose to decrease in the experimental group but, again, not in the controls. We had predicted that hospital readmissions would be lower in the experimental group but, in fact, there were only two admissions throughout the year of the trial – one from each group.

The Relatives: Our initial hypothesis was that an increase in the overall level of family support would reduce the well-described high levels of minor psychiatric morbidity in the carers. This reduction was observed in the experimental relatives but not in the control group. In fact, our consumer satisfaction data indicated that experimental group relatives were increasingly happy with the service they received – with the practical advice given, the information and knowledge obtained about the illness, the emotional support offered and the overall service-coordination.

The Community Psychiatric Nurses: We piloted a simple measure of CPN function for use in this study because we wanted to know, as far as possible, how undertaking psychosocial intervention changed the role of the CPN (if at all). We established that psychosocial intervention is more time-consuming than control intervention with families. Not surprisingly perhaps, the proportion of CPN caseloads consisting of sufferers from schizophrenia increased. There was an improvement in relationships with consumer groups, day-centres and in-patient unit coordination (also commented on by the relatives). Finally, we observed a valuable extension of CPN role in relation to the minimum therapeutic level of neuroleptic medication required by clients.

The final report to the Department of Health which will describe the outcome of the main study, is currently being prepared and the findings are just as encouraging as those of the pilot study. We feel certain that psychosocial intervention presents an important framework for CPN practice with families caring, not just for those with schizophrenia, but probably all those suffering from long-term mental illness. The next crucially important step is to disseminate the skills required to deliver psychosocial intervention. This will involve the training of 'trainers'.

Researchers

Charles Brooker and Professor Tony Butterworth

Department of Nursing, University of Manchester, Medical School, Oxford Road, Manchester M13 9PT. (061 275 5346; FAX 061 275 5584)

Publications

Chapters:

Brooker, C., Tarrier, N., Barrowclough, C., Butterworth, C., and Goldberg, D. (1992) 'Skills for CPNs working with the seriously mentally ill: Report of a pilot trial of psychosocial intervention', in C. Brooker, and E. White (eds), *Community Psychiatric Nursing: A Research Perspective (Vol II)*, London, Chapman and Hall.

Articles:

Brooker, C. (1990) 'The health education needs of families caring for a relative with schizophrenia', *Journal of Advanced Nursing*, **15**: 1092–1098.

Brooker, C. (1990) 'Expressed emotion and psychosocial intervention: a review', *International Journal of Nursing Studies*, **27**, 3: 267–276.

Brooker, C. (1990) 'The application of the concept of expressed emotion to the role of the community psychiatric nurse: a research study', *International Journal of Nursing Studies*, **27**, 3: 277–285.

Brooker, C. (1990) 'A new role for the community psychiatric nurses in working with families caring for a relative with schizophrenia', *International Journal of Social Psychiatry*, **36**, 3: 216–225.

Brooker, C., Barrowclough, C., and Tarrier, N. (in press) 'An evaluation of the outcome of training community psychiatric nurses to educate relatives caring for a relative with schizophrenia', *Journal of Clinical Nursing*.

Brooker, C., and Butterworth, C. (1991) 'Psychosocial intervention and schizophrenia: the evolving role of the community psychiatric nurse', *International Journal of Nursing Studies*, **28**, 2: 189–200.

Brooker, C., Tarrier, N., Barrowclough, C., Butterworth, C., and Goldberg, D. (in press) 'Training community psychiatric nurses for psychosocial intervention: report of a pilot study', *British Journal of Psychiatry*.

Interprofessional Collaboration in Mental Health Care

Study 1 – Where Do People with Psychosocial Problems go for Help?

GPs
Resources
Outcomes

Ninety-five per cent of the population are registered with a GP. In the first study, a sample of people aged between 25 and 75 was drawn from one general practice. These patients were sent a postal questionnaire to ascertain whether they had had a psychosocial problem in the last ten years, and in whom they had confided. Of the 396 respondents, 281 (71 per cent) admitted to having had a problem, which included significantly more women. Of these 281 individuals, 94 per cent had confided in someone, mainly friends and relatives, 47 per cent had consulted one or more professionals or agencies and 39 per cent had confided in their GP. Although the majority had found the contact with the agency or professional helpful, those with depression or anxiety or child-care problems were less likely to feel that they had been helped. The provision of practical advice, sympathy and support were most often mentioned as being helpful.

The study indicates the important role of the GPs as confidants. They were more likely to be consulted than any other professional, with 43 per cent of women and 27 per cent of men with problems confiding in them. The doctor was more likely to be a confidant among the older age groups rather than the younger, particularly among the men. The findings underline the importance of close collaboration between GPs and other community workers so that they can refer patients to these agencies when appropriate.

Study 2 – Which Professionals are Collaborating with GPs in the Field of Mental Health?

The White Paper 'Caring for People' recognizes the key role of GPs and stresses the importance of collaboration between health and social services in the management of community care. But despite widespread agreement on the need for inter-disciplinary collaboration, it has generally been found difficult to achieve in practice. Barriers have included structural barriers, a lack of common objectives, poor communication, ignorance of respective roles, mutual suspicion, professional insecurity and professional jealousy.

In this study, six District Health Authorities in England and Wales were randomly selected. Each general practice was sent a questionnaire to elicit details of mental health professionals who were in contact with the practice either through employ-ment, attachment, liaison schemes or because they used the same building as a base. The results are shown in tables 4.7 and 4.8.

Two of these districts were chosen for more intensive study. Questionnaires were sent to all the professionals based in the community who were involved in providing mental health services. These included GPs, social workers, community psychiatric nurses and clinical psychologists.

Table 4.7: *Contact with Practice: by Profession, and Nature of Link*

% Practices	Nature of Link				Some link	Planned link
	Employment	Attachment	Liaison	Base		
Community Psychiatric Nurse	0.0	20.7	24.9	2.3	47.9	1.9
Social Worker	0.0	3.4	15.7	1.9	21.0	0.4
Clinical Psychologist	5.0	2.7	6.5	0.8	15.0	1.9
Psychiatrist	1.1	3.1	9.2	2.3	15.7	0.0
Counsellor	5.0	4.2	6.9	0.8	16.9	1.9

Table 4.8: *Contact with Practice: by District, and Profession*

% practices some link	Community Psychiatric Nurse	Social Worker	Clinical Psychologist	Psychiatrist	Counsellor
All districts	**47.9**	**21.0**	**15.0**	**15.7**	**16.9**
Chester	59.3	14.8	14.8	22.2	44.4
Maidstone	55.2	27.6	13.8	13.8	17.2
Tower Hamlets	39.4	15.2	48.5	27.3	21.2
West Birmingham	41.4	28.6	12.9	11.4	8.6
Barnet	38.3	18.3	1.7	8.3	15.0
Hull	66.7	16.7	11.9	21.4	11.9

Analysis of the questionnaires sent to the GPs is now under way. Preliminary results indicate that doctors were more likely to refer problems to those professionals who were linked in some way to the practice, and were more satisfied with the services provided by them. However, many doctors pointed out that any complaints they had were not usually directed at the professionals themselves but were due to overstretched staffing and inadequate resources. Low levels of funding meant that in many cases the waiting-lists for treatment were very long or that the professional's involvement was considered to be inadequate.

Study 3 – Client Outcome and Satisfaction

This study will investigate whether inter-professional collaboration has an effect on client outcome and consumer satisfaction. Four general practices have been identified, representing a wide range of levels of collaboration.

Twenty-five women with chronic severe depression/anxiety, who have young children 'at risk', will be interviewed. All clients will have had some contact with other community services or psychiatric services in the previous six months.

Information will be collected on their views of and satisfaction with the primary care services, social services and other community psychiatric services which may be involved. An assessment of the mental health problems will be made using the Clinical Interview Schedule[16], and a social assessment will also be made.

Details will also be collected from all the agencies in contact, on:–

(a) services and help received;

(b) attendance rates of patients and number of home visits made by the various agencies involved;

(c) attendance rates of other family members;

(d) any collaboration between the professionals involved;

(e) treatments given including drugs prescribed.

These details will be recorded over a period of nine months after the interview, in order to make a simple assessment of outcome. A follow-up interview will also be undertaken. The patient's mental health and social problems will be reassessed using the same instruments and the doctor and key-workers will be asked for a brief assessment of the physical and mental health of the client and any social problems.

Researcher

Dr R. Corney

Institute of Psychiatry, De Crespigny Park, Denmark Hill, London SE5 8AF. (071 703 5411)

Publications

Corney, R. (1990) 'A survey of professional help sought by patients for psychosocial problems', *British Journal of General Practice*, **40**, 365–368.

---

[16] Goldberg, D., Cooper, B., Eastwood, M., Kedward, H., and Shepherd, M. (1970) 'A psychiatric interview suitable for using in community surveys', *British Journal of the Society of Preventive Medicine*, **24**: 18–26.

Nafsiyat: a Psychotherapy Centre for Ethnic Minorities

The Nafsiyat Inter-Cultural Therapy Centre was established in North London in 1983 to provide short-term psychotherapy for members of ethnic minority groups. Between 1986 and 1989 the then DHSS funded a research team to evaluate the Centre.

Assessment
Inter-cultural therapy
Outcomes

Research was carried out in four stages. The first three stages involved: a retrospective study; the choice and development of the assessment instruments and questionnaires; and piloting the instruments.

The fourth stage comprised the major prospective study with which this report is principally concerned. In the prospective study, 157 patients – *the referred group* – were assessed on demographic and referral variables, of whom 52 – *the treatment group* – completed therapy and all the research instruments. They were assessed before and after therapy with the General Health Questionnaire (GHQ), the Present State Examination and new questionnaires concerned with case history, social history, and eventual self-report. The therapists completed a Centre psychiatric symptom checklist, a therapy action schedule, and a therapy profile.

The treatment group were similar to the original referral group in terms of sex ratio (2.3 compared with 1.7), origin in North London (65 per cent and 66 per cent), general practitioner referral (21 per cent compared with 19 per cent), and psychiatric referral (11 per cent and 9 per cent). Men were more likely to be referred by doctors than women. Few patients in either the referral or treatment group requested a therapist of the same ethnic origin. The major origins of the patients in the referral group were 1/5 UK, 1/5 West Indies, 1/6 Africa, 1/6 South Asia; the treatment group were similar except that only a tenth were African. In total, there were 38 different countries of origin specified.

Of the treatment group, a high proportion had completed secondary education but nine were unemployed. The most common presenting complaints as reported by patients were depression, a general inability to cope and identity problems; 25 per cent of the women reported rape or other sexual abuse. Seventy-three per cent had not previously been offered psychotherapy. Forty-two per cent of patients received 12 or less therapeutic sessions. On the initial PSE, two patients were assessed as having schizophrenic symptoms, two hypomania and four non-specific psychosis (15 per cent of the total treatment group); 42 had the Syndrome Check List category of Simple Depression and 46 per cent had other SCL depressive syndromes. Only 7 patients had an initial GHQ score of less than 12. After therapy, 38 had scores of less than 12. Of the 40 patients with initial GHQ scores in the 'high' range, six remained in this category after therapy. Ninety-one per cent of patients described a 'good outcome' to their therapy. There was no association between ethnicity and symptom pattern or improvement.

Correlation between the different outcome measures has not yet been carried out, nor have more sophisticated multi-variate analyses of the results necessary to determine which factors might predict good outcome. These results can therefore only be considered as preliminary, and more detailed analysis is continuing.

The most striking conclusions are the high level of psychiatric morbidity in this population, their readiness to use the Centre and the efficacy of highly cost-effective psychotherapy for relatively severe psychopathology. A further detailed study could usefully examine (a) long-term efficacy and social adjustment, and (b) whether the process of treatment is specific to the psychotherapeutic assumptions of the therapists. The efficacy of this type of therapy also suggests that the currently-reported high rates of psychiatric illness among some British minorities cannot be readily attributable to a biological aetiology or to genetic predisposition.

Researchers

Sharon Moorhouse, Sourangshu Acharyya, Roland Littlewood and Jafar Kareem

Nafsiyat, Inter-Cultural Therapy Centre, 278 Seven Sisters Road, Finsbury Park, London N4 2HY. (071 263 4130)

Publications

Acharyya, S., Moorhouse, S., Kareem, J., and Littlewood, R. (1989) 'Nafsiyat: A Psychotherapy Centre for Ethnic Minorities', *Psychiatric Bulletin*, **13**, 7: 358–360.

Conference Proceedings: 'Assessment and Treatment Across Cultures' (Conference held in Eastbourne, January 1987), Nafsiyat.

Moorhouse, S. 'Quantitative Research in Intercultural Therapy: Some Methodological Considerations', in J. Kareem, and R. Littlewood (eds), *Intercultural Therapy: Themes, Interpretations and Practices*, Oxford, Basil Blackwell.

Primary prevention of Depression and Anxiety – Literature Review

The review will consider the literature within the following framework:

1. *Prevention*
   The use of the concept in health and health care. Primary, secondary and tertiary prevention: the focus of this review is on the first, with some necessary overlap into secondary prevention.

   Macro- and micro-level approaches, the first involving whole populations and the second specifically aimed at identified 'risk'-groups.

   The importance of research in planning and evaluating interventions.

2. *Social factors and the aetiology of depression and anxiety*
   Adversity, stress, personal resources and health outcome: discussion of the various theoretical perspectives.

   The role of social support in aetiology: direct effect upon sources of stress or buffering effect upon health outcome.

   The identification of vulnerable groups, in which social factors have been shown to enhance risk of depression and anxiety.

3. *Prevention strategies in vulnerable groups*
   Outline of government policy, including the implications of community care legislation.

   Mobilizing social support to vulnerable groups and evaluating outcomes. Specific examples will include:
   * pregnancy and early motherhood
   * parents of handicapped children
   * families of mentally ill adults
   * isolated elderly people
   * widows
   * informal carers of dementia sufferers.

   Particular emphasis will be given to the growing research literature on the last group, from which a series of research studies will be developed.

Researcher

Joanna Murray

Institute of Psychiatry, De Crespigny Park, Denmark Hill, London SE5 8AF. (071 703 5411; FAX 071 703 5796)

Chapter 5

Learning Disabilities

Learning Disabilities

Planning in health and social services will, in future, be based on assessing population needs. Some of the projects summarized in this Chapter are directly relevant to needs assessment in the field of learning disabilities: one, for example, is about predicting future trends in the numbers of children with severe learning disabilities. Others have investigated the prevalence of challenging behaviour or the degree of psychiatric and physical morbidity among people with learning disabilities. Individual assessment has also been the subject of research – in particular, the development of ways of assessing individuals with psychiatric disorders in addition to learning disabilities.

The running down or closure of particular long-stay hospitals has been studied: the process of closure, the type of accommodation to which people moved, their comparative quality of life, and the implications for staff in terms of recruitment, management, training and morale. Other work has focused on services provided in the community, whether for ex-hospital residents or young adults who have grown up since community care policies were first implemented: for example, different forms of domiciliary and day-services.

Two programmes of work reported on in this Chapter are concerned with evaluating various aspects of the All-Wales Mental Handicap Strategy, initiated in 1983. The Strategy had as its aim the development of locally-available, community-based residential, day, family support, respite and professional services. This work, as well as some of the other studies of local authority services and their users, includes information about comparative costs and quality. A number of these projects are also concerned with the needs of carers (both paid and informal).

Other entries in the Chapter concern clinical research and evaluation, looking at different methods of helping particular groups: for example, adults with severely challenging or self-injurious behaviour, and children.

Predicting Future Trends in Severe Learning Disability

THE STUDY

Service planning

Severe learning disability stemming from birth or early childhood is found in association with a very large number of different conditions. This type of disability usually makes an independent existence impossible, and leads to a need for life-long care. There is therefore a requirement for local authorities, whether in the health, social service, or educational field to plan ahead for the services that will be needed by those affected.

> The work summarized here was aimed firstly at predicting the incidence and age-specific prevalence of severe learning disability in the birth cohorts derived from conceptions between now and the end of the century, taking account of the effects of likely changes in demography and advances in medical care. Methods comprised a review of available data, a survey of researchers to identify likely new developments over the period concerned, and a synthesis of the findings in the form of predictions for populations of different demography or risk status. The second aim was to present these predictions in the form of a guidebook to be used by local authorities for extrapolation to their own local situation, for the planning of likely relevant medical, social and educational service needs over the next 30 years.

For this exercise, it was decided that the term *severe learning disability* should be taken to mean individuals whose mental disability was likely to bring them to the attention of service agencies; and that the study should focus on trends in the major contributory causes. These comprise Down's syndrome, which accounts for about one-third; cerebral palsy with mental disability, which we estimate accounts for about one-fifth; and the relatively recently-described mental retardation linked to the X-chromosome, which may account for about one-tenth. The large group of different single gene defects accounts for another tenth; the remainder is made up of rare syndromes, including autistic disorders, malformations, and those for whom the cause remains unknown.

Any major trends in the prevalence of these conditions will be reflected in the overall prevalence of severe retardation. Those who plan for the care of affected individuals will need to know what the trends are likely to be, and how this will be expressed in the relative proportions of each in the overall population under consideration, for each group has different needs.

RESULTS

Down's Syndrome

Over the next decade, the projected rise in births, especially to older mothers, will lead to an increase in the number of conceptions with Down's syndrome, many of which will be lost naturally in early pregnancy. Those that are born with this condition will have a longer expectation of life than in the past, so that potentially there could be a marked increase in prevalence up to adult life. However, this will probably be checked, if not reversed, by the predicted uptake of the improved prenatal screening and diagnostic tests for the condition, and the likely high proportion of parents who will choose to terminate an affected pregnancy. Advances in ultrasound, in particular, may allow the diagnosis of a high proportion of Down's syndrome foetuses with complications such as congenital heart disease, leading to offers of pregnancy termination. This would mean that those children born affected may be less often physically disabled than in the past.

Cerebral Palsy

In the case of cerebral palsy, there are a large variety of causes. Overall, about 35 per cent will have severe learning disability, as well as disorders of movement, often communication, and other sensory problems. It seems that the recent marked rise in the survival of the very immature or low birthweight births, comprising about half the cases, has already led to a small increase in birth prevalence of this condition. This is likely to continue, given the present trends in birthweight distribution and survival. Since many of the affected children seem to have been damaged early in pregnancy, the hope that the majority of cases might have been prevented by excellent obstetric and neonatal care has not been substantiated. Only in the group due to post-natal causes, such as infections and accidents, is there real hope for a reduction in the near future. It seems that in all birthweights the degree of severity of those affected is unlikely to be less than in the past, and there is every chance that even those with severe associated defects are likely to survive longer than in the past.

X-Linked Syndromes

Over the last year, there have been remarkable advances in our understanding of the genetic background of the most important of these conditions – Fragile-X syndrome. From our enquiries it seems that these will not lead to immediate opportunities for prenatal diagnosis, although for some families this is already a possibility. However, it seems that within the next decade there may be a real breakthrough in this field, which could have a substantial impact on the birth prevalence of the condition. Those affected seem to have few associated defects and a normal life expectancy.

Other Causes

Perhaps the most remarkable success story in this area has been the reduction in the prevalence of neural tube defects. The success has been partly due to prenatal screening and termination of affected pregnancies; partly due to an overall fall in incidence, perhaps as a result of improved diet. We now know that the administration of folic acid around the time of conception will considerably reduce the risk of recurrences, and possibly even the first such case in a family. Children with these conditions who require substantial medical and other care now contribute very little to the overall burden of severe learning disability. There is a vast number of other genetically-caused relevant conditions which contribute little individually, but are important taken together. There are constant advances in this field, many of which will provide help for individual families, but none that are likely to have an important numerical impact in the next decade, except possibly an increase in their survival.

In summary, the changes we have outlined are likely to cancel each other out, so that the prevalence rate of severe mental retardation overall is likely to remain stable over this decade, but the number will fluctuate with the annual number of births. The 'guidebook' being prepared for local authorities will indicate the likely numbers in a given population in cohorts born up to the turn of the century.

We consider that the group as a whole will need increased medical and paramedical care, as the proportion of the relatively lightly handicapped individuals with Down's syndrome may decrease, and those more handicapped – such as the group with cerebral palsy – are likely to increase. These changes will be reflected in the need for parental support and appropriate educational provision. Social service and educational authorities should become aware of provision of prenatal diagnostic and counselling services in the areas for which they are responsible, as these could have an impact on local patterns of need for long-term care.

Researchers

Professor Eva Alberman and Dr Amanda Nicholson

Department of Environment and Preventive Medicine, Wolfson Institute of Preventive Medicine, The Medical College of St Batholomew's Hospital, University of London, Charterhouse Square, London EC1M 6BQ. (071 982 6269; FAX 071 982 6270)

Publications

Papers in press or submitted:

Nicholson, A., and Alberman, E. (in press) 'Cerebral palsy – an increasing contributor to severe mental retardation?', *Archives of Disease in Childhood*.

Nicholson, A., and Alberman, E. (in press) 'Prediction of the number of Down's syndrome infants to be born in England and Wales up to the year 2000 and their likely survival rates', *Journal of Mental Deficiency Research*.

Nicholson, A. 'Information to help the planning of medical facilities for Down's syndrome children and adults' (in preparation).

Nicholson, A. (submitted) 'Future prevalence of severe mental retardation due to x-linked mental retardation', *Journal of Paediatric and Perinatal Epidemiology*.

Report of project to the Department of Health – May 1992

Guide Book to help local authorities plan services for those with severe learning disabilities is in preparation and should be available after July 1992.

Darenth Park Project: an Evaluation of a Hospital Closure

THE STUDY

Costs
Staff moral
Service
quality

The Darenth Park Project was the earliest attempt by a Regional Health Authority to close a large, 100-year-old hospital for people with learning disabilities and to provide services for all the residents in local communities. In the past, the hospital had housed 1,500 people and served a large area of south-east England.

The study monitored and evaluated the clsoure process over seven-and-a-half years, following events from the planning stage through to the time, in August 1988, when the hospital actually closed. The researchers had access to meetings and documents, conducted extensive interviews with staff and managers as well as with a sample of nearly 100 residents who had moved. An economic analysis of the costs of 're-provision' was undertaken, and compared with the cost of running the old hospital. It was the first comprehensive study of its kind in the United Kingdom.

THE RESULTS

In brief, the study showed that it is possible to provide alternative services outside a hospital setting in smaller and far less institutional surroundings, and to do so for all the residents, even those with the severest handicaps. It also showed that to do so properly is a highly complex task which takes a long time to plan and execute, and that it costs money – more money than it takes to house such residents in a large, old hospital.

Regional Leadership

Given the wide area from which residents were drawn, sustained Regional Health Authority leadership was required over a long period to bring the venture to a successful conclusion. Many districts and local authorities, housing associations and voluntary organizations had to be mobilized.

Financial Incentives

The Project began in the 1970s following assumptions about the way to plan services which were current at the time. It relied on a top-down approach, which assumed that all the participants and local agencies would follow the Region's lead and interpretation of what was needed. It was also assumed that local authorities would be ready to collaborate and expand services without receiving more money to do so. Both assumptions proved incorrect. Regional officers developed a system of financial incentives which paid agencies and districts to provide services on a per-patient basis, to replace the beds lost in the hospital. Increasingly, this NHS money was supplemented by making deals with housing associations, which could draw on social security benefits for residents and on Housing Corporation grants. Housing associations became the most effective vehicle for providing alternative small scale provision in the later stages of the project. Social security and Housing Corporation money was crucial to this process.

The Costs of Closure

A sample of residents who left the hospital were followed up. Details were collected about the facilities in which they were living and the services they were using in the community – day-centres or the local GP, hospital and social work services, the cost of any drugs and so on. An assessment was then made of the way in which these services and facilities were paid for, so that the total cost of the new forms of community care could be estimated.

The findings were striking. First, the annual average costs per resident, excluding capital costs, in the new facilities varied enormously. At one extreme were residents with limited handicaps who were placed in a small hospital or in large homes. At the other extreme were severely- and multiply-handicapped people in small specialist-care facilities.

Expressed in 1987–8 prices, costs for some people in the first group totalled about £10,000 a year, but on average the cost was £15,500 a year. Costs for some of the most disabled people were over £40–50,000. The average cost to public funds of those living in the most successful environments – group homes – was £25,500 a year, if the cost of social security, housing subsidies and local services are included. By comparison, housing people in the old and poorly staffed hospital when it was working at full capacity had cost an average of about £12,500 a year.

In the group facilities, over 60 per cent of the cost of care came from the NHS, but 27 per cent was met out of social security benefit funds, and 6 per cent from the Housing Corporation grants. Local authorities met less than 3 per cent of the costs.

Care in the Community – a Continuing Process

Acquiring houses in the community and moving people into them was comparatively easy. We observed the difficulties that were experienced in continuing to provide a stimulating environment, in keeping staff morale high in small isolated environments, in monitoring standards and in achieving any real integration with the local residents and community groups. The task of sustaining the quality of the new services had only just begun.

Researchers

Professor H. Glennerster and Nancy Korman

London School of Economics, Houghton Street, London WC2A 2AE. (071 405 7686)

Publications

Glennerster, H. (1990) 'The Costs of Hospital Closure', *Psychiatric Bulletin*, **14:** 140–143.

Glennerster, H., and Korman, N. (1990) 'Normalisation is not Easy', *Community Care*, 3 May 1990.

Glennerster, H., and Korman, N. (1990) 'Success Costs Money', *Community Care*, 26 April 1990.

Korman, N., and Glennerster, H. (1985) *Closing a Hospital: The Darenth Park Project*, Occasional Papers in Social Administration, London, Bedford Square Press.

Korman, N., and Glennerster, H. (1990) *Hospital Cosure: a Political and Economic Study*, Milton Keynes, Open University Press.

Several articles were published in the *Health and Social Services Journal* as the project proceeded, in the years 1984 to 1988.

Evaluation of Care in the Community for Adults with Learning Disabilities Leaving Hospitals in the Northern Region

The main aim of this three-year descriptive study was to evaluate the process of selection for and transition to community care of adults with learning disabilities in long-stay hospitals. A second objective of the project was to describe the views of paid care-staff about their work and jobs, as well as towards resettlement.

From among the people selected by community projects to leave hospital, we compared the characteristics of those who actually went to live in the community with those who remained behind. Using a broad lifestyles approach, we compared life in hospital with that in the community over a minimum of the first nine months. We described the organization and management of the projects and carried out a survey of the characteristics and attitudes of care staff in the three hospitals as well as the seven community projects included in the study.

At the outset, the projects were all managed by statutory authorities. Social services took the lead in all but two which were joint health and social service managed. One project was managed in the short term by the health authority but was transferred to the voluntary sector. Charitable and housing associations became involved only after the project teams had carried out assessment and preparation for discharge with hospital residents.

The 'Leavers'

From plans submitted to the RHA it was clear that just over 200 people in hospital were intended to be resettled to community living in the five local authorities included in the study between 1989–90. In the event, 84 people were identified as potential leavers for funded projects and, of these, 46 people actually left hospital over an 18-month period. None were resettled into private care.

The 84 who were selected as potential leavers were at the more able end of the ability continuum among hospital residents. Age was not a barrier to leaving and neither was gender. However, those who left were more independent in functional abilities associated with hygiene and mobility, had better communication skills, were more sociable and less likely to be described as presenting management problems for hospital staff. Delay in leaving hospital, and deselection, was associated with inadequate funding which resulted in insufficient physical and staff resources to enable community living.

Of the 46 people who left hospital, we were able to interview all but seven both in hospital and in their new homes. For some, we used signing as well as speech and modified questions according to their understanding and communication skills. We also went on outings with them and spent time in their homes: those who could not be interviewed were able to demonstrate aspects of their lifestyle in both settings. Carers were also interviewed about residents in both settings and a diary of activities was completed over one week in both settings.

Consumer views
Quality of life
Staff views

Experience in the Community

None of the people who left hospital wanted to return there to live, although one ultimately did so. Some demonstrated typical grief responses at separation from friends and staff, as well as activities which they missed. Carers assessed that half the leavers had demonstrated problems settling into their new homes. There was also an increase in what staff described as unacceptable behaviour: objectively, behaviour appeared to change little.

Since just over two-thirds of the leavers had been in hospital for more than 20 years, and ten for more than 40 years, it is not surprising that some of them experienced difficulties. Nevertheless, there were a larger number of positive comments and fewer negative comments about life in the community compared with hospital. At the simplest level, people enjoyed the greater privacy, control over their own possessions, and relaxation of institutional regulations. Thirty-five residents lived in ordinary houses of five or fewer people.

While staff reported greater and more flexible family contacts, this was not the perception of residents, although they used the telephone more to inititate contact themselves. Overall, there was no change in the amount of activity outside of the residence, but a wider **range** of activities was involved, and more included people without learning disabilities. Several new friendships had been established and some neighbours visited. However, only one person was in open employment and for several, there was less structured activity out of the home than had been available to them in hospital. This was offset by an increase in domestic work at home, as well as shopping for provisions and using other community facilities.

On balance, life in the community offered several improvements over hospital care, including attention to long-standing health problems. While some of those who moved were disappointed by the absence of meaningful occupation and by the lack of interest shown by family members, for most, lives and self-concept had been transformed for the better.

The Views of Care Staff

A postal survey of 1,200 care staff in the three hospitals and community projects in the five local authorities found that community staff, on the whole, were less experienced: only 3 per cent of senior staff had more than three years' experience, compared with a third of those in hospital. Fourteen per cent of the community staff had a statutory qualification related to mental handicap. Community staff were more likely to work extra hours for which they were paid overtime, had time in lieu, or were not paid at all. They also showed a greater orientation to community options for residents than hospital staff.

Using scales developed in a similar study by Allen, Pahl and Quine[17], we found that there was no difference in overall job satisfaction or role conflict between hospital and community staff. However, community staff were more uncertain about the components and limits of their job, felt less sense of a hierarchy and a greater sense of participation in decision making. Hospital staff, on the other hand, had higher burn-out scores. There were also fewer differences between community senior and unqualified staff than between qualified staff in hospitals and care assistants.

---

[17] Allen, I., Pahl, J., and Quine, L. (1990) *Care Staff in Transition*, London, HMSO.

Acknowledgement

This study was funded jointly by the Northern Regional Health Authority and the Department of Health.

Researchers

Dr Senga Bond, Mrs Monica Smith, Mrs Kathleen Pitcairn

Centre for Health Services Research, University of Newcastle, 21 Claremont Place, Newcastle upon Tyne NE2 4AA. (091 222 7045)

Publications

Bond, S., Smith, M., and Pitcairn, K. (1992) *Community Resettlement from Hospital of People with a Mental Handicap*:

Vol. 1	'Moving On – A chance to leave'
Vol. 2	'Moving On – It's asking a lot'
Vol. 3	'Moving On – A different world'
Vol. 4	'Service Staff in Hospital and Community'
Vol. 5	'An overview of the study'

Centre for Health Services Research, Report No. 53.

Care in the Community for People with Learning Disabilities: North Warwickshire Study

BACKGROUND

The objective of this study was to evaluate new developments in residential care in the community for people with learning disabilities. The study was based in the North Warwickshire Health District and focused on the transfer of hospital patients, together with others currently living with their families, to a series of small supervised residential homes. The aim was to monitor transfers to each new unit and to assess the outcomes of the move for the individuals involved, taking account of the perspectives of both clients and their carers. The study also investigated the financial costs.

The work was designed to run in parallel with the relevant transfers; but in the event, this proved impossible. Delays in funding meant that four of the five facilities to be evaluated had become operational before the investigation began; and one of the facilities refused to participate. Finally, a major hospital from which the clients were transferred was closed abruptly, effectively limiting observation of the 'run-down' period.

The loss of the 'before and after' comparison, the administrative problems, and the limited cooperation received, effectively reduced the numbers covered by the study. In these circumstances, the descriptive data which were collected, drawing on the views of clients, staff and carers, assumed a greater importance than originally planned.

Despite the small numbers finally available and the limitations of the study, an attempt was made to assess adaptive change following transfer from one form of institution to another and to separate these effects from the characteristics on which selection for transfer was made.

RESULTS

- There was evidence from retrospective histories, taken from staff, that there had been marked improvements in skills and abilities, and in other behavioural measures, in the period immediately after relocation. The changes observed by the research workers later in the course of the study were less significant, but did indicate a continuing improvement which confirmed the retrospective record.
- There were substantial differences between the different community residential facilities. Three of the four clearly enriched the patients' lives, and a fourth one did not. In the three more successful homes, the residents were encouraged and helped to pursue individual interests and hobbies, and to develop active and varied social lives. This was less evident in the fourth home. However, part of the observed difference may have been due to the way in which the residents were selected for relocation: the residents of the less successful facility included a high proportion who needed nursing care as well as simple residential care.
- There was evidence that people who moved into another hospital suffered damage to their skills and abilities; social behaviour also deteriorated. This was probably due to the fact that these moves occurred with no individual planning.

Consumer views
Quality of life
Costs

The patients were moved within 48 hours of the decision being made, and more in accordance with the availability of floorspace than personal needs. However, for almost all other moves there was clear evidence of immediate benefit.

● The research highlighted the need for a number of guidelines for relocation policy at the personal level. For example, there was evidence that mixing long-term and short-term residents within a single home was detrimental to the quality of the life of the long-term residents. It was also important, in smaller institutions, to pay particular attention to personal preferences and relationships between residents. Both in hospital and in community residences, staff had not always thought through issues relating to residents' sexual relationships and activities, or provided appropriate counselling and protection.

● As regards cost, the limited economic data available suggested that the costs amounted to about £20,000 per resident per annum in the new facilities – rather more than that for hospital residents. There is therefore no evidence that these policy changes can be justified in terms of cost savings in respect of clients already in hospital care. They must be justified in terms of the degree to which they improve standards.

Researchers

Jenny Summerfield, Amanda Gatherer, Professor E. G. Knox

Department of Public Health and Epidemiology, The University of Birmingham, The Medical School, Edgbaston, Birmingham B15 2TT. (021 414 6755; FAX 021 414 4036)

Quality and Costs of Residential Services for Adults with Learning Disabilities

This four-year study was designed to investigate and explain the costs and quality of community residential services for adults with learning disabilities. The first two years of the work were concerned with costing different services for people with learning disabilities and developing the research proposal for the costs and quality project.

The study drew together two previously independent strands of work, one concerned with costing care, the other related to the quality of service provision. In addition to cost data, a battery of measures was used to assess the quality of the services provided in a sample of staffed facilities in England (outside London).

A sample of 150 facilities from four different sectors of provision in NHS, local authority social services departments, voluntary and private sectors was included in the study, and visited by the research team. The facilities varied in size from 2 to 31 beds.

Costs

Quality measures

Staff morale

Variations in the Quality of Care

Significant differences were found between the agencies. Facilities run by the private and voluntary sector are more attractive, and provide more individualized accommodation than statutory facilities. In private facilities, clients are less likely to be involved in activities relating to daily domestic life, and care regimes are generally less individually-orientated than homes in other sectors. Opportunities for clients to make decisions abut their own lives are frequent in all homes, but local authority and voluntary facilities provide most opportunity to do this and private sector homes, least. The use of community amenities is uniformly low.

Staffing

Staff morale is lowest in the public sector homes and is higher where communication among staff is satisfactory. Attitudes to people with learning disabilities are positive in all types of home, but are more positive among facility managers than direct-care staff.

Differences in Client-Mix

The mean age of residents is similar across homes in all sectors. In total, one-third of residents have previously been living in hospital and one-third have been living at home. Health authority facilities have the largest proportion of residents with additional physical handicaps and sensory impairments. Levels of personal and social sufficiency are highest in the voluntary sector and lowest in the health authority facilities. A number of private homes specialized in accommodating people with mental health problems in addition to their learning disability and, as a result, the residents of private sector homes are on average less competent than those living in local authority facilities.

Differences in Costs

Mean total cost is £38 per resident-day and ranges from £16 to £95 per day. On average, health authority facilities are the most expensive. Those in the independent sector are least costly. Structural differences in the type of building in which facilities are located, or the quality of the physical environment, have no significant effect on costs. Size variables are also insignificant, suggesting there are no economies of scale within the size-range of facilities surveyed, and therefore no cost disadvantages in smaller facilities. The most significant explanatory variables relate to *case-mix*, that is the mean age and dependency of residents. Facilities providing accommodation for younger, older and least competent residents cost more per resident-day. Since the four measures of service quality were all closely correlated with one another, it was possible to construct a composite quality variable. This measure was positively and significantly associated with costs, indicating that *higher quality of care in community facilities costs more*.

Two substantial pieces of analysis still remain to be completed. The first of these is aimed at explaining differences in the quality of care amongst facilities. This will go beyond inter-sectoral differences to assess the impact of facility size, and structural design, client characteristics and staffing. The second area will develop the cost-function analysis, to allow for more sophisticated modelling of the relationship between costs and the quality of care.

Researchers

Norma Raynes, Catherine Pettifer (University of Manchester); Alan Shiell, Ken Wright (CHE, University of York)

Centre for Health Economics, University of York, Heslington, York YO1 5DD. (0904 433646; FAX 0904 433644)

Publications

Shiell, A., Pettifer, C., Raynes, N., and Wright, K. G. (1990) 'The economic approaches to measuring quality of life: conceptual convenience or methodological straitjacket?', in S. Baldwin, C. Godfrey, and C. Propper (eds), *The Quality of Life: perspectives and policies*, London, Routledge, 105–119.

Shiell, A., Pettifer, C., Raynes, N., and Wright, K. G. (1990) 'Watching the pounds', *Insight*, **5**, 16: 24–25.

Shiell, A., Pettifer, C., Raynes, N., and Wright, K. G. (1992) 'The Costs of Community Residential Facilities for Adults with a Mental Handicap in England', *Mental Handicap Research*, **5**, 2: 115–129.

Shiell, A., Wright, K. G., Pettifer, C., and Raynes, N. (1990) 'Keep up the small talk', *Health Service Journal*, **100**, 5212: 1149.

Shiell, A., Wright, K. G., Raynes, N., and Pettifer, C. (1991) 'Attitudes to clilents with mental handicap', *Nursing Standard*, **5**, 20: 25–27.

A Demographic Study of Older People with Severe Learning Disabilities

The survey was undertaken in a single Local Authority/District, Oldham Metropolitan Borough, in the North West of England. This borough is within the North Western Regional Health Authority (NWRHA) in which the national policy of developing a community care service (including hospital closure) is at present being implemented.

Service planning
Informal care

Aims

- To establish the prevalence of people with severe learning disabilities over the age of 50 and to determine sex and age structure of this population.
- To determine the characteristics of the population in terms of intellectual level and adaptive behaviour.
- To collect detailed information on services and informal support received by individual clients.
- To investigate the relations between client characteristics, (age, sex and adaptive behaviour) and levels of specific services and informal support received.
- To develop a set of questionnaires and procedures which can be used as a complete package by other local authorities wishing to a) make an accurate characterization of their own population of older people with severe learning disabilities, and b) survey the levels of services and informal support they are receiving.
- To provide a well-defined sample to explore further research issues relevant to ageing in this population in the community.

The study included two major survey components: (1) an agency survey in which people with severe learning disabilities over the age of 50 years were included; (2) an 'outreach' exercise in which individuals meeting the stated criteria but not in contact with the Community Mental Handicap Team (CMHT) were included.

In defining the population, criteria related to severe learning disabilities were specified, with an intelligence quotient of approximately IQ=50 being taken as a guide to inclusion. Individuals 50 years or older were included, since the aim was to look at 'older' rather than exclusively at *elderly* people.

Questionnaires were prepared which covered personal details, residential information, history of residential relocations and planned resettlement, employment and day services, education and training, leisure, informal social networks and legal aspects. Detailed information on the lives of population members living at home with relatives was also collected.

The core population on which analyses were undertaken was 122, 74.6 per cent from CMHT, and 25.4 per cent from outreach.

Results

1. The Characteristics and Context of the Group

— A recurrent finding in the present study was the association between receipt of services and the degree of antisocial behaviour exhibited.

— Increasing age was not related to intellectual functioning, nor was there any relation between age and competence **or** maladaptive behaviour. Given the present life-expectation of people with severe learning disabilities which is lower than average, we do not anticipate the emergency of a fragile elderly population of declining intellectual and functional abilities, though those providing services will inevitably encounter **some** people with these characteristics.

— Adaptive behaviour and intellectual ability were significantly related, particularly in relation to community competence.

— Members of this population were found in a variety of settings. For purposes of analysis, five classes of residential accommodation were defined:
  (a) hospitals;
  (b) independently resident;
  (c) hostel/Part III accommodation;
  (d) sheltered accommodation;
  (e) family home.

— The difference in mean age of residents in the various types of accommodation was significant. The oldest were in sheltered accommodation (68.3 years), followed by those in hospital (66.8 years), in hostels/Part III accommodation (65.7 years), independently resident (58.4 years), family resident (57.6 years).

— Assessments of intellectual ability and community competence tended to be related to the characteristics of different residents in a consistent fashion. Those in sheltered residences and those living independently were the most able with respect to all measures of such abilities. Those living with their family tended to be least competent, with hostel and hospital residents occupying an intermediate position. By contrast, the measure of personal/social competence presents a different picture. Here, family residents were **most** competent, followed by hostel/Part III residents. Independent and sheltered residents occupied an intermediate position, with hospital residents least competent in these respects. No difference emerged with respect to maladaptive behaviour in the various residential categories.

— In all areas of social provision – that is, individual treatment programmes, education and leisure – members of the CMHT sample received more, despite no difference in the functional levels of the two samples.

— Those moving into independent accommodation were significantly younger than those moving into sheltered accommodation, (by 11 years). However, competence level or the degree of difficult behaviour did not predict resettlement destination. Taken together, these findings reflect a tendency for younger, rather than older, people to be resettled from hospitals, typically moving into an independent residential setting.

— A picture emerged of a population of people highly vulnerable to enforced moves, both as a result of formal resettlement policy, and the coping difficulties of ageing families. In the period 1983–1988, a substantial majority will have moved their home.

2. Service Support

— Over half the people in touch with the CMHT had contact three times a year *or less*. People living alone or in group houses without 24-hour staffing received the majority of the CMHT's input; support was intensive for people who had been resettled from hospital to community.

— In many cases, individual programme plans were provided by residential staff, rather than by members of the CMHT. There was a very wide variation in the extent to which specific areas of activity were the subject of those plans.

— Activities counted as 'continuing education' included those designed to teach skills or impart knowledge; leisure and individual intervention programmes were specifically excluded. Overall, only 12 per cent of the population received any educational input.

— Service providers generally showed a concern with provision of leisure to members of this population. In particular, 90 per cent of the population were reported as going on day trips, although the frequency varied from several times a week to once or twice a year.

— Apart from Adult Training Centres (ATCs), the level of employment within the population was *extremely small*.

3. Medical, Para-Medical Services and Use of Aids

— The great majority of the population (88 per cent) had seen a GP in the past two years.

— A substantial proportion of the population (14 per cent) were reported as receiving psychiatric treatment.

— Hospital residents received a greater level of medical input and use of aids than people living in the community.

4. Informal Networks

Models of informal networks typically describe a continuum of informal care ranging through families, friends, neighbours and wider community contacts. The degree and nature of commitment decreases throughout the continuum. Results of this project were in accordance with this model.

— Contact with relatives was independent of a number of factors which might have been likely to demonstrate significant effects, including client's age, functional level, or category of residence.

— Unlike the findings for contact with relatives, patterns of friendship were found to be closely linked to residential category. People most likely to have a non-handicapped friend were those living in the community, or in group housing. In addition, people receiving services for the elderly population, rather than mental handicap services, were more likely to have non-handicapped friends.

5. Questionnaires

The questionnaires developed for the survey are intended for wider use. This study has shown that relevant information can be provided by those involved in services, and can be analysed in such a way that the pattern of services and the individuals' situations can be clearly defined. The questionnaires could now be refined and shortened in the light of the key factors emerging from our data analysis.

Researchers

James Hogg, Steve Moss, Michael Horne, Helen Prosser

Hester Adrian Research Centre, University of Manchester, Manchester M13 9PL (061 275 3340; FAX 061 275 3333)

Publications

Hogg, J., and Moss, S. (1987) 'Survey of people with Mental Handicap over 50 Years of Age: Version of Questionnaire for Use in the Community', University of Manchester, HARC.

Hogg, J., and Moss, S. (1987) 'Survey of People with Mental Handicap over 50 years of Age: Version of Questionnaire for Use in Hospital', University of Manchester, HARC.

Hogg, J., and Moss, S. (1989) 'A Demographic Study of Older People with Mental handicap in Oldham Metropolitan Borough, Part 2', University of Manchester, HARC.

Hogg, J., and Moss, S. C. (1992) 'The applicability of the Kaufman Assessment Battery for children (K-ABC) with older adults (50+ years) with mental retardation', *Journal of Mental Deficiency*.

Horne, M. (1989) 'A Demographic study of older people with mental handicap in Oldham Metropolitan Borough, Part 4', University of Manchester, HARC.

Horne, M. (1989) 'Identifying 'hidden' populations of older adults with mental handicap: Outreach in the UK', *Australian and New Zealand Journal of Development Disabilities*, **15**: 207–218.

Kiernan, C., and Moss, S. C. (1990) 'Behavioural and other characteristics of the population of a mental handicap hospital', *Mental Handicap Research*, **3**: 3–20.

Moss, S. C., Goldberg, D. P., Patel, P., and Wilkin, D. (1992) 'Physical morbidity in older people with moderate, severe and profound mental handicap, and its relation to psychiatric morbidity', *British Journal of Epidemiology and Community Health*.

Moss, S. C., and Hogg. J. (1989) 'A cluster analysis of support networks of older people with severe intellectual impairment', *Australian and New Zealand Journal of Development Disabilities*, **15**: 169–188.

Moss, S. C., and Hogg, J. (1992) 'A factorial and hierarchical cluster analysis of the Adaptive Behaviour Scales (Part I & II) in a population of older people (50+ years) with mental retardation', *Australian and New Zealand Journal of Developmental Disabilities*.

Moss, S. C., Hogg, J., and Horne, M. (1989) 'A Demographic Study of Older People with Mental Handicap in Oldham Metropolitan Borough, Part 2', University of Manchester, HARC.

Moss, S. C., Hogg, J., and Horne, M. (1992) 'Demographic characteristics of a population of people with severe mental handicap over 50 years of age: Age structure, IQ and adaptive skills', *Journal of Mental Deficiency Research*.

Moss, S. C., Hogg, J., and Horne, M. (1992) 'Individual characteristics and service support of older people with moderate, seer and profound learning disability with and without Community Mental Handicap Team support', *Mental Handicap Research*.

Moss, S., Simpson, N., and Hogg, J. (1988) 'A Demographic Study of Ageing and Elderly People with Mental Handicap: Physical and Mental Health Data Collection, A Research Proposal submitted to the DHSS', University of Manchester, HARC.

Prosser, H. (1989) 'A demographic study of older people with mental handicap in Oldham Metropolitan Borough, Part 3', University of Manchester, HARC.

Psychiatric and Physical Morbidity in Older People with Severe Learning Disabilities

Background

'PAS-ADD' instrument

Service planning

The broad aim of the project was to determine the mental health of a population of people over 50 years of age with severe learning disabilities and to relate this to their physical health and intellectual level. An additional aim was the development of an appropriate structured clinical interview as a response to the problems of detecting psychiatric symptoms in this population. This interview – the Psychiatric Assessment Schedule for Adults with a Development Disability (PAS-ADD) – is to undergo further clinical trials and refinements, leading to the eventual publication of the instrument and accompanying glossary.

The project studied a community sample of 105 people with severe learning disabilities over the age of 50 years, living in or originating from Oldham Metropolitan Borough. Although the majority of sample members were identified through mental handicap services, the sample also included people who were not in current contact, or had never been in contact with the Community Mental Handicap Team. An extensive outreach exercise ensured that almost 100 per cent of people fulfilling the age and ability criteria were included in the study.

All the physical and mental health assessments were carried out by a psychiatrist of senior registrar level. Psychiatric interviewing was conducted with both subjects and informants using the specifically modified semi-structured interview. Physical assessments used a combination of physical examination and informant interviewing.

Probable cases of dementia were identified by a combination of subject and informant interviewing, based on established clinical procedures. In addition, repeat assessments of functional behaviour were conducted on all suspected cases, enabling estimates to be made of cognitive and functional change occurring over a three-year period.

Findings

1. Psychiatric Morbidity

Twelve individuals out of a total sample of 105, were identified as psychiatric cases – an overall prevalence rate of 11.4 per cent excluding dementia. Most cases were of depression and anxiety.

Nine of these cases were *not* receiving appropriate treatment, but in the majority of cases the key informants were aware of the symptoms.

Table 5.1: *Diagnoses of the 12 Identified Psychiatric Cases*

Diagnosis	number of cases
Mania	1
Generalized anxiety disorder	2
Panic disorder with agoraphobia	1
Agoraphobia without panic attacks	1
Major depression	4
Major depression superimposed on long-standing panic disorder with agoraphobia	1
Depressive neurosis	1
Dysthymia	1
TOTAL	12

2. The Psychiatric Assessment Schedule

- Sixty-two per cent of the subjects were able to complete at least the 'core' items of the PAS-ADD (i.e. the items identified as the minimum necessary for case identification).
- Fifty per cent of the indentified psychiatric cases involved subjects who had *not* been able to give a fully adequate clinical interview.
- Only 50 per cent of the identified cases were detected by patient interview only, i.e. with no recourse to data from informants.

Table 5.2: *Physical Health of Subjects*

Physical disorder	no.	percentage
Hearing problem requiring aid	19	18.1
Eye disorder requiring medical treatment	24	22.9
Chronic respiratory disease	17	16.2
Cor pulmonale	2	1.9
Arthritis	53	50.5
Arthritis with restricted mobility	21	20.0
Hypertension	9	8.6
History of stroke/Cardio-Vascular Accident (CVA)	4	3.8
Congestive cardiac failure	5	4.8
Angina/Ischaemic heart disease	5	4.8
Epilepsy	16	15.2
Parkinson's disease	3	2.9
Drug-induced Parkinsonism	4	3.8
Tardive dyskinesia	3	2.9
Diabetes – Insulin dependent	3	2.9
Diabetes – Maturity onset	8	7.6
Biochemical hypothyroidism	5	4.8
Thyroid goitre	1	0.9
No disorder needing medical intervention	35	33.3

3. Dementia

Twelve cases of dementia were identified clinically and confirmed by assessments of change in functional ability over a three-year period – a prevalence rate of 11.4 per cent. People with Down's syndrome were particularly at risk, five of the nine individuals in the total being included in these 12 dementia cases.

Physical health was generally good, and comparable to non-handicapped people of the same age.

There was no relation found between *psychiatric and physical morbidity*.

CONCLUSION

Although there has been an increasing interest in the detection and diagnosis of psychiatric disorders in people with learning disabilities, there has been little progress in the development of objective criteria with which to guide these processes. This project focused on the development of instrumentation and the investigation of the performance of currently available diagnositc algorithms. The close attention to sampling and clinical information, coupled with the care taken to distinguish behaviour problems from genuine psychiatric disorders, lends confidence to the overall prevalence rates reported here. The detection of dementia – a particularly difficult task for the clinician – was aided by the availability of functional assessment data taken at two points in time, separated by a three-year gap.

Overall, the study supports the view that, with appropriate training and expertise, it is possible to undertake psychiatric interviewing with people whose development level is relatively low.

Although lower than in many published studies, a prevalence rate of 11.4 suggests a significant number of diagnosable psychiatric cases in this population, most of which (75 per cent) had not been drawn to the attention of specialist psychiatric services. In the majority of identified cases not receiving treatment, however, informants were aware of the problem; and this highlights the important role of care staff in the identification of potential psychiatric morbidity, and the need to provide them with adequate training to ensure that they make appropriate referrals.

Researchers

Steve Moss, David Goldberg, Neill Simpson, Pradip Patel

Hester Adrian Research Centre, University of Manchester, Manchester M13 9PL. (061 275 3340; FAX 061 275 3333)

Publications

Hogg, J., and Moss, S. (1989) 'A Demographic Study of Older People with Mental Handicap in Oldham Metropolitan Borough', University of Manchester, HARC.

Health Care Delivery to Residents of Community Facilities for People with Learning Disabilities – Preliminary Findings

Individuals with learning disabilities have the same health care needs as others, including the need for preventive care and treatment for acute and chronic illness. They also experience a greater number of health problems than the rest of the population. Many are dependent on others to monitor their health and ensure that they receive appropriate care: this is particularly the case where people cannot conceptualize or communicate their health problems.

GPs
Collaboration
Carers

This two-year study was designed to examine the delivery of health care, particularly primary health care, to people with learning disabilities living in the community. The study was based in one district health authority (Bristol and Weston health district) and focused on the following questions:

◆ How is health care organized for people with learning disabilities moving from hospital to the community?

◆ What are the health care needs of people with learning disabilities living in the community?

◆ Are there any differences between the health care needs of people with learning disabilities and the rest of the population?

◆ How effective is the service offered by the primary health care team and in particular, the GP, to people with learning disabilities?

◆ What part should preventive medicine play in services for people with learning disabilities?

The following findings are based on data relating to 90 people with learning disabilities. Analysis is not yet complete, and this summary is therefore partial and provisional.

GENERAL PRACTITIONERS

(1) Resettlement, and Contact with the Mental Handicap Services

(a) Very few GPs had been consulted about the resettlement of individuals from mental handicap hospitals to the community. Many would have liked the opportunity for some discussion of the practical implications of such changes.

(b) We asked GPs whether professionals working in the learning disability field were working with their patients and whether they had any contact with those professionals.

(c) Half the GPs thought that improvements could be made to the mental handicap services. The lack of communication between themselves and the services was cited most frequently as an area ripe for improvement. The need for the mental handicap services to have greater resources was also mentioned.

Table 5.3: *Number of Patients in Contact with Health or Social Services Professionals*

Consultant psychiatrist in mental handicap	20
Social Worker	15
Community Mental Handicap Nurse	8

Number of patients where GP and professional are in contact		How helpful GP finds contact	
		Very	Quite
Consultant	15	9	6
Social Worker	8	2	6
Community Mental Handicap Nurse	4	1	1

2. GP's Responsibilities and Skills

(a) GPs clearly felt that they were the most appropriate people to care for the medical needs of their patients with learning disabilities.

(b) Less than a quarter of GPs felt that they had any expertise in dealing with patients with learning disabilities. Their perception of expertise arose mainly from experiences as clinical assistants in mental handicap hospitals, voluntary work or through having relatives with learning disabilities.

(c) None of the GPs thought that their undergraduate medical training had provided them with any expertise, and only two mentioned postgraduate training in this context.

(d) Two-thirds of GPs thought that a caring attitude and an awareness of services was more important than training, when treating people with learning disabilities; whilst just under half the GPs agreed that they had sufficient numbers of such patients to justify training.

3. Consultations

(For comparative purposes, people with learning disabilities – 'subjects' – were matched with control patients of the same age and sex registered with the same GP.)

(a) More subjects than controls had consulted their GPs in the previous year. Thirty-five subjects and 36 controls had between one and four consultations in the previous year.

(b) The medical problems brought to the attention of GPs differed between subjects and controls. The subjects presented more diseases of the central nervous system, (usually epilepsy), more gastro-intestinal problems, (usually abdominal pain), more psychiatric problems and more skin problems, (usually eczema). The controls had more musculo-skeletal problems, especially back pain, and more gynaecological problems.

4. Health Promotion and Screening Services

(a) Forty per cent (31) of the sample were women, of whom 71 per cent were eligible to be invited to have a smear test. Virtually all controls had been given smear tests whilst very few subjects had. Reasons cited for not giving smear tests to subjects were their refusal to have the test, that they were not considered to be sexually active or that such a procedure would cause them unnecessary distress.

(b) Most women over 40 (both subjects and controls) had not been given breast palpation. Self-examination may not be an option for some women with learning disabilities, who may therefore have increased need for breast palpation from a GP.

(c) Slightly less than half the subjects, but just over two-thirds of controls, had had their blood pressure recorded over the previous five years.

(d) Nine subjects and 16 controls were known by GPs to be smokers. Four subjects and 13 controls received advice about giving up smoking from their GP. GPs did not have information about whether 28 subjects and 31 controls smoked or not.

(e) Half the subjects with Down's syndrome had been screened for atlanto-axial instability and half had been screened for thyroid function. Not all GPs considered screening for thyroid levels in patients with Down's syndrome to be appropriate.

5. Behavioural Difficulties or Problems During Examinations

(a) A small number of subjects presented behavioural problems during consultations or whilst waiting in the surgery. Problems in getting the patient to understand advice or have physical examinations were more common.

(b) Fewer than half the GPs thought that their practice had been affected by resettlement.

(c) Fewer than half the GPs thought that they should receive a higher capitation fee for looking after patients with learning disabilities.

CARERS

(Although we have collected information about 90 individuals, we only have information from 81 carers, since some subjects were living independently.)

(1) About two-thirds of carers were either satisfied or highly satisfied with all aspects of GPs' communication skills with subjects, and considered that the GPs treated their patients with learning disabilities with due respect.

(2) About one-third of carers thought that GPs needed guidance or help to improve the way in which they dealt with people with learning disabilities. Carers believed that the GPs needed to be more understanding of the needs and capabilities of people with learning disabilities. Fewer in this group were as satisfied with GPs' communication skills.

(3) About one-quarter of carers thought that subjects would benefit from health screening or health promotion, for example, a general health check, a smear test or breast screening. It is likely that their opinions about the need for these may have been stimulated by questions about the tests or procedures subjects had already received.

(4) Over half the carers had received some advice or training in dealing with the health or psychiatric problems of people with learning disabilities. These tended to be paid carers rather than informal carers such as relatives. Two-thirds of the carers who had not been given training or advice saw no need for any such guidance. More relatives than paid carers held this opinion.

THEMES FROM PRELIMINARY ANALYSIS

- Overall, GPs had little contact with professionals working in the learning disabilities services. They would clearly have liked greater involvement with those professionals.
- There were differences between subjects and controls in the type of medical problems they experienced and although fewer control patients had consulted their GPs in the previous year, they were more likely to be offered preventive health care.
- Carers were generally satisfied with the care GPs provided to individuals with learning disabilities, although further data analysis should provide answers about whether carers' satisfaction stemmed from a lack of knowledge of what constitutes good quality health care for people with learning disabilities.
- Although some patients with learning disabilities did present GPs with additional work, most GPs were willingly treating such people in the community.
- Future work will concentrate upon developing procedures within primary health care teams to ensure that health care needs are systematically monitored – for example, through the use of treatment guidelines. Raising awareness amongst individuals with learning disabilities and carers about the components of good health care, including preventive health care, would also be valuable.

Researchers

Joan Langan, Dr Oliver Russell, Dr Michael Whitfield

Norah Fry Research Centre, University of Bristol, 32 Tyndall's Park Road, Bristol BS8 1PY. (0272 238137)

Refining Measures of the Quality of Community Residence for People with Learning Disabilities

PROGRESS REPORT

Quality
measures
Choice
Inspection

Background

Concern about the quality of institutional care initiated a debate which has continued to the present over what is meant by the terms 'quality of care' and 'quality of life'. It also initiated a process of reform whereby community alternatives to hospital care have been provided, in the expectation that the quality of the service will be improved. The need to evaluate the changing design of residential services has resulted in a considerable number of attempts to define quality in measurable terms. The usefulness to service operation of defining and monitoring quality, so that staff have feedback on the level of achievement of the service has become recognized; and valid, practical and standardized ways of measuring quality will be required by the 'arms-length inspection units' set up under the new community care arrangements.

The project

The primary concern of this research is to investigate practical, yet systematic, measures to quantify the quality of residential services. It involves applying a number of quality measures, taken from the research literature, to 14 staffed community residences for adults with learning disabilities, over the course of two years. The selected measures represent a number of measurement approaches, including various interview scales and methods of establishing a direct record of activity. The scales we are using appear in figure 5.1.

Direct assessment of activity or behaviour has been adopted to ascertain the frequency and variety of social and community events, the level of participation of residents in daily life, staff interaction with residents and resident progress.

Measures have been selected which appear to relate to a number of dimensions that have gained broad acceptance as important to our understanding of service quality. These dimensions are the extent to which service users:

Figure 5.1: *Quality-Measurement Scales Used in the Project*

Index of Community Integration

Index of Participation in Domestic Life

Group Home Management Scale

Characteristics of the Treatment Environment Scale

Community-Oriented Program Environment Scale

Program Analysis of Service Systems

Physical Quality Scale

- have opportunities to experience ordinary community life and be part of the community they live in,
- are able to maintain a social network and enjoy a variety of social relationships,
- are able to participate in the full range of activities of ordinary life and to grow in experience and competence over time, and
- have opportunities for choice and are able to exercise choice.

The project aims to explore the correlation between measures, to establish what quality dimensions are being tapped, and to identify how practical and efficient they are. The end product will be a package of usable measurement approaches, which can be recommended to people monitoring or managing services.

The research will have a direct application to the strong emphasis given to monitoring and inspection in the new community care arrangements. Continued research on the determinants of the quality of services is also clearly relevant to the specification of contracts between purchaser and provider agencies. Further research which clarifies the connection between service design, the way services are operated and the eventual quality of outcome can help to shed light on the kind of relationship needed between purchasers and providers, as well as help those providers committed to quality to improve the services offered.

Researchers

Dr David Felce and Mr Jonathon Perry

Mental Handicap in Wales: Applied Research Unit, 55 Park Place, Cardiff CF1 3AT. (0222 226188; FAX 0222 641871)

Publications

Beswick, J., Zadlick, T., and Felce, D. (1987) *Evaluating Quality of Care*, Kidderminster, BIMH Conference Series.

Evans, G., Felce, D., and Hobbs, S. (1991) *Evaluating Service Quality*, Cardiff, Standing Conference of Voluntary Organizations.

Felce, D., and Evans, G. (1990) 'Assessing the quality of service outcomes: Refining a set of usable and valid measures applied to community residence', in D. Felce, and others (eds) *Research Proposals, 1990–1994*, Cardiff, Mental Handicap in Wales: Applied Research Unit.

Citizen Advocacy for People with a Learning Disability in Wales

Consumer
views
Volunteers

The 1990 NHS and Community Care Act implies the need to empower users, and to make provision on the basis of individual needs within a mixed economy of care. For many disabled and disadvantaged persons, the ability to exploit the opportunities of this system of provision will depend not only on their care managers, but also on the interest of other groups such as parents, friends and associates. Given that there may be a number of competing agendas amongst service-providing agencies, and parents and informal carers, it is important to ensure that the *voice of the user* is also heard.

Citizen advocates are volunteers who, working independently of direct service-providing agencies, provide long-term friendship and support, and practical help on a one-to-one basis to disabled and disadvantaged people. They aim to support the rights of their partners in their day-to-day social, recreational, health and other life spheres, by speaking up on their behalf as if their partner's problems were their own. There are presently five projects in Wales which seek to provide a citizen advocacy service for people with a learning disability, and a further project which is in the process of being set up.

This research is designed to examine the structures and processes of three elements of the citizen advocacy (CA) projects: the management committees, the work of the advocacy office, and the CA partnerships themselves.

Given the independence of the advocates from service-providing agencies, and their singular commitment to their partner, the research will also investigate how other groups, such as statutory service providers and family carers, have reacted to the citizen advocate. From a consideration of the structure and processes outlined above, an evaluation will then be made of the outcomes of the citizen advocacy input for the user; for example in terms of the growth of community integration for the user, the increase in life choices, improvements in their quality of life, the securing of relevant services, and the growth of their own ability to speak for themselves.

The five CA projects under study are:

(1) South Glamorgan
(2) Torfaen
(3) Bryn-y-Neuadd
(4) Montgomeryshire
(5) West Glamorgan

Primary findings

The methods of selecting users for CA differ between the projects. Citizen Advocacy in South Glamorgan had a number of prospective users, identified by a member of its steering group during the commissioning stages of the project; but contacting prospective users in the local hospital has proved more difficult. Torfaen

CA initially took one person from each of 12 villas in the local hospital and, through visits to a number of community establishments, has identified a number living in the community.

In contrast, the Bryn-y-Neuadd project was set up to provide not only a CA scheme, but also self-advocacy groups, two of which are now operational, and a professional advocacy service where the coordinators act as advocates themselves. More recently, this project has also set up a Users' Council, which has representation on the hospital's Management Group. With access to the hospital, the coordinators of this project use their knowledge of residents to identify potential partners. No referrals are taken and the identification of prospective users is left to the project coordinators: given the vast possible user-group, this process is inevitably rather hit or miss. The main reason for this is that there is a limit to the number of CA partnerships which can be supported by any one project. The Montgomeryshire CA project, which is funded through the hospital's resettlement programme, seeks to provide for those being resettled under this programme, and therefore has a 'ready-made' user-group. The West Glamorgan Lay Advocacy Project differs from the other four in a number of ways. Not only is it generically organized, but it also takes referrals from local voluntary groups.

Most projects have now been in operation for over two years. Two have 12 partnerships, one 16, and another 17. By contrast, the West Glamorgan project has provided support for 45 people during the past year, by moving away from the strict model of CA. The advocacy provided is designed to be primarily short-term and aimed at problem-solving, unless it is felt that the friendship and support element is specifically relevant. The citizen advocates are therefore 'recycled' to a number of users over a short time-period.

The projects' independence from statutory service-providing agencies remains a problem. At present, and despite the official policy intent that the projects should be set up through voluntary organizations, four of the projects are funded out of Strategy funds directed through social services county-planning groups. These groups will obviously hold allegiance to their own service providers, and this presents a possible conflict of interest and threat to the independent functioning of the CA projects.

Despite these difficulties, there is evidence that the CA input has, in some cases, quite radically affected the lives of its users. For example, after a family crisis and the recommendation of rehospitalization for one resettled user, the advocate was able to argue the case for keeping their partner out of hospital and, further, went on to organize this with other services. A number have benefited from increases in welfare benefit payments; others have been able to organize social activities in integrated community settings, which some partners now attend on their own, and there has been a strong presence of citizen advocates with their partners in meetings regarding future plans for service provision.

Researcher

Mr Paul Ramcharan

Centre for Social Policy Research and Development, University of Wales, Bangor, Gwynedd LL57 2DG. (0248 351151)

Publications

Ramcharan, P. (1991) *A PASS for the Welsh Citizen Advocacy Projects?*, Bangor, Centre for Social Policy Research and Development, University of Wales.

Day Services for Adults with Learning Disabilities: Changing Policies and the Evolution of Service Design

Integration

Supported employment

Policies on day services have, at different stages, emphasized occupation in the form of segregated contract work, training for competitive employment, continuing social education, work experience and involvement in community activities. Sheltered work was criticized for its monotony, low wages and total segregation. The move to a work-training function was criticized for its ineffectiveness. More recent attempts to develop a social and recreational curriculum have also failed to gain universal support. The primary role of large, segregated activity centres in the organization of day services has been a consistent feature throughout these changing emphases in policy; but a fundamental redesign of service infrastructure is now being debated.

Existing Services in Wales

The number of places in adult training centres, including special needs provision, rose from 2,997 in 1983 to 3,192 in 1988, with the average unit size decreasing from 81 to 76 places. There has been an increase in sessional attendance with a complementary expansion in alternative forms of day occupation, particularly opportunities for work experience and access to colleges of further education. A major survey of services in four districts in 1990 illustrates the predominance of centre provision. Four-fifths of adults in the sample who attended some day service did so at an adult training centre, social education centre, hospital day-centre or some other form of centre. A quarter of the adults received no day service, and only about one in ten was involved in some form of employment – either sheltered work, open employment or voluntary work. Colleges of further education were attended by 7 per cent of the adult sample, mostly on a part-time basis.

What do Adult Training/Social Education Centres Offer?

A survey of all centres (approximately 30) in Wales has shown the wide range of activities undertaken under the day-centre umbrella. Arts and crafts, personal development, sports and work experience each occupied between a quarter and a twelfth of the person-hours timetabled. However, there was great variation between centres in the extent of time given to each activity, as there was in how much time was spent by service users engaging in activities taking place within or away from the centre.

Figure 5.2: *A Typology of Day-Centres for Adults with Learning Disabilities*

Number of centres	Emphasis of centre
9	Arts & Crafts, then Sports and Personal Development
12	Personal Development and Arts and Crafts, then Sports
5	Mainly provided Contract Work, with Arts & Crafts
3	Work Experience and Outside Employment

The centres could be classified into a typology, based on the balance of activity.

This variation in emphasis of centres cannot be explained in terms of County policies, and must reflect differences in orientation, persuasion and experience of local day-service staff. The All-Wales Mental Handicap Strategy suggested that variety of day-service alternatives may be a means of promoting individual choice and the flexibility to match service delivered to individual need; the variation from centre to centre found in the survey should not be confused with choice. There appears to be little consensus over what options may be most beneficial to service users; and this implies the need for clearer, higher-level policies on the purposes and nature of day services.

Supported Employment

Supported Employment services differ from traditional provision in that systematic steps are taken to find a pool of real, entry-level job vacancies: these are then matched with people with disabilities needing jobs. The person begins work with support and structured training on the job from a job coach. This support is gradually phased out as the individual learns to do the job independently, or with the help of colleagues. Supported Employment is focused on achieving real employment in ordinary workplaces, where people with disabilities work alongside their peers and earn regular payment for the job.

Our research on day services includes an action programme to establish and evaluate a Supported Employment service in Cardiff, in collaboration with purchasing and provider agencies. The service – QUEST – was established in 1991 with a coordinator and the equivalent of two-and-a-half job coaches. Currently, seven people are supported in part-time or full-time employment and the service is about to expand with the addition of a specialist job finder and a further two job coaches. The evaluation will describe processes, and compare outcomes with those achieved in existing day services. Measures collected will include intensity and length of job coach involvement; task attainment; hours worked; payment earned; level of integration of the worker with a disability in the workplace; employer satisfaction; family satisfaction; the individual's satisfaction and their involvement in purposeful activity. A number of other similar schemes are in operation in England and Wales and the research unit is collaborating in a national survey to establish a database of services involved in supporting people in open employment. This will provide a means of tracking the development of this emerging service form.

The Future of Day Services

Further changes in the nature and design of day services can be expected, with a new emphasis on employment through the expansion of supported employment projects, small businesses and other collaborative ventures between the commercial and service worlds. The new arrangements for contracting services will be implemented in an area which is itself changing. Purchaser agencies will need to be aware of and learn from successful local initiatives throughout the country. There are opportunities under the new arrangements for the stimulation of a variety of provider agencies, the creation of genuine choice, and the ability – through systems of care-management – to match day services more closely to individual needs and preferences. Opportunities also exist for the separation of the multiple functions of existing day services, and the specification of separate contracts for different service components – perhaps with several specialist provider agencies. This will enable purchaser agencies to be more specific in each contract about the quality of the contracted service, and this in turn will clarify the basis for monitoring service quality.

Researchers

Dr Stephen Beyer, Mr Mark Kilsby and Dr David Felce

Mental Handicap in Wales: Applied Research Unit, 55 Park Place, Cardiff CF1 3AT. (0222 226188; FAX 0222 641871)

Publications

Beyer, S. (1991) 'Employment and People with a Mental Handicap', in R. Jenkins (ed.), *Changing Approaches to Mental Handicap*, Occasional Paper No 23, Swansea, University College of Swansea School of Social Studies.

Beyer, S., and Kilsby, M. (1992) *What do ATCs Offer? A Survey of Welsh Day Services*, Cardiff, Mental Handicap in Wales: Applied Research Unit.

Beyer, S., Todd, S., and Felce, D. (1991) 'The implementation of the All-Wales Mental Handicap Strategy, 1983–1988', *Mental Handicap Research*, **4**, 2: 115–140

Lowe, K., Beyer, S., Kilsby, M., and Felce, D. (in press) 'Activities and engagement in day services for people with a mental handicap', *Journal of Intellectual Disability Research* (also available as a report from Mental Handicap in Wales: Applied Research Unit, Cardiff).

Comprehensive Community-Based Ordinary Housing Services for Adults with the Most Severe or Profound Learning Disabilities:
Lessons from the Andover Project, and the Evaluation of NIMROD

Two projects in the early 1980s tested whether it would be feasible to provide ordinary living in the community for adults with the most severe or profound learning disabilities, including people with severely challenging behaviour. The evaluation of the projects centred on comparing the benefits and costs of the new housing services with existing forms of residential care.

Challenging behaviour

Costs

Outcomes

The Houses and the Residents

Two 8-place houses, each occupied during the initial years by only six people, were established in Andover to serve adults with the greatest levels of handicap or challenging behaviour requiring a service, from a catchment area with a total population of 60,000. Five 4- to 6-place houses and one group of three flats for five people were set up within the NIMROD service to cater for a wider group from a similarly-sized catchment area in Cardiff. Houses were ordinary residential properties, and normal domestic standards and characters were maintained. Each house was intensively staffed to match the level of disability of residents, with the ratio of residents to total staff establishment averaging approximately 1:1.7.

The Andover houses served 14 people during the three-year evaluation period. At admission, all needed help to feed, wash or dress, and most lacked language or had command of a few words only. Nine (64 per cent) had some form of severely challenging behaviour, with an average of more than four different types of problem behaviour per person. About half of the NIMROD residents were similarly severely handicapped but the other half could feed, wash and dress independently. Just over half could speak in sentences. Fourteen of the 22 people who moved from hospital (64 per cent) had severely challenging behaviours, with an average of three different types of behaviour problem per person. Most residents of both schemes had many years of institutional care behind them and some moved straight from specially designated wards or facilities for people with the most challenging behaviour.

Working Methods and Staff Training

Although the emphasis was on ordinary living, both services were organized in a structured way, based on behavioural psychology principles and practice. Set ways of working were developed for staff to follow, which covered how to implement individual programming, teach, organize activities, support resident involvement and monitor outcome. Staff were given tailor-made induction and in-service training on the use of these methods, which were also documented in a handbook or procedural guide.

Benefits and Costs

The evaluation of benefits focused on the level of resident involvement in daily activities; the level of interaction among staff and residents; the development of skills; the level of family and friendship contact; and, the extent of community integration. Taking the results of the Andover and NIMROD research together, there is good evidence that house residents made significantly better progress in skills than comparison groups did, in hospital or family homes. There were greater opportunities and support for participation in household, leisure and social activities than in hospital or larger community units. Staff–resident interaction was significantly greater in the houses. Family and friendship contact was significantly greater for those residents moving back to be near families from distant hospitals; but there were no significant differences when compared with other local but larger settings. However, house residents used community amenities significantly more than comparison groups did, in hospitals or larger community units, even though some of these facilities were based in the community.

Formal evaluation of the impact of the services on challenging behaviour was not undertaken in the Andover houses, and research on the NIMROD houses gives no evidence of challenging behaviours reducing. In fact, a higher proportion of people were reported as having challenging behaviours at the end of the evaluation period than at the beginning, which is consistent with research demonstrating the chronicity of such behaviour. Nonetheless, both services showed a capability to cope with people with the most challenging behaviours.

The costs of the Andover houses were compared with those for two hospitals and several larger community units. All settings were operated by District Health Authorities within Wessex and standard cost returns were used to compare expenditure in 1984–85. The large community units were, on average, cheapest at £11,330 per person per year, compared with the average for the two hospitals of £13,514 and that for the two houses of £15,283. Greater staff costs in the houses compared with the hospitals were partly offset by economies in administrative, utility and estate management costs. Moreover, house costs were below the average for the two hospitals when occupancy levels were taken into account. Annual costs per place averaged £12,246 for the hospitals, £9,905 for the larger community units and £11,611 for the houses. Some account should also be taken of the higher average dependency of the house residents compared with the total hospital population. NIMROD house costs ranged from £18,883 to £26,009 per person per year at 1986/87 prices, inclusive of DSS benefits and externally arranged day-care. Direct comparability with the Andover data is difficult because of differences in how cost estimates were derived. However, it is possible to show that average staff costs per person were equivalent between the schemes after taking appropriate account of cost inflation. Staff costs are a high proportion of total costs in intensively staffed residential provision; the NIMROD evaluation therefore lends support to the earlier conclusion that the costs of community housing for people with severe or profound learning disabilities can be approximately similar to those in existing hospitals.

Service Design and Costs in Relation to Quality

The slightly higher-costing community housing services have been convincingly shown across a number of measures to produce better outcomes than hospital or larger community unit provision. Staffed, ordinary housing is not only a feasible option – it produces beneficial outcomes in a way that can be described as cost-effective.

However, it is important to remember that both services laid great emphasis on designing working methods to make high-quality staff performance more likely and thus achieve beneficial outcomes for residents. It cannot be assumed that similar outcomes, or the ability to cope with people with severely challenging behaviour will be a feature of all community housing services unless *equal care is taken in their design*. The methods of working, training and monitoring, as well as the basic structure of the service must be replicated if the quality demonstrated within these two projects is also to be repeated.

As early examples of staffed housing services, the Andover and NIMROD houses are larger than many which have been provided since. The costs of these larger ordinary housing schemes compared fairly favourably with average hospital costs. However, still smaller services may involve higher staff–client ratios, and therefore higher staff costs per person.

This and other research demonstrates the variation in cost within both community provision and hospitals – a variation which is not always possible to explain by reference to client needs or the quality of outcome. The rather arbitrary judgements which often determine staffing levels in services may be the explanation. Research on the relationship of staff–client ratios to patterns of care and resident activity, conducted as part of the Andover and NIMROD evaluations, suggests that services which allocate increasingly higher levels of staffing will not necessarily achieve a higher standard of quality. Instead, **the key is to secure the best return from the investment in staff by attention to specific working methods, effective staff training and effective monitoring and management**.

CONCLUSION

The research underpins and validates the broad direction of the care in the community policy in terms of providing locally available, community-based housing for the vast majority of people with severe learning disabilities, including those with severely challenging behaviours, who previously have had residential care in long-stay hospitals. The determinants of quality and outcome for services like these are complex, and go beyond the obvious factors included in traditional service planning. This, in turn, has considerable implications for the nature of service planning and the detail required in future contracts between purchaser and provider agencies.

Researchers

Dr David Felce and Ms Kathy Lowe

Mental Handicap in Wales: Applied Research Unit, 55 Park Place, Cardiff CF1 3AT. (0222 226188)

Publications

A bibliography of over 30 publications on the NIMROD and Andover Project research can be obtained from the above researchers.

Felce, D. (1988) 'Behavioural and social climate in community group residences', in M. P. Janicki, M. W. Krauss, and M. M. Seltzer (eds), *Community Residences for Persons with Development Disabilities: Here to Stay*, Baltimore, Paul H Brookes.

Felce, D. (1989) *The Andover Project*, Kidderminster, BIMH Publications.

Felce, D. (1991) 'Using behavioural principles in the development of effective housing services for adults with severe or profound mental handicaps', in R. Remington (ed.), *The Challenge of Severe Mental Handicap: a Behaviour Analytic Perspective*, Chichester, John Wiley and Sons.

Felce, D., Lowe, K., and de Paiva, S. (in press) 'Ordinary housing for people with severe learning disabilities and challenging behaviours', in E. Emerson, P. McGill, and J. Mansell (eds), *Severe Learning Disabilities and Challenging Behaviour: Designing Quality Services* London, Chapman and Hall.

Felce, D., Repp, A. C., Thomas, M., Ager, A., and Blunden, R. (1991) 'The relationship of staff : client ratios, interactions, and residential placement', *Research in Developmental Disabilities*, **12**, 3: 315–331.

Lowe, K., and de Paiva, S. (1991) *NIMROD: An Overview*, London, HMSO.

Domiciliary Support Services for People with Severe Learning Disabilities: Lessons from the NIMROD Evaluation and Research on Family Aide Schemes in Wales

The majority of people with severe learning disabilities live with their families and continue to do so far longer into adulthood than is typical for the general population. Community care policy has highlighted the vital role parents play as carers, and emphasized the provision of effective support to individuals in their own localities and homes. Researchers and practitioners have long recognized the importance of the informal support which families with handicapped members may receive from their communities or relatives: domiciliary support services can be seen as a supplement or substitute for this.

Carers
Family aides
Service planning

Models for domiciliary support services in a variety of areas have existed for some time, and elements of all of these approaches can be seen in the domiciliary support services for families and individuals with learning disabilities developed in Wales in the last decade. They are an extremely popular form of service with families and, despite their rapid expansion, provision may still be at a lower level than families would prefer.

NIMROD Community Care Workers

An early example of domiciliary support was established in the NIMROD service: two community care workers worked with people living in family homes in each neighbourhood of approximately 15,000 total population. The original idea was that the workers would focus on teaching skills to people of all ages. They quickly, however, moved on to a wide range of other tasks including accompanying individuals to appointments, classes and social activities; supporting their use of amenities in the local community; and teaching skills outside the home.

The Growth of Family Aide Services in Wales

Domiciliary support services have become widespread in Wales, growing rapidly from 41 individuals/families served in 1983 to 1,840 by 1988. Three-quarters of the families received support from workers organized in teams varying in size from 5 to 60 members. Each team supported between 7 and 90 families, and each worker was involved with between 2 and 12 clients. No set management arrangements for these new services has yet emerged: workers are predominantly female, and pay and conditions are typical of low status employment. Arrangements like these create the impression that the service is still marginal in terms of service agency priorities.

Operation of Domiciliary Support Services

The work undertaken by support workers covers four main areas:

— providing assistance to carers by working directly with the person with a disability in the home;

— providing respite to carers by taking the family member with a disability out, or by offering a sitting-in service;

— promoting independence of the individual with a disability by structured teaching and by providing opportunities to use everyday self-help, social, community, domestic or leisure skills; and

— encouraging integration by accompanying the person with a disability to a range of community amenities or events.

In practice, these tasks are not mutually exclusive; but may have conflicting priorities. One focus is on providing support and respite to carers, another is to broaden the experience and aid the development of the individual with a learning disability. The role of the support worker is not clear cut and expectations concerning the function of the service may differ between different parties. The particular difficulties encountered by workers may point to the need for greater specialization, as well as for a higher status, better paid and better trained workforce.

Effective ways of targeting domiciliary support services have still to be developed: a process for assessment of need and individualized care-management is essential. Current evidence suggests that individual planning is routinely undertaken for **only a third** of potential clients in Wales, and it is not clear on what basis support workers are deployed. When the resource first became available, there was a tendency to offer it on demand rather than in relation to eligibility criteria or extent of need. Appropriate targeting may also be undermined by using support workers to plug gaps in the service system – for example, by providing additional activities for people in residential care, or working with people attending day services.

Evaluation of Domiciliary Support Services

The NIMROD evaluation showed that the provision of the community care worker service had a small impact on the rate of skill acquisition and the use of community amenities by individuals with disabilities. Both increased slightly more than for a comparison group who received no domiciliary service. However, the difference in the scale of change was not great – a result which was in keeping with the relatively low level of the intervention. Research in Wales more generally has shown such services to be very popular with families: both families and clients saw them as contributing new opportunities, and a source of companionship. There were criticisms from parents concerning the availability and continuity of services, but these further emphasize how welcome such services are, and there is still considerable scope for expansion.

It is not known whether the greater availability of domiciliary support extends family home care, and lowers the requirement for residential provision.

More detailed evaluation of family aide services has involved direct observation of sessions. Those directed towards support or respite for carers were clearly meeting their aims. Support workers have a clear assignment to fit into the family routine and substitute for the primary parental carer, doing whatever needs to be done in much the same way as the parent would have done it. However, less evidence of success was found for sessions where the purpose was to promote development of community integration. These are ambitious goals, and support workers were often given very little guidance about how to set about achieving them. Domiciliary support services are currently providing an excellent source of help to families, but may be achieving little in terms of changing the fundamental situation of the individual with a disability.

Researchers

Ms Kathy Lowe, Dr Stephen Beyer, Mr Stuart Todd, Mr Gerry Evans and Dr David Felce

Mental Handicap in Wales: Applied Research Unit, 55 Park Place, Cardiff CF1 3AT. (0222 226188)

Publications

Beyer, S., Todd, S., and Felce, D. (1991) 'The implementation of the All-Wales Mental Handicap Strategy, 1983–1988', *Mental Handicap Research*, **4**, 2: 115–140.

de Paiva, S., and Lowe, K. (1988) *Community Care Workers Part 3*, Cardiff, Mental Handicap in Wales: Applied Research Unit.

Evans, G. (1989) *A Review of the North Powys Family Aide Service*, Cardiff, Mental Handicap in Wales: Applied Research Unit.

Evans, G. (1989) *Providing Support to individuals at Home and in their Locality*, Cardiff, Mental Handicap in Wales: Applied Research Unit.

Evans, G., Felce, D., de Paiva, S., and Todd, S. (1992) 'Observing the delivery of a domiciliary support service', *Disability, Handicap and Society*, **7**, 1: 19–34. (A fuller account is also available as a report from the Mental Handicap in Wales: Applied Research Unit, Cardiff, under the title 'An observational study of domiciliary support services'.)

Evans, G., Todd, S., Beyer, S., Felce, D., and Perry, J. (1992) *Assessing the Impact of the All-Wales Mental Handicap Strategy: A Survey of Four Districts*, Cardiff, Mental Handicap in Wales: Applied Research Unit.

Humphreys, S., Lowe, K., and de Paiva, S. (1986) *Community Care Workers Part 1*, Cardiff, Mental Handicap in Wales: Applied Research Unit.

Lowe, K., de Paiva, S., and Humphreys, S. (1987) *Community Care Workers Part 2*, Cardiff, Mental Handicap in Wales: Applied Research Unit.

Lowe, K., and de Paiva, S. (1991) *NIMROD: An Overview*, London, HMSO.

Aggressive Behaviour by People with Learning Disabilities

The project was conducted in two stages: the aim of the first stage was to document the nature, extent and circumstances of aggressive behaviour among people with learning disabilities; the second stage was concerned with evaluating the effectiveness of services and interventions.

Challenging behaviour

Service evaluation

Consumer views

Stage 1 – the Nature, Extent and Circumstances

A survey was conducted in a single health district with a general population of about 370,000. At the time of the survey, the mental handicap register for the district recorded 1,362 people as having a learning disability.

The survey identified 168 people as presenting aggressive behaviour, of whom 26 were pupils attending school. Given the available base-population data, the overall prevalence rate of aggressive behaviour for people with learning disabilities from the district was 17.6 per cent. The lowest rate was identified amongst day facilities (9.7 per cent) and the highest in hospitals within the district (38.2 per cent). The prevalence rate amongst those attending schools for children with severe learning disabilities was 12.6 per cent.

Range and Incidence of Aggressive Behaviour

Sixty-nine per cent of the 168 people identified were said to have engaged in at least one act of physically aggressive behaviour during the past month. Hitting-out at others (i.e. 'punching/slapping/pulling people') was the most frequently reported type of behaviour, about half the group were said to have engaged in this type of interaction during the past month. There was a much lower incidence of behaviour such as biting (12.6 per cent) head-butting (7.1 per cent) and using weapons (6.5 per cent).

Table 5.4: *Frequency of Aggressive Behaviour*

Behaviour	Past month %
Hitting	50.6
Kicking	23.4
Pinching	21.4
Scratching	20.2

Details of other types of challenging behaviour were also collected and it was found that self-injury, withdrawn, stereotypical and ritualistic behaviours were also common (table 5.5).

Table 5.5: *Frequency of Other Challenging Behaviours*

Behaviour	Past month %
Self-injury	35.7
Withdrawn	38.1
Stereotypical	36.3
Ritualistic	35.1

Injury to Others

Table 5.6 shows the number of people involved in incidents resulting in injury to others. About 40 per cent of the group had never injured anyone. On the other hand, serious injuries (requiring medical attention) and very serious injuries (resulting in stays in hospital or certified absences from work) were accounted for by eight people. It was clear that two of these people no longer presented problems of aggression, and the last serious incident had occurred a number of years ago. The six remaining people were reported to have been involved in recent incidents resulting in severe injury to another person.

Table 5.6: *Number of People Involved in Incidents Resulting in Injury to Others*

	N	%
No injury	67	39.9
Minor injury	45	26.8
Moderate injury	48	28.6
Serious injury	6	3.5
Very serious injury	2	1.2
	168	100.0

CONCLUSIONS

The number of people who were reported as presenting aggressive behaviour was quite high; however, the risk of a serious injury to another person was low. Six people were identified as having been involved in recent incidents which resulted in severe injury. They represented less than one per cent of the total population of people with learning disabilities from the district.

The people identified as presenting serious problems of aggression tended to have a long history of challenging behaviour. Traumatic life-events, lack of control over their environment, insecurity and anxiety were hallmarks of their development. Aggressive behaviour often began during early childhood, tended to become more unmanageable in the teenage years and continued into adulthood. In the past, they have usually been referred to secure accommodation in hospital settings. This approach contained the problem, but offered few opportunities for satisfactory development for the individuals concerned.

The research found little evidence of demand for more secure accommodation: instead, there was seen to be a need for new and effective services within community settings. A crucial task for these services would be to intervene early to develop the person's adaptive skills, increase his/her quality of life and reduce aggressive behaviour.

The research at this stage suggested that the causes and maintenance of aggressive behaviour are inextricably bound up with the person's quality of life. In general, supportive, compensatory and normalizing environments help to eliminate aggressive behaviour, whereas deprived, stressed and poorly stimulated circumstances tend to exacerbate early difficulties.

Stage 2 – Evaluating Services and Interventions

This stage had three parts. The first was a detailed study of the progress of four people with very challenging behaviour and the services which support them. The second part was a follow-up study of five people with aggressive behaviour who moved from a hospital to a community setting. The final part was a pilot study evaluating the effect of communication training for three people with severe communication difficulties and aggressive behaviour.

Measuring progress

The effectiveness of services and intervention procedures was evaluated by measuring not only changes in the frequency, severity and management difficulty of aggressive behaviour but also the effect on other behaviour, for example, adaptive skills, as well as the person's quality of life. The degree of personal and organizational support available to staff working in these services was also measured.

Preliminary findings

Initial analyses of the data have suggested the following general findings:—

1. Progress for service users must be defined in terms of quality of life and development of adaptive skills, as well as changes in aggressive behaviour. The project findings indicate that *service users were more likely to make progress in community rather than hospital settings*. There were clear indications that life experiences were much reduced in hospital settings and that there were fewer opportunities to use and develop adaptive skills. In some cases, there was a marked reduction in aggressive behaviour after relocation from hospital to the community. In other cases, the frequency and severity of aggression did not appear to change significantly, but staff in the new settings were less likely to perceive the behaviour as presenting major management problems. There was little evidence of increases in aggressive behaviour after transferring to a community setting. Participation in decision-making and control over events by service users appeared to be important factors in making progress.

2. Progress is most likely to take place in environments which are *responsive to the needs and wants of service users*. Staff were found to be the most important resource in this respect: adequate numbers, appropriate training and sufficient staff support were all necessary. The research suggested that staff were likely to be more satisfied and less stressed at work if they were clear about their roles, received regular and specific feed-back about their performance, and had guidelines about what to do if something went wrong. The availability of practical help in crisis situations and having someone to talk to in times of difficulty were found to be important.

3. The research indicated the necessity of clearly distinguishing between *crisis interventions* and interventions designed to bring about individual development. Crisis interventions are simply emergency procedures which provide sufficient and temporary control of dangerous situations to ensure that no one gets hurt. They should not be seen as a substitute for more positive measures.

4. Interventions designed to bring about a *wide variety* of (sometimes unspecified) changes were more evident in practice than were *single interventions* designed to bring about specific changes in aggressive behaviour. They included the relocation of individuals from hospital to community settings, increased opportunity for choice, greater access to preferred events, skills training and staff training. The focus was on changes in lifestyle with the intention of increasing positive behaviour and decreasing aggression. Psychotropic drugs were used in both community and hospital settings. There was little evidence of agreed, written behaviour-modification programmes, but where they were in use they were focused on the development of skills, rather than the reduction of aggressive behaviour. Other types of intervention included the use of relaxation, massage and the use of Snoezelen-type sensory rooms.

5. Controlled conditions are required to demonstrate the effectiveness of single interventions. The relationship between communication and aggressive behaviour was the focus of a pilot study. Existing research has demonstrated an inverse relationship between communicative ability and the level of challenging behaviour. There is some evidence that aggressive behaviour can be reduced through communication training. Whereas most of the intervention work in this area has focused on the person's *expressive skills*, by developing new ways to communicate needs and wants, the pilot study suggested that *receptive communication skills* are also important in understanding aggressive behaviour and in bringing about change.

Researcher

Philip Harris

Norah Fry Research Centre, University of Bristol, 32 Tyndall's Park Road, Bristol BS8 1PY. (0272 238137)

Now at: Faculty of Health and Community Studies, Cardiff Institute of Higher Education, Llandaff Centre, Western Avenue, Cardiff CF5 2YB. (0222 578084)

Publications

Clarke-Kehoe, A., and Harris, P. (1992) '. . . it's the way that you say it', *Community Care*, 9 July, 21–22.

Emerson, E., Cambridge, P., and Harris, P. (eds) (1991) *Evaluating the Challenge. A guide to evaluating services for people with learning difficulties and challenging behaviour*, London, King's Fund.

Harris, P. (in press) 'The nature and extent of aggressive behaviour amongst people with learning difficulties (mental handicap) in a single health district', *Journal of Intellectual Disability Research*.

Harris, P., Humphreys, J., and Thomson, G. (submitted) 'A Checklist of Challenging Behaviour: assessing aggressive behaviour attributed to people with learning difficulties', *Mental Handicap Research*.

Harris, P., and Russell, O. (1989) 'The nature of aggressive behaviour among people with learning difficulties (mental handicap) in a single health district: second report', University of Bristol, Norah Fry Research Centre.

Harris, P., and Russell, O. (1989) 'The prevalence of aggressive behaviour among people with learning difficulties (mental handicap) in a single health district: interim report', University of Bristol, Norah Fry Research Centre.

Harris, P., and Russell, O. (1990) 'Aggressive behaviour among people with learning difficulties – the nature of the problem', in A. Dosen, A. van Gennep and G. J. Zwanikken (eds), *Treatment of Mental Illness and Behavioural Disorder in the Mentally Retarded*, Leiden, The Netherlands, Logan Publications, 367–374

Harris, P., and Russell, O. (1990) 'Rising to the challenge? The lives of five people with very challenging behaviour: third report', University of Bristol, Norah Fry Research Centre.

Harris, P., and Russell, O. (1992) 'How to meet a challenge', *The Health Service Journal*, 8 October, 28–29.

Harris, P., and Thomson, G. (accepted) 'The Staff Support Questionnaire: a means of measuring support among staff working with people with challenging behaviour', *Mental Handicap*.

Harris, P., Thompson, G., and Russell, O. (1992) 'An evaluation of services for four people with learning difficulties and aggressive behaviour: final report', University of Bristol, Norah Fry Research Centre.

Harris, P., and Thorp, C. (submitted) 'Staff support groups: an antidote for stress', *Community Living*.

Knowles, J., and Harris, P. (1991) 'Shifting the focus – new ways of working with people with learning difficulties and challenging behaviour', *Community Care*, 4 April, 20–22.

Behaviour Problems Project

Introduction

Self-injury
Staff stress
Collaboration

The programme had *four inter-related components*. First, an epidemiological survey was undertaken across seven representative health districts in the area covered by the North Western Regional Health Authority. This first stage was designed to identify all people aged 5 or more years who were using, or were excluded from, mental handicap services and who showed behaviour problems to the extent that additional resources were consumed by, or required for, their care.

Three related studies complemented the epidemiological data: first, a study of policy and practice across the Districts consisting of the analysis of documents and interviews with managers in relevant health and local authorities; second, a study of the experiences and views of parents caring at home for young adults who showed behaviour problems; third, a small number of qualitative case studies which focused on particular individuals and the care system which surrounded them. More detailed reports on all these studies are available: this summary will concentrate on the main findings.

Rates

The epidemiological survey investigated the numbers of people who were administratively defined as having learning disabilities, **and** who showed behaviour problems such that additional resources were required for, or already consumed by, their care.

In all, 701 people were identified. One in four were aged 19 or less; the remaining three-quarters were equally divided into adults living in the community and adults living in hospital. Half of those identified were between the ages of 15 and 30. Nine people were identified who were excluded from services.

The probability that a person would be living in the community, and – in particular – in the family home, decreased very sharply with increasing age. Fifty-eight per cent of those over 25 years old were living in hospital, compared with 25 per cent of adults aged 19 to 25. Over two-thirds of children (68 per cent) lived in their family home, but less than half (46 per cent) of young adults lived at home, and only one in eight of those aged over 26 lived at home. Around one-third of adults living away from home had little or no contact with their families. No one under 18 was found in hospital, although a small minority (7.4 per cent) were out-District placements.

Characteristics

The majority of the population identified were mobile (around 90 per cent) with good sensory abilities and relatively low prevalence of epilepsy. However, their communication skills were highly variable: around 40 per cent were reported as having good communication skills. The non-mobile group were likely to have additional impairments and epilepsy. They were also likely to have poor communication skills.

A minority (14.7 per cent of adults and 6.8 per cent of children) were said to have been diagnosed as suffering from a psychiatric disorder. The overwhelming majority of people with psychiatric disorders were mobile and had good communication skills. Difficulties were reported in gaining access to community-based psychiatric services.

Behaviour problems

The most common serious behaviour problems reported overall were physical attacks (23.2 per cent), non-compliance (22.8 per cent), and temper tantrums (20.9 per cent). Self-injury was shown by 17.2 per cent of adults and 12.9 per cent of children.

Table 5.7: *Serious Management Problems Among Mobile Adults*

Communication skills	Problems (in order of prevalence)
Good	verbal abuse (27.6 per cent); temper tantrums, non-compliance, anti-social behaviours and physical attacks (24.0 per cent)
Poor	physical attacks (24.8 per cent); destructive behaviour, temper tantrums, self-injury, and non-compliance (17.2 per cent)
None	self-injury (23.8 per cent); physical attacks, destructive behaviour, non-compliance and eating non-food objects (19 per cent)

Self-injury was by far the most common management problem in the non-mobile group (40.5 per cent), followed by physical attacks, verbal abuse, smearing, and non-compliance (9.5 per cent). It is important to note that, for mobile people, *over half* were reported as having more than one serious management problem.

Similar patterns were shown by children and young people up to the age of 19 years.

Consequences of Behaviour Problems

Disruption caused by problem behaviour lasted up to an hour or longer for over 50 per cent of the population. Staff were often involved in calming other clients, and – in 50 per cent of cases – the disruptive individual was excluded from group activities at least once.

For around one-third of the group, problem behaviour was seen as the main factor preventing their transfer to a less restrictive setting. However, for around half of people where relocation was felt to be desirable, staff felt that this should be to a more intensive treatment setting.

The commonest causes of *staff stress* were that behaviour problems were very wearing over time (88.6 per cent); they lowered the quality of life for others (78.7 per cent); and there were no effective ways of dealing with them (72.5 per cent).

Service responses

Although it is policy in the North Western Region for all people with mental handicap to have *Individual Programme Plans*, only around 40 per cent of this population of people with behaviour problems were reported as having such plans. A further 27 per cent had 'some written plans'. Around one-third of adults and half of the children and young people identified were said to be subject to *behaviour modification programmes*. Such programmes were more likely to be reported for individuals showing a range of serious and controlled problems.

Adults living in hospital were more likely to be given anti-psychotic drugs (63 per cent), than those in hostels (43 per cent), or with their families (28 per cent). *Variations in prescription practices* between different districts suggest the need for further investigation.

Service responses to people with severe problem behaviour across districts vary considerably in their use of *community-based services*, with some districts making much greater use of hospital care, both for people with learning disabilities in general, and for people showing behaviour problems. The presence or absence of a long-stay hospital in the district, and the state of development of community-based services, including the degree of progress on the settlement are important factors. There was evidence from all aspects of the research programme of the existence of a *two-tier service*, with people who had never been admitted to hospital, especially those remaining in their family home, relatively deprived in terms of services, compared with those who had been discharged from hospital.

The epidemiological study suggests that, over the next few years, a number of factors will combine to produce increasing demands on community-based services from people with problem behaviour. **All parts of the research programme cast considerable doubt on the capacity of existing community services to respond adequately to additional numbers.** Even in terms of conventional provision there was a considerable shortage of long-term and short-term residential care in the community for adults with behaviour problems and a need for more and better-structured day-care services. Voluntary and private sector provision was minimal. Service managers suggested that when there was low availability of residential accommodation, 'less problematic' clients were preferred; that lack of residential accommodation could lead to challenging behaviour in the home; and that priority access to special services led to problem clients being 'clumped' and reduced service quality.

Parental Perspectives

Interviews with parents suggested that almost all of the young adults will eventually become the *entire responsibility of the formal sector*. The majority of parents (87 per cent) felt that they had never received useful advice from professionals on handling behaviour problems at home, and substantial numbers believed that professionals had no real conception of the problems they faced.

Psychological distress in mothers was found to be related to factors which were distinct from those which led them to want to give up caring. Improvements in services designed to reduce *psychological distress* should concentrate on relieving the 'daily grind' of extra domestic work and night-time disturbance. The desire to give up might be reduced by services which would enable parents to make up for some of the costs of caring – lost employment for mothers, financial costs and foregone social activities.

Planning for the Future

On average across the seven districts, there were 32 people aged between 15 and 30 identified per district as showing behaviour problems, of whom 10 would be rated serious by our criteria. Service managers across all districts recognized that it was essential to devise some appropriate response, and most were convinced that some kind of *specialist service* would have to be developed. Service planning and development were undeniably hampered by the variety of conflicting models for a specialist service, the lack of knowledge and information about the effectiveness of different models, and the precise way in which to decide on the appropriate client group to benefit from the service.

Although there were exceptions, *coordination* between health and service agencies in relation to this group was not impressive. There was even less evidence of collaboration between Education Services and other agencies. A few had jointly considered the needs of individuals likely to be transferring to adult services in the near future but this was not a regular procedure in the seven districts covered by the study.

Finally, the possibility of *preventive work* with younger age-groups is inhibited by a lack of information about the long-term effectiveness of techniques to control behaviour. There is also little systematic information about whether and how parents' child-rearing practices may in some instances unnecessarily generate or reinforce unacceptable behaviour. Varying responses were found in different Districts; one Education Department had a specialist team which worked in schools with pupils identified as showing challenging behaviour, another district had a separate special school for children with complex learning disabilities. Both these services were perceived as in some measure successful but neither had been subject to systematic long-term evaluation.

Researchers

Professor Chris Kiernan, Hazel Qureshi

Hester Adrian Research Centre, University of Manchester, Manchester M13 9PL. 061 275 3340; FAX 061 275 3333)

Challenging Behaviour in the Community: The Effectiveness of Specialist Support Services

PROGRESS REPORT

Service evaluation
Quality of life

Specialist Teams

The design of services for people with severely challenging behaviour is central to the achievement of comprehensive community care. The Andover Project and NIMROD services (see above) demonstrated the potential for maintaining people with severe or profound learning disability, and severely challenging behaviour in the community. Subsequent work in South East Thames Region has confirmed the conclusion that community care for this group can be comprehensive, if services are sufficiently well designed and operated. However, the level of specialism required to design and operate high quality services is still daunting and is generally regarded as being a scarce supply.

Specialist professional teams, concentrating knowledge on how to work with people with severely challenging behaviour, have been developing rapidly in recent years as a response to these issues. Their brief is generally to help such people regain or maintain their places in mainstream settings in the community. Their remits vary, but can involve working with a broad spectrum of clients – those with profound through to borderline learning disabilities, those with or without additional mental illness, children or adults – in a variety of settings: family home, school, day service, community residence or hospital. No standard model of support service exists. They vary in size, professional composition, working methods, agency affiliation, and authority over other services and resources. However, they all tend to be relatively expensive, working with relatively few clients at a time.

The Evaluation

This research is examining the effectiveness of specialist support services developed recently in two counties. New referrals between November 1990 and October 1992 are being assessed before and after involvement from the specialist services and at a six-month follow-up. A comparison group who do not receive specialist support is being established.

The first aim is to investigate which people are referred as having severely challenging behaviour, and what factors might determine their being viewed as 'the most challenging'. Data on the prevalence of particular challenging behaviours suggest a greater number of potential clients than would generally be expected for such intensive services. The first set of questions therefore relates to the basis of selection of specialist-service clients: whether they differ from other people also seen as having challenging behaviour, or whether the key distinction lies in the quality of settings in which people with challenging behaviour live or spend part of their day.

The second aim is to describe the behaviour of individuals in their existing settings, prior to intervention from the specialist support services, and to characterize broad environmental conditions, such as activity programmes and the nature and frequency of staff interaction.

The third aim is to evaluate change as a result of specialist intervention: whether the existing setting becomes more effective, whether the individual's challenging behaviour decreases and their appropriate activity increases, and whether there are other changes to the person's quality of life.

Preliminary Findings

The clients of the two services show considerable variation in characteristics, in terms of profundity of learning disability, and psychopathology. This diversity has implications for the required competencies of specialist services; the scope for variation in target clients, therapeutic orientation, working methods and practical competence is considerable. **The idea that a single additional resource, such as a specialist support team, is an adequate planning response to meet the problem may prove to be an over-simplification**.

Secondly, a high proportion of referred clients currently live in or go to settings which do very little to encourage them to occupy their time appropriately. The fact that these settings are sometimes barren, chaotic, badly organized and poorly staffed presents the specialist services with a considerable task of service reform – one which may be beyond their powers or resources. Even where settings are reasonably well organized, much of the effectiveness of an external advisory input is necessarily dependent on the willingness and ability of the setting and its management to implement recommendations and maintain them beyond the period of specialist involvement.

Researchers

Ms Kathy Lowe, Ms Danute Orlowska and Dr David Felce

Mental Handicap in Wales: Applied Research Unit, 55 Park Place, Cardiff, CF1 3AT. (0222 226188; FAX 0222 641871)

Publications

Lowe, K., Felce, D., and Orlowska, D. (in press) 'Evaluating services for people with challenging behaviour', in I. Fleming, and B. Stenfert-Kroese (eds), *People with Severe Learning Difficulties who also Display Challenging Behaviours in the UK*, Manchester, Manchester University Press.

An Evaluation of Behavioural Interventions for Severe Self-Injurious Behaviour in People with Learning Disabilities

The development of interventions which are effective in reducing self-injurious behaviour (SIB) in people with learning disabilities presents a major challenge to services for this client group. From prevalence statistics, it can be estimated that approximately 10,000 people in the UK currently show SIB, and that only 200 may be receiving interventions which have proved to be effective.

The aim of this project was to provide intensive behavioural interventions for a group of the most severely self-injurious people and to compare their progress to that of controls (people with equally severe SIB, living too far away for the intensive treatment to be possible).

At the beginning it was agreed that the behavioural intervention should be of the highest quality possible, and should be based on existing research findings:

◆ interventions were always undertaken in the client's day and/or residential placement;
◆ the use of painful, distressing or dehumanizing procedures was avoided;
◆ a full functional analysis using a variety of techniques was employed for every subject;
◆ local psychologists were involved where possible, and training was always provided to the subject's care staff.

For the control group, general training in self-injury was provided but no specific suggestions on how to deal with a particular subject's services were given. Staff were always free to ask local services for help.

Staff stress
Training
Systems

PRELIMINARY FINDINGS

The results of the project are still being evaluated, but there are a number of preliminary findings which can be reported:

1. The functional analysis of subjects' SIB proved to be extremely difficult in some cases. This was due in part to the high frequency and intensity of self-injurious responding which was too dangerous to be allowed to continue. The analysis was often brief or consisted only of interviews and questionnaires.

2. Interventions often took longer to develop and implement than was anticipated, (possibly related to 1 above); and programmes required constant modification when the functional analysis had been incomplete or inconclusive.

3. The interventions were generally successful. Subjects in the intervention group showed lower levels of SIB during the intervention compared with baseline, and generally lower levels than matched controls. However, for some subjects the intervention was, in effect, for only a limited period during the day, so that there was only a limited impact on the individual's overall well-being.

4. All gains from interventions were fragile, and liable to wear out over time. Some subjects quickly became immune to the prompts designed to divert them from SIB; in other cases, suitable prompts which could out-motivate the SIB could not be identified. Other causes of intervention failure were unrelated to the subject: in one case, a successful programme was employed less and less by staff and was eventually discontinued – partly as a result of difficulties over staffing levels.

5. During the interventions, the degree of support needed by staff – both by the client's day/residential staff and by project staff – turned out to be enormous. The stress of working with profoundly disabled, extraordinarily challenging clients, day after day, sometimes without seeing any progress, was very high.

CONCLUSION

■ It became clear when assessing care-staff's knowledge about the causes of, and interventions for, SIB that they had received very little direct training in this area.

■ Functional analysis has undoubtedly contributed to an increased understanding of the determinants of SIB, but it is not always possible to reach firm conclusions when considering high-frequency-and-intensity SIB.

■ Those who work with individuals who are extremely challenging require support, encouragement and recognition of the task that they undertake.

■ Interventions may prove to be more robust and thus more cost-effective when the *systems* that determine their long-term effectiveness are acknowledged to be influential.

Researchers

Dr Glyn Murphy, Dr Chris Oliver, D. Head, Scott Hall, and J. Hales.

Institute of Psychiatry, De Crespigny Park, Camberwell, London SE5 8AF. (071 703 5411)

Publications

Hall, S., and Oliver, C. (in press) 'Differential effects of severe self-injurious behaviour on the behaviour of others', *Behavioural Psychotherapy*.

Oliver, C. (1988) 'Self-injurious Behaviour in people with a Mental Handicap', *Current Opinion in Psychiatry*, **1**: 567–571.

Oliver, C. (1989) 'Self-injurious Behaviour: The lost cause', in V. Cowie, and V. J. Harten-Ash (eds), *Current Approaches: Mental Retardation*, Southampton, Duphar.

Oliver, C. (1991) 'The Application of Analogue Methodology to the Functional Analysis of Challenging Behaviour', in B. Remington (ed.), *The Challenge of Severe Mental Handicap: A behaviour analytic approach*, Chichester, Wiley and Sons.

Oliver, C., and Head, D. (1990) 'Self-injurious Behaviour in people with Learning Disabilities: Determinants and Interventions', *International Review of Psychiatry*, **2**: 99–114.

Oliver, C., Murphy, G. H., Crayton, L., and Corbett, J. A. (in press) 'Self-injurious behaviour in Rett's syndrome: Interactions between features of Rett's syndrome and operant conditioning', *Journal of Autism and Developmental Disorders*.

Differential Effects of Severe Self-Injurious Behaviour on the Behaviour of Others

Case Study

Research into the factors which stimulate self-injurious behaviour (SIB) in people with learning disabilities has largely concentrated on the effects that the behaviour of others may have in reinforcing the occurrence of SIB.

In this single case study, the effects of SIB of differential severity on the behaviour of others are considered. **The results of continuous, direct natural observations show social contact to be more likely to follow long bursts of SIB than short bursts, and to be presented intermittently during and following long bursts of SIB**. The implications of this finding for the functional analysis of SIB and the long-term maintenance and development of severe SIB are discussed and related to the elements which determine the behaviour of the participants in the interaction.

Researchers

Scott Hall and Dr Chris Oliver

Department of Psychology, Institute of Psychiatry, De Crespigny Park, Camberwell, London SE5 8AF. (071 703 5411; FAX 071 708 3497)

Publications

Hall, S., and Oliver, C. (1992) 'Differential Effects of Severe Self-Injurious Behaviour on the Behaviour of Others', *Behavioural Psychotherapy*, **20**: 355–356.

The Functional Analysis of Self-Injurious Behaviour: A Comparison of Methods

Effective intervention

Recently there has been increased interest in the functional analysis of the challenging behaviour – particularly self-injurious behaviour (SIB) – sometimes shown by people with learning disabilities. This interest has been stimulated by the need for more effective behavioural interventions, and by the desire of many practitioners to use techniques which do not depend on aversion. Currently, a number of methods of functional analysis are employed in empirical studies and the applied field. These methods include direct natural observation, interview and, more recently, analogue methodology (an experimental technique which tests specific stimuli of SIB). The importance of applying these methods is widely recognized, but there has been little research into how useful they are in relation to effective intervention, or agreement between the conclusions which may be drawn from applying them.

In this study, the methods of direct natural observation, interview and analogue methodology were used to conduct a functional analysis of five subjects' severe self-injurious behaviour. Each method was employed by a different investigator who then attributed function(s) to each aspect of each subject's SIB.

Analysis showed that there was a *high level of disagreement* between the three methods used. Interview attributed significantly more functions to the detailed elements of self-injury than direct natural observation, which in turn attributed more functions to elements of self-injury than analogue methodology. These results reflect the fact that analogue methodology necessarily restricts analysis to a limited number of variables, while the other two methods are able to sample a greater range of situations and potentially influential stimuli. On the basis of these findings, it is recommended that interviews and natural observations provide useful screening strategies which can clarify potential causes of SIB, which may then be subjected to the experimental tests offered by analogue methodology.

Researchers

Dr Chris Oliver, Dr Glyn Murphy, Lissa Crayton, John Clements and Adrian Burgess.

Institute of Psychiatry, De Crespigny Park, Camberwell, London SE5 8AF. (071 703 5411)

The Current Education, Treatment and Handling of Autistic Children and Adults in England and Wales

This research, which was funded jointly by the Department of Health and the Department for Education, was designed in two stages; the first stage descriptive and the second evaluative. Stage 1 began in May 1987 and the second stage is due for completion in April 1993. This abstract presents the aims, methods and main findings of *Stage 1*.

The *aims* were to identity facilities and services which cater for autistic children and adults and to obtain detailed information on the current education, treatment and handling of children and adults with autism.

Questionnaires were sent to all local education authorities, social services departments and health authorities to obtain data on the facilities and services provided or funded for children and adults with autism. Questionnaires were then sent to establishments set up specifically for autistic children and adults, and to those with mixed populations which had experience of autistic children and adults. Visits were made to 56 schools, units, centres, hostels and communities to talk with staff and to observe some of the work being done.

Specialist provision
Integration
Outcomes

1. General Findings

- Lack of separate records made it very difficult for professionals in health, education and social services to provide data, firstly, on how many autistic children and adults they had in their authority and, secondly, on where they were placed. Even at the level of an individual establishment, it was not easy to obtain accurate data. Some professionals were not in favour of using diagnostic labels, and would not categorize people in this way.

- Four options exist for a child or an adult with autism (as for people with other special needs):

  — **specialist and segregated provision** – provision set up specifically in response to the problems of a particular condition, which is physically separate and where all the children or adults are autistic;

  — **specialist and integrated provision** – provision in a setting set up specifically to deal with the problems of that particular condition, but where children or adults with other types of special need also attend;

  — **provision which has been designed for an individual child or adult taking into account his/her autism** – for example, placement in a mainstream school, with outreach support; or placement in a Social Education Centre, with support from staff of communities which specialize in working with autistic adults;

  — **provision in a setting where staff do not consider it is necessary or important to know that the person is autistic** – for example, placement in a school or in a Social Education Centre, where staff might have little knowledge of autism.

These options differ in relation to a number of variables, including staff expertise and experience; staff–client ratios; one-to-one work; the curriculum; interaction between peers; distance from home; parental involvement; residential or day; integration; and access to information on autism. These variables will be given different weighting by different professionals and parents depending on their own experiences and views; thus very different recommendations may be made for quite similar autistic children or adults.

- The research showed that professionals have very different views on autism and the provision required. The policies, practice and provision varied a great deal from one area to another.
- There are often substantial differences between children with autism (and the same is true for adults with autism and also for other conditions) such that a variety of provision is likely to be necessary in any one authority. However, an autistic child or adult in one area might have a *range* of options, whilst a similar autistic person elsewhere might be offered no alternative to placement in a school for children with severe learning disabilities or, as an adult, placement at a Social Education Centre.
- It was often difficult for parents to obtain a diagnosis of autism for the following reasons:

  — the professional to whom the child or adult is referred may not have the expertise or confidence to make the diagnosis;

  — autism can be unclear – especially where the person is mildly autistic and has some high-level skills, or where the person has very severe learning disabilities;

  — a small minority of professionals were not convinced autism existed;

  — the diagnosis might have resource implications;

  — the 1981 Education Act encourages professionals to describe a child in terms of his/her special educational needs, rather than on the basis of diagnostic label, and this was used to justify withholding the diagnosis altogether.

- Principals and headteachers felt there was often insufficient reviewing of specialist placements for both children and adults. Most sponsoring author-ities relied on staff and parents to evaluate the placement, and indicate any need for a change in provision.
- Very few staff had evaluated their work in any formal sense. Many believed that the changes they observed in a particular child or adult were directly due to the type of approach they had used, but had not tested this.

2. Provision for Children with Autism

- There is a total of 29 schools and 26 units specifically for autistic children. Fifteen of the schools are run by LEAs (10 of which have children with other types of special need on roll) and 14 schools are run by either the National Autistic Society (NAS)(7) or a Local Autistic Society (LAS)(7). All 26 units are run by LEAs. Ten per cent of LEAs funded no specialist provision at all, and placed their autistic children within their own schools for children with moderate or severe learning disabilities.
- In total, there are approximately 1,000 places in units or schools which specialize in teaching children with autism; approximately one autistic child in every eight (12.5 per cent) attends a special school or unit. The majority of autistic children attend specialist autistic schools and units with a mixed special needs population.

- Four distinct approaches to the education and treatment of children with autism (although not limited to this population) were identified by the research team: behavioural approaches which focus on the development of skills without giving priority to any one area; behavioural approaches which give priority to the development of social relationships, communication skills and social skills; the Geoffrey Waldon approach, which focuses on the development of the child's general understanding; and holding therapy, which focuses on reinforcing the bond between mother and child. All four of these are being evaluated in Stage 2 of the research.

3. Provision for Adults with Autism

- In total, there are approximately 450 places in 24 homes or communities run by the NAS (3) or LAS (21) specifically for adults with autism. There are also one LAS day and one NAS residential training centre, and a unit specifically for autistic adults within a Social Education Centre funded by a social services department. Less than 2 per cent of adults with autism attend facilities which specialize in working with autistic adults; the vast majority are offered places in establishments with mixed special needs populations.
- For adults, the approaches used were largely behavioural. They focused on the development of independence and life skills, and on day activities designed to accommodate the particular needs, skills and interests of individual adults with autism.
- There was little evidence of either social services departments or health authorities setting up provision which specializes in working with adults with autism, and it seems likely that parent groups and Local Autistic Societies will continue to be the principal initiators of specialist provision in the future.

Stage 2 aims to identify the main characteristics of some of the approaches identified in Stage 1, and to evaluate the effects of these approaches on the behaviour and skills of young autistic children over a two-year period.

Researchers

Glenys Jones and Professor Elizabeth Newson

Child Development Research Unit, Department of Psychology, University of Nottingham, University Park, Nottingham NG7 2RD. (0602 484848 x 3259)

Publications

Gilby, K., Jones, G., and Newson, E. (1988) 'Autistic children in ordinary mainstream schools: Summary Report', Unpublished report. Child Development Research Unit, Nottingham University.

Jones, G., and Newson, E. (1991) 'Final report to the Department of Health and Department of Education and Science on the current education and treatment of children and adults with autism in England and Wales: Stage 1', Unpublished report. Child Development Research Unit, Nottingham University.

Out of Hospital

INTRODUCTION

Children

Staff attitudes

Management

This survey of 30 centrally-funded domestic-scale health schemes, designed to get children with learning disabilities out of hospital, covered a wide range of topics. Every scheme is unique, each representing a specific local response to a unique combination of recurrent challenges. Each scheme has to balance the independence, privacy and 'homeliness' of the home with the need to learn from the experience of others and contribute to the development of policy.

A major lesson to emerge from the research is that the most successful of the schemes are those in which the philosophy and aims, and their practical implications, are understood and accepted at all levels.

Secondly, there is encouraging evidence from the survey of the ability of staff to respond effectively to the new environments provided by the homes, and take on board the challenges and possibilities in them. Positive staff attitudes and staff development depends on the support of management.

FINDINGS

Homes and Residents

41 homes in use at time of research visits

23 homes provide only long-stay places (+ one more planned) ie overall,
   112 long-stay places

17 homes provide a mix of short- and long-stay places ie 76 long-stay places
                                                     33 short-stay places

1 home provides only short-stay places, ie six short-stay places

Totals: **227 places** are provided overall
              188 long-stay places
               39 short-stay places

25 homes provide a **'Homes for Life'** for long-stay residents

Of these: 17 are long-stay only homes
                  8 homes are mixed long- and short-stay

15 homes are age-limited

Of these: 1 is short-stay only
              5 are long-stay only
              9 are mixed long- and short-stay

One District has not decided its policy in this respect
Two Districts are reviewing their policy

Approximately **186** of the long-stay places were occupied at the time of the research. Of these residents, approximately **180** had handicaps of severity equivalent to Wessex Scale IV. **More than 50** of them presented severely challenging behaviour.

Three homes exclusively accommodate residents presenting challenging behaviour; 12 homes have no residents who present challenging behaviour. All the rest accommodate a mixture of residents with and without challenging behaviour (of various degrees of severity).

Improvements in the health and well-being of nearly all the young residents were reported, documented and observed in the course of this survey. The profound handicaps experienced by residents included double incontinence, inability to feed themselves, or even to eat solid food, inability to walk or communicate verbally. Despite this, considerable and sometimes dramatic improvement in mobility, communication and basic social skills has often been achieved. Better diet has led to better health: improved digestion and less dependence on emetics; weight and height gain; increased energy and physical well-being. Better sleep patterns have generally been established, with reduced dependence on tranquilizing or sleep-inducing drugs; epilepsy is under better control, and where patterns change, there is rapid response and usually successful alleviation of any new problems. The opportunity to exercise choice over what food they eat means that residents enjoy it more; and staff concern for the personal appearance of the young people ensures that they dress in very much the same way as their peers.

These changes have been possible as a result of the concentrated and expert attention which is available. In most cases, key-worker schemes have been adopted, and staff work with groups as small as six young people. Staff appreciate this ratio, although smaller groups would be better still. Everyday routines are generally devised flexibly in response to the individual needs of residents.

Only one home has not adopted a formal skill-learning programme for residents: all other schemes have individual programme plans, with written records of varying degrees of sophistication. Written records were not always properly maintained, but home staff seemed to be extremely familiar with all aspects of the lives of the young people they are looking after. The outcome of the individual residents' training programmes inevitably varied.

How do the Schemes Fit into the Whole Picture of Mental Handicap Services?

The new initiatives provide an opportunity for the needs – physical, social, emotional and educational – of individuals to be central in the planning and delivering of services. But problems remain: the inadequacy of community resources and some joint planning; the growing number of multi-disciplinary 'teams' of various kinds; the lack of short-term care facilities in nearly all Districts; and the lack of provision for young people who present severely challenging behaviour. The research suggests that it is damaging to try to accommodate young people whose behaviour is challenging in a setting where physically frail children are also living; but – with this proviso – the intensive, specialized care available in the homes can produce remarkable results.

The Planning Process

This can provide a valuable opportunity to generate shared understanding and underpin the development of the schemes.

The early involvement of supplies departments, works officers and finance officers was found to be particularly valuable and the involvement of residents' parents from the very start helped to ensure their support and participation in the life of the homes. The opposition which may be provoked by public consultation about the introduction of a scheme into a neighbourhood, is not usually encountered when a low-key, matter-of-fact approach is adopted. Generally speaking, participation of lay people was not highly developed – even professional representation amounted to a very few, interested individuals.

Regulations governing the setting-up of schemes of this kind should be clarified, so that unnecessary delays are minimized. In particular, fire regulations governing traditional Health Service premises are often inappropriate for these small-scale, intensively-staffed schemes.

The planning process is most productive when key individuals with a sound understanding of the issues and a firm commitment to the aims and intentions of the schemes occupy positions of sufficient seniority to be able to steer them to successful implementation.

Physical Settings

The most successful physical settings demostrate the effectiveness of sensitive planning. In the majority of schemes, ordinary family houses in ordinary streets have proved best: they succeed in being homely and comfortable as well as convenient without obtrusive institutional or clinical features. New-build schemes are generally less successful in achieving an ordinary, non-institutional ambience.

The most successful schemes have imaginatively-adapted buildings, well-chosen in relation to the group of residents, to ensure that they can be involved to the limits of their capabilities in all the day-to-day activities of their home. The need for office space has been met discreetly and unobtrusively. Nearly all the schemes have been able to provide residents with a bedroom either to themselves or shared with only one other person, demonstrating in a practical way the value put on residents' need for privacy and independence.

Staffing and Management

A high level of staff commitment at all levels is an indispensable ingredient in the success of the schemes, as well as a style of management which promises open communication and avoids the rigid hierarchical atmosphere common in some large-scale organizations. Sensitivity and flexibility are essential for the full development of the schemes, and to give staff the necessary support in achieving them.

The competence of staff with nursing qualifications and hospital experience is a source of reassurance for parents and inexperienced staff. Anxiety about career development possibilities for staff at all levels is an issue that needs to be resolved. Several Districts have developed management styles and in-service training schemes which could provide models here.

The ideal range of care is not yet in place. Short-term care and provision for young people with challenging behaviours is scarce; there is not enough back-up professional help, like speech therapy and physiotherapy; fostering as an option has hardly been developed; cross-liaison has still a long way to go, as have liaison and skill-sharing with parents. But the survey found that the 41 homes in operation provide many grounds for optimism. The young people living in the homes have clearly and almost without exception benefited from the innovation, and the schemes have proved to be flexible and resilient.

Researcher

Mr John Brown

Department of Social Policy and Social Work, University of York, Heslington, York
YO1 5DD. (0904 433494)

Publications

Leonard, A. (1991) *A Home of their Own*, Aldershot, Gower.

A Study of the Process of Adaptation in a Cohort of Children with Down's Syndrome and their Families

BACKGROUND

This study continued the longitudinal work with the Manchester Down's Syndrome Cohort – a representative sample of children with Down's Syndrome and their families. At the time of the investigation, it contained 127 families.

The aims of the study were:

(i) to provide contemporary and normative descriptive data on the families and children;

(ii) to identify variables related to the well-being of the family and the child, as well as factors associated with risk of low quality of life, stress, poor child-development and behaviour difficulties; and

(iii) to identify specific areas requiring further investigation.

Data were collected on a wide range of variables from mothers, fathers, teachers and assessors, through the use of detailed questionnaires, checklists, interviews and standardized texts. The comprehensive approach chosen for the study emphasized the importance of seeing the family as a complete system of transactions, in which all the components interact and influence each other. Multi-variable analyses were used to determine the important factors relating to child and family well-being.

One hundred and twenty-three families participated in the study. Child assessments and teacher checklists were obtained for all children; 99 per cent of mothers were interviewed and 97 per cent returned questionnaires; 87 per cent of fathers were interviewed and 78 per cent returned questionnaires. Data on over 3,000 variables were coded for each family. The reliability and validity of these data were carefully investigated and proved satisfactory.

Indices of outcome measures were constructed, reflecting the child's cognitive, academic, independent and social functioning, and behaviour problems and stress and quality of life for the parents and family. Longitudinal data were also available from previous studies on important outcome measures.

RESULTS

The main findings indicated both those factors relating to poor outcome for the children and families, and those relating to successful functioning. In this summary, the factors will be described from the point of view of *risk of poor outcome*.

Those relating to *low child functioning*, in terms of low mental age, IQ, academic abilities or self-sufficiency, were: parental educational level; a boy's father viewing the family as lacking in cohesion; the father having a low 'locus of control' score, i.e. taking the view that he could not control events; low use of practical coping strategies by the mother; the child attending an SLD school; high excitability in the child; high levels of child behaviour problems.

Child development
Stress
Quality of life

Those relating to high levels of *child behaviour problems* were: low child functioning; health problems, in terms of recurrent infections; poor parent–child relationships; socio-economic factors, particularly inadequate housing; low family cohesion.

Those relating to *low quality of life* and *high levels of stress* in families were: parental personality – high neuroticism scores; lack of family cohesion; marital dissatisfaction; parental coping strategies – low use of practical coping/high use of passive acceptance in dealing with child-related problems; lack of active-recreational involvement in the family; lack of strong moral/religious emphasis in the family; socio-economic factors including unemployment, lack of a car, inadequate housing; low child functioning; high excitability in the child; high behaviour problems; high levels of strain from current life-events.

The children's appearance, and health and disability did not appear to be major factors influencing their development and functioning. Important differences between mothers and fathers were found throughout the study, implying that they had different effects on, and reactions to, the child: these differences require further investigation.

Most of the factors relating to child and family functioning apply to many families, not only those with children with disabilities. This finding confirmed the earlier work done with the cohort and underlined the need for services to focus – not on pathology and handicap – but on families as systems functioning within normal limits, with the child's disability as a factor within the system which may create extra needs.

The *variety of factors* which were relevant to outcome underlined the importance of coordination of services to families. It also indicates the need for a comprehensive method of family assessment to identify vulnerability and needs and to target resources. The techniques developed in this study provide the basis for developing such a method.

Researchers

P. Sloper, C. C. Cunningham, C. Knussen and S. Turner

Hester Adrian Research Centre, University of Manchester, Manchester M13 9PL. (061 275 3340; FAX 061 275 3333)

Publications

Cunningham, C. C., Turner, S., Sloper, P., and Knussen, C. (1991) 'Is the appearance of children with Down's syndrome associated with their development and social functioning?' *Developmental Medicine and Child Neurology*, **33**: 285–295.

Sloper, P. (1989) 'The Manchester Down's Syndrome Cohort Study', *Manchester Medicine*, **4**, 6: 9–11.

Sloper, P., and Cunningham, C. C. (1991) 'Home–school links for children with Down's syndrome: mothers' views', *Educational Research*, **33**, 1: 42–54.

Sloper, P., Cunningham, C. C., Turner, S., and Knussen, C. (1990) 'Factors related to the academic attainments of children with Down's syndrome', *British Journal of Educational Psychology*, **60**: 284–298.

Sloper, P., Knussen, S., Turner, S., and Cunningham, C. C. (1991) 'Factors related to stress and satisfaction with life in families of children with Down's syndrome' *Journal of Child Psychology and Psychiatry*, **32**: 655–676.

Sloper, P., Turner, S., Knussen, C., and Cunningham, C. C. (1990) 'Social life of school children with Down's syndrome', *Child: Care, Health and Development*, **16**, 4: 235–251.

Turner, S., Sloper, S., Knussen, C., and Cunningham, C. C. (1990) 'Health problems in children with Down's syndrome', *Child: Care, Health and Development*, **16**: 83–97.

Turner, S., Sloper, P., Knussen, C., and Cunningham, C. C. (1991) 'Factors relating to self-sufficiency in children with Down's syndrome', *Journal of Mental Deficiency Research*, **35**, 1: 13–24.

Turner, S., Sloper, P., Knussen, C., and Cunningham, C. C. (1991) 'Socio-economic factors: their relationship with child and family functioning for children with Down's syndrome', *Mental Handicap Research*, **4**, 1: 80–100.

The Croxteth Park Project: Evaluation of Dr Barnardo's Intensive Support Unit in Liverpool for Children with Severe Learning Disabilities

CONTEXT

Costs
Collaboration
Informal sector

In the early 1980s, Ministers accepted a commitment to move all children with learning disabilities out of long-stay institutional facilities, such as mental handicap hospitals, into community-based facilities. Children with severe learning disabilities presented a special challenge. They were often 'medically fragile' and therefore needed nursing and/or medical care, which had traditionally been provided within mental handicap hospitals.

In 1983, the Department of Health provided special funding for Barnardo's to establish and run an 8-bedded Intensive Support Unit in Croxteth Park, Liverpool. This Unit took children with a profound learning disability out of hospital in the Liverpool area. A multi-disciplinary research team based at the University of Hull, and led by Dr Alaszewski, undertook an evaluative study of the Croxteth Park Project from 1983 until 1986.

FINDINGS

Children with severe learning disabilities who are medically fragile can be successfully moved from a hospital environment into a unit located in ordinary housing on a new owner–occupier estate, managed by a social work agency and staffed by residential workers. Despite the poor prognosis for such children, the children in the Project thrived. In many cases, the children experienced a substantial initial 'burst' of development that laid the foundation for subsequent steady expansion of their skills and abilities. Many children did so well that they were able to move to foster families.

High quality units do not need to cost more. An analysis of the costs of the Croxteth Park Project showed that, even though it operated as two, 4-bedded sub-units, the costs for providing care for each child were comparable to those of providing care in 24-bedded NHS units, when assessed over a three-year period. The intensive initial investment of resources in the Project enable children to move on to lower-cost foster family placements.

Research has an important role to play in the development of services. Evaluative research into small community-based units is intensive and absorbs both staff and management resources; but there are major benefits, particularly in an experimental and innovative project. Researchers can document the development of the project so that funders can judge the success of the project and other agencies and practitioners can learn from the experience. It also enables managers to identify the successes and shortcomings of the project and provide rapid remedial action.

Forward planning is essential. It is important to invest resources in planning, especially in a new development. Identification and establishment of suitable facilities, recruitment and training of staff and identification of potential clients must all be carefully planned and adequate time and resources made available. The considerable investment in recruiting and training staff, and the involvement of frontline staff in key decisions, played an important role in the success of the Project, as did the careful selection and sensitive conversion of the houses.

Caring is often emotionally demanding. If staff are provided with sensitive support and adequate opportunities for expressing their anxieties, they will respond by providing high levels of commitment. Coercive styles of management favoured in some traditional facilities are less effective than the styles developed and used Croxteth Park, which gave explicit encouragement to emotional investment by care staff in specific children.

Effective and sensitive management is a vital component in the development of a successful residential unit. There is a shortage of adequately trained managers, especially first-line managers. Middle and senior managers therefore have a crucial role to play in the development and training of first-line managers. They can act as role models, and through supervision and appraisal they can enhance the development of first-line managers. Effective communication depends on the development of a close and mutually supportive relationship between first-line and middle managers.

Effective collaboration is essential for the successful development of community-based units. While institutions attempt to provide a comprehensive service for their residents, community-based units concentrate on a limited range of services. The Croxteth Park Project needed support from a range of agencies, services and practitioners to provide a comprehensive service for its children. It acted as the lead agency in developing a package of services. In many respects the Project leader acted as a case or care manager for the children in the Project. S/he needed to develop a range of different relationships and use a variety of resources to ensure that the children experienced a consistent pattern of care.

The informal sector of care has a crucial role to play in the development of effective community care but it is also difficult to integrate into more formal structures of care. While the children were in institutions, the informal sector of care played a very limited role – the children received occasional visits from relations and/or volunteers. In the Croxteth Park Project, Barnardo's actively encouraged the involvement of the informal sector – especially relatives, volunteers and neighbours. The involvement of the informal sector had important benefits for the children. It enriched their lives and provided experiences that would be difficult, if not impossible, for agency employees to provide. In some cases, it provided preparation for and a bridge into ordinary family life. Despite its obvious advantages, the informal sector is by definition difficult to control. Project staff needed to act as advocates for the less attractive children and to encourage the development of contacts so that all the children had some relationship within the informal sector.

Community-based units need explicit policies for dealing with risk. Children with severe learning disabilities are often medically fragile and therefore more vulnerable to the dangers of everyday living. Institutions, such as mental handicap hospitals, attempted to minimize the risk to which these children were exposed; but in doing so, they removed many of the experiences of everyday life that provided a natural stimulus to child development. Community-based units, such as Croxteth Park, provide the stimulus of everyday life, and the Project clearly demonstrated that these stimuli enhanced the development of even the children with the most profound problems. To ensure that the children received the benefits of everyday living and were not exposed to excessive risk, it was important to develop explicit procedures for managing risks.

Researcher

Dr Andy Alaszewski

Department of Social Policy and Professional Studies, University of Hull, Hull HU6 7RX. (0482 46311; Direct line 0482 465895)

Publications

Books:

Alaszewski, A., and Ong, B. N. (eds) (1990) *Normalisation in Practice: Residential Care for Children with a Profound Mental Handicap*, London, Routledge, xviii, 299.

Pamphlets:

Alaszewski, A., and Chappell, A. (1986) *The development of Community Relations on a new Owner– Occupier Housing Estate*, Barnardo's, iii, 53.

Alaszsewski, A., and Hayes, S. (1987) *Setting up a Community Unit: Sessions from the Dr Barnardo's Intensive Support Unit in Liverpool*, Barnardo's, ii, 53.

Alaszewski, A., Ong, B. N., and Lovett, S. (1987) *Residential Care for Children who are Profoundly Mentally Handicapped*, Barnardo's, 34.

Wright, K., and Shiell, A. (1987) *Assessing the Economic Costs of a Community Unit: The Case of Dr Barnardo's Intensive Support Unit*, Centre for Health Economics, University of York, Discussion Paper 31, 32.

Book Chapters:

Alaszewski, A., Dodson, G., and Ong, B. N. (1990) 'Providing Child Care', in A. Alaszewski and B. N. Ong (eds), *Normalisation in Practice*, London, Routledge, 118–139.

Alaszewski, A., and Hayes, S. (1990) 'Lessons from the Croxteth Park Project', in A. Alaszewski and B. N Ong (eds), *Normalisation in Practice*, London, Routledge 265–281.

Alaszewski, A., and Ong, B. N. (1987) 'Community Care for Profoundly Mentally Handicapped Children', in N. Malin (ed.), *Reassessing Community Care*, Croom Helm, 116–142.

Alaszewski, A., and Ong, B. N. (1990) 'Researching the Croxteth Park Project', in A. Alaszewski and B. N. Ong (eds), *Normalisation in Practice*, London, Routledge, 30–56.

Alaszewski, A., Ong, B. N., and Roughton, H. (1990) 'Staff Management and Support', in A. Alaszewski and B. N. Ong (eds), *Normalisation in Practice*, London, Routledge, 140–160.

Alaszewski, A., and Roughton, H. (1990) 'The Development of Residential Care for Children with a Mental Handicap', in A. Alaszewski and B. N. Ong (eds), *Normalisation in Practice*, London, Routledge, 12–29.

Chappell, A., and Alaszewski, A. (1990) 'Relatives, Neighbours and Volunteers: Mobilising the Informal Sector of Care', in A. Alaszewski and B. N. Ong (eds), *Normalisation in Practice*, *ibid.*, 140–160.

Lovett, S. (1990) 'The Psychological Development of the Children', in A. Alaszewski and B. N. Ong (eds), *Normalisation in Practice*, *ibid.*, 205–226.

Morris, A., and Alaszewski, A. (1990) 'Education and Health: Coordinating Services' in A. Alaszewski and B. N. Ong (eds), *Normalisation in Practice*, *ibid.*, 183–205.

Ong, B. N., and Alaszewski, A. (1990) 'The Selection and Transfer of the Children', in A. Alaszewski and B. N. Ong (eds), *Normalisation in Practice*, *ibid.*, 57–75.

Ong, B. N., and Alaszewski, A. (1990) 'The Selection and Training of the Staff', in A. Alaszewski and B. N. Ong (eds), *Normalisation in Practice*, *ibid.*, 76–96.

Ong, B. N., and Alaszewski, A. (1990) 'The Selection, Purchase and Conversions of the Bungalows', in A. Alaszewski and B. N. Ong (eds), *Normalisation in Practice, ibid.*, 97–117.

Ong, B. N., Eccles, N., and Alaszewski, A. (1990) 'The Children's Quality of Care', in A. Alaszewski and B. N. Ong (eds), *Normalisation in Practice, ibid.*, 228–249.

Shiell, A., and Wright, K. (1990) 'The Economic Costs', in A. Alaszewski and B. N. Ong (eds), *Normalisation in Practice, ibid.*, 249–266.

Articles:

Alaszewski, A., and Ong, B. N. (1988) 'Nurses no longer required', *Nursing Times*, **84**: 41–3.

Alaszewski, A., and Dodson, G. (1991) 'Real Lives: Dylan's Story', *Social Work Today*, **23**: 14–15.

MacLachlan, R. (1986) 'Martin: A Success Story', *Community Care*, 11th June.

Shiell, A., and Wright, K. (1988) 'The economic costs of a normal life: the case of Dr Barnardo's Intensive Support Unit', *Mental Handicap Research*, **1**: 91–101.

Videos:

The Art of the Possible (1988) 24 mins, Barnardo's

A Very Special Relationship (1988) 20 mins, Barnardo's

Managing Care: A Positive Choice (1990) 21 mins, Barnardo's

Respite-Care for Children and Young People with Learning Disabilities

INTRODUCTION

The study focused on three main areas:

1. the availability of respite services and how far these matched users' needs;

2. the reasons why some young people stay on waiting-lists for services;

3. non-users of services and likely take-up rates.

Three local authorities were selected to provide a contrast in terms of social and demographic variables and to include a range of respite services: these were Sheffield, Croydon and Somerset. In each area, all respite facilities were studied: family-based schemes, local authority residential units, holiday centres and health service provision, including general and special hospitals.

Waiting-lists
Take-up
Consumer views

PROVIDERS, CONSUMERS AND PATTERNS OF USE

Main Findings

► Health, social services and education records tended to be inaccurate and not cross-checked.

► Mental Handicap Registers were of variable quality, using different criteria for inclusion in each area.

► Thirty-one children (5.5 per cent of the total group), many of whom had multiple disabilities or challenging behaviour, received some level of respite-care within a hospital setting – mainly on paediatric or orthopaedic wards.

► Some children experienced a respite-care admission which became long-term (anything between 8 months and 3 years).

► A considerable number of children were going to residential schools outside their own area, and many of them were also receiving respite-care during school holidays.

► Between 18 per cent and 21 per cent of users in each area were receiving respite-care from more than one source.

► The evidence suggests that minority ethnic and economically disadvantaged groups were less likely to use family-based services and more likely to use institutional forms of care.

► Children were still on waiting-lists after 12 months. Factors leading to difficulty in placing them included: age (older children are more difficult to place), challenging behaviour, and 'difficult parents' who might be problematic to link to another family.

► Demand exceeds supply for respite in all areas.

FINDING OUT THE CONSUMER'S VIEW

Characteristics of Families and Children Using Different Respite-Care Services

1. Children using family-based services tend to be from more affluent, 'younger' families, to be younger themselves and to have more health problems, but of a less serious nature. They also have fewer mobility problems and quite low levels of dependency (6.3). (*This is assessed using a 10-point scale – one point is scored every time a child is reported by parents to need help with specific aspects of daily living such as washing, dressing, feeding and getting around.*)

2. Children using local authority homes tend to be from a range of social classes, but most commonly from social class III, to be older, to weigh more, to have an average dependency-rating (7.1) and to be described as exhibiting anti-social behaviours.

3. Children using health service units tend to be from lower socio-economic backgrounds, to be slightly older, to have a variety of serious, long-term health problems which require regular medication. They also have higher levels of dependency (8.6) and experience mobility problems. They tend to be described by parents as either 'content/easy-going' or 'passive/introverted'.

Main Findings

▶ The need to obtain a break from caring and a chance to relax were most frequently cited as reasons for using respite-care services.

▶ Twenty-one families reported feeling under pressure to use respite-care services, e.g. from teachers, social workers, doctors.

▶ Families perceived that local authorities can provide a reliable break, whilst family-based services promised a better environment, but less instant availability.

▶ Eighty-nine per cent of children had been linked with a family within six months of applying for family-based respite.

▶ Families using institutional services rarely had to wait more than a month for a service.

▶ In each group of children, there was a significant proportion for whom no attempt was made at preparation prior to using a service. In three cases (11 per cent), children were left for two weeks or more the first time they had respite-care in a health authority facility.

▶ Seventy-five per cent of local authority hostel users had to give at least one month's notice to obtain a booking (41 per cent had to give six months' notice). In contrast, in the family-based service, 37 per cent had to give at least one month's notice and 8 per cent six months' notice. The majority of parents appeared satisfied with booking arrangements as they stood.

▶ The majority of families had no contact with a social worker.

▶ A major concern for users of family-based services was the number of children being cared for at any one time.

▶ Parents using buildings-based services were concerned about the behaviour of other children, especially when they saw their child as vulnerable.

▶ At least a third of all user groups felt that the amount of respite-care they received was too little.

▶ The average amount they received varied according to the type of service they used. An average of 31 days per year was available through family-based schemes, 47 days in local authority residential units and 56 through health service provision (1989 figures).

- The need for more information about service provision generally was apparent, irrespective of which service was used.
- Respite-care does not always have a beneficial effect on the child or the family. For a minority of families there was an acknowledgement that **they** were the only beneficiaries and that their child only tolerated his/her stays away from home.

THE EXPERIENCE OF FAMILIES ON WAITING-LISTS

This part of the study concerned families who had been on waiting-lists for family-based and residential units for at least six months.

Main Findings

- Twenty-two per cent (6/27) of families on a waiting-list for family-based respite-care had been waiting for over a year, 18 per cent (5/27) for over two years.
- Thirty per cent of children waiting for family-based respite-care came from black and minority ethnic groups.
- There is a higher incidence of 'anti-social' behaviour among children on waiting-lists. Three particular behaviours were associated with difficulty in finding links for children, namely: disruptiveness, a tendency to run off and destructiveness.
- Other factors associated with a long wait for family-based respite-care are a) a high level of physical dependency when combined with being older, bigger and less mobile; b) attendance at residential school; c) being older.

THE NON-USERS OF RESPITE-CARE

Families who were eligible to use respite-care services, but who were not doing so at the time of the study, were sent a postal questionnaire.

Main Findings

- Children using no services had a lower dependency level (5.1), and a lower number of long-term health problems.
- These children were described as having a very similar range of behaviours to children receiving family-based respite-care.
- The main reasons for not using services at present were, in order of importance: lack of perceived need, insufficient information (20 per cent), inaccessible services and a preference to keep child-care responsibilities within the home.
- Twenty-five per cent of respondents who lacked information were black. However, black and Asian mothers were twice as likely as white mothers to express a need for support.
- Children's services are often withdrawn at the age of 16, and provision for adults is often much more limited.

Researchers

Dr Carol Robinson, Dr Oliver Russell, Dr Kirsten Stalker

Norah Fry Research Centre, University of Bristol, 32 Tyndall's Park Road, Bristol BS8 1PY. (0272 238137)

Publications

Robinson, C., and Stalker, K. (1989) *Time For a Break*, an Interim Report to the Department of Health, Norah Fry Research Centre, University of Bristol.

Robinson, C., and Stalker, K. (1990) *Respite Care – The Consumer's View*: second Interim Report to the Department of Health, Norah Fry Research Centre, University of Bristol.

Robinson, C., and Stalker, K. (1991) *Regional Analysis*: fifth Interim Report to the Department of Health, Norah Fry Research Centre, University of Bristol.

Robinson, C., and Stalker, K. (1991) *Respite Care – Summaries and Suggestions*: final Report to the Department of Health, Norah Fry Research Centre, University of Bristol.

Stalker, K., and Robinson, C. (1991) *Out of Touch – The Non-Users of Respite Care Services*: third Interim Report to the Department of Health, Norah Fry Research Centre, University of Bristol.

Stalker, K., and Robinson, C. (1991) *You're on the Waiting-List: Familes Waiting for Respite Care*: fourth Interim Report to the Department of Health, Norah Fry Research Centre, University of Bristol.

Chapter 6

Physical Disabilities and Sensory Impairment

Physical Disabilities and Sensory Impairment

The very varied range of projects documented here covers both strategic issues such as integration, and the views of young consumers with disabilities, as well as a number of detailed studies.

Services relevant to the needs of people with a variety of disabilities or sensory impairments – people who are deaf, blind or partially sighted, suffer a combination of sensory impairments and learning disabilities – as well as to different age-groups are considered in this Chapter. One group of projects analyses the prevalence and management of incontinence, examines services and evaluates training techniques for professionals. Other studies relate to the management of pain, rehabilitation after head injury, and the provision of communication aids and physiotherapy in the community.

A separate stream of work focuses on the difficulties of people with visual impairment: their adjustment and spatial awareness, and the approaches to their training that are likely to be most successful.

Evaluation of UK Participation in the HELIOS Programme

Summary

Fifteen rehabilitation centres and 'local model activities', from across the UK, have participated in the EC's HELIOS Programme, aimed at promoting the social and economic integration of people with a wide range of disabilities. The UK HELIOS Evaluation is assessing the value at a national level of participation in the programme. An Interim Report, focusing on the views and experiences of the local projects, has been produced half-way through the study period.

Integration
Innovation

The HELIOS Programme seeks to promote the social and economic integration and independent living of people with a wide range of disabilities. Four EC-wide networks, one of rehabilitation centres and three of 'local activities' – in the fields of economic integration, social integration and independent living, and integration in schools – constitute a central element of the Programme. There are 15 participating projects in the UK. These are widely-spread geographically and assist people with a variety of disabilities. The Programme was formally approved in April 1988 and finally terminated on 31 December 1991.

The European Commission hoped for evaluation at EC, national, and individual project levels. Britain is one of a very few member states which has commissioned an independent study at national level. The 'UK Evaluation', funded by the Department of Health on behalf of the UK HELIOS Coordinating Committee:

  starts from a central, but not exclusive, focus on the four networks of rehabilitation centres and local model activities;

  explicitly conceives the participating projects as development initiatives, involved, both through HELIOS and in a sense independently of the Programme, in a continuous process of innovation, learning, dissemination and exchange; and

  focuses clearly upon the tasks appropriate to an overall national appraisal, as opposed to a series of local evaluations.

The principal aim of the evaluation is to identify the extent to which the projects function as a focus for learning from good practice, and the ways in which participation in HELIOS influences this. Interviews, direct observation, and documentary material are combined in the research approach. Other important aspects of the HELIOS Programme which bear on its overall success, are the organizational contexts of the projects' HELIOS activities, both at UK and EC levels, including the roles of various officials; and the role of 'non-governmental organizations' (NGOs). These are also covered in the study.

The research is designed to throw light on the value – at national level – of participation in the Programme; and on the extent to which – at EC level – HELIOS has succeeded in contributing to the development of policy and practice. The formal, detailed objectives of the research are to examine:

- the nature and extent of innovative work and active learning on the part of the participating UK centres and projects;
- the extent to which this has been shared between and among them and their European counterparts within HELIOS, and how this has been done;
- the nature and extent of wider dissemination of such information and learning, both at national and international level;
- the contribution of the HELIOS Programme to these activities.

Interim Findings

The Interim Report, produced roughly half-way through the 18-month evaluative study, gives a preliminary account of the local projects' own experience of HELIOS. It draws mainly on data collected on a first round of visits to each local project in the UK. Local HELIOS coordinators were interviewed and the day-to-day work of the projects was observed first-hand.

The preliminary findings of the evaluation are presented under the headings:

— organizational issues,

— participation in HELIOS activities, and

— different uses of HELIOS.

These sections deal respectively with the management and coordination of the programme at EC and UK levels; the projects' experiences of taking part in EC-wide conferences, seminars, study visits and training exchanges; and the variety of ways in which the projects can be seen to have made use of the opportunities provided.

The report offers some preliminary comments, based on the partial data so far analysed, on a number of issues needing further attention in the proposed second HELIOS Programme, (HELIOS II, due to start in 1992). These include the structure of the networks, the role(s) of local coordinators, coordination at national (UK) level, the nature of participative learning, and the participation of people with disabilities.

A more detailed examination of the extent and nature of innovation and active learning on the part of the projects, and their approach to various forms of dissemination, are major topics for the final phases of the study. The projects' views and experiences will be set alongside those of key informants at national level – officials in government departments and appropriate representatives of non-governmental organizations who have been involved in HELIOS. Centrally-held documentation will also be examined.

Researchers

Robin Lovelock, Jackie Powell

Centre for Evaluative and Developmental Research, Department of Social Work Studies, University of Southampton, Highfield, Southampton SO9 5NH. (0703 592614/592565/593569)

Publications

The full reference to the Interim Report is:

Lovelock, R., Powell, J., and Stack, E. (1991) *Evaluation of UK Participation in the HELIOS Programme – Interim Report*, Southampton, CEDR, Department of Social Work Studies, University of Southampton.

This has only been distributed to a very limited extent, mainly to the participating projects and to those closely involved in Government Departments and at the European Commission.

The Final Report on the evaluation is scheduled for September 1992. It is anticipated that a book based on the research will be published by Gower in due course. Articles will also be produced for professional and academic journals.

National Survey of Young People with Disabilities

There are some developmental needs common to all adolescents, and many of the social and practical problems they experience – drawing away from dependence on parents, forming new relationships, finding a job, setting up a home of their own, possibly marrying and having children – are the same for all. But for some, the road to adult life can be particularly difficult. Disabled young people for example often face difficulties additional to those experienced by young people in general.

Consumer views
Independence
Adult status

The principal aim of this research was to investigate the extent to which young people with disabilities attain an independent adult life. A secondary aim was to help assess the adequacy of services as they move to adult provision. The study was based on a follow-up survey of 13–21-year-olds, drawn from the national surveys of children and adults with disabilities living in private households carried out by the OPCS. All the young people were interviewed in 1987. The study sample represents almost 200,000 young people with disabilities in Great Britain – around 3 per cent of all young people aged 13 to 21. Most have multiple disabilities and a third are severely disabled.

As well as looking at their circumstances, lifestyles, and personal satisfaction, we also gathered the views of a comparable group of young people in the general population matched by age and location.

For most of the disabled young people we talked to, their circumstances, relationships and activities are no different from those of young people in general. However, a minority – around 30 to 40 per cent – face difficulties. Whether we define independence or adult status in personal, financial, social or in other terms, the findings show that:

- young people with disabilities have less independence and autonomy than young people generally. Many feel restricted by their disability and are less than satisfied with their lives;
- the disparity between disabled young people and their non-disabled peers widens with increasing age, suggesting that the experience of disability prolongs or limits the transition to a more adult life; and
- severely disabled young people are most disadvantaged in attaining adult status.

SELF-ESTEEM

The experience of disability in adolescence is associated with feeling helpless and inadequate. Young people with disabilities have lower self-esteem and less sense of control over their own lives than young people in the general population. Those who attended or had attended a special school or college for disabled pupils are more likely to feel negative about themselves. By contrast, young people with severe disabilities who go on to an ordinary school, or who had been to one, are more like their non-disabled peers in having a generally positive view of themselves. Further, while feeling good about oneself and having a sense of personal control generally increase with age among young people, there is no evidence of such a trend among disabled young people.

LEISURE

Young people with disabilities engage in fewer social and leisure activities on average than their non-disabled counterparts. The differences are often substantial. In relation to social activities that take place outside the home – such as visiting friends, going out for a drink or a meal, going to the cinema, discos or parties – the differences between young people with and without disabilities are particularly striking. Disabled young people's participation in many spare-time activities also declines with age and, for the more popular social activities, the gap between them and young people generally widens as they grow older. Young people with disabilities are more likely to engage in activities centred on the home with their families. However, more severely disabled young people belong to youth clubs and other formally constituted groups, though these often segregate them from their non-disabled peers.

FRIENDS

The depth and scope of the friendship networks of young people with disabilities are strikingly different from those of young people in the general population. More disabled young people than their non-disabled peers are disadvantaged in such things as contact with friends, the presence of a confiding relationship (including special friends of the opposite sex), difficulties making new friends and social isolation. Young people with disabilities who are attending or had attended special school or college are least likely to have a satisfactory network of friends.

INDEPENDENCE

The barriers facing many of these young people to achieving the personal and social goals of transition to adult life underline the need to promote a sense of control over their own lives through self-advocacy. There are clear links here with community care policies which aim to promote autonomy, independence, choice and partnership between people with disabilities and service providers. Parents play a crucial part in fostering their children's independence, but will often need help to 'let go' and redefine their roles as their sons and daughters enter adult life.

WORK AND MONEY

Unlike their non-disabled peers, who are mostly in paid work, the majority of disabled young people either are not engaged in any regular weekday activity, or attend day-centres after leaving full-time education. Many young people with disabilities never make the transition to adult employment, or do so much later than young people in the general population. The poor employment prospects of school- and college-leavers with disabilities are a particular cause for concern: many need practical help and continuing support to find and keep a job.

The sharp contrast in employment prospects between disabled and non-disabled young people is reflected both in their income levels overall and amounts of income from different sources. Young people with disabilities often rely on social security benefits as their main source of income after leaving school or college. When they do find a job, these young people earn less than their counterparts in the general population. The findings show that the financial disadvantages of being disabled from birth or in early childhood begin soon after leaving full-time education.

Taking into account levels and sources of income, patterns of expenditure and control over money reveal that financial independence generally increases with age for all young people. However, young people with disabilities have much less financial independence overall than young people in general, and the more severely disabled young people the least. This disparity also widens with increasing age.

MEDICAL CARE

We found no evidence of major shortcomings in the provision of medical care. Young people with disabilities who have a recent history of regular contact with hospital services are generally unconcerned about whether anyone takes overall responsibility for their medical care, or whether oversight is transferred to a GP when hospital appointments cease. Whether seeing a hospital or family doctor, however, disabled young people are less likely than their non-disabled peers to be treated as adults and to be seen on their own.

COMMUNITY SERVICES

Contact with community health services declines as young people get older. These services are mostly concentrated on those with severe disabilities, particularly those whose disabilities have a physical origin. This implies that community health services are targeted on those with greatest need. Nonetheless, a substantial minority of young people with disabilities lose contact with, for example, speech therapists, psychologists and hearing therapists for reasons unrelated to their health needs or to the problems for which help was originally provided. A framework for coordinating, at a local level, the health and social services that some young people with disabilities require is long overdue; arrangements for transferring young people with disabilities from children's services to adult provision are also required.

Researcher

Michael Hirst

Social Policy Research Unit, University of York, Heslington, York YO1 5DD. (0904 433608)

Publications

Flynn, M. C., and Hirst, M. A. (1992) *This Year, Next Year, Sometime . . .? Learning Disability and Adulthood*, London, National Development Team.

Hirst, M. A. (1989) 'Transition to dependence', *Cash & Care*, **6**: 1–2.

Hirst, M. A. (1990) 'Financial independence and social security', *Children & Society*, **4**, 1: 70–78.

Hirst, M. A. (1991) 'Dissolution and reconstitution of families with a disabled young person', *Developmental Medicine and Child Neurology*, **33**: 1073–1079.

Hirst, M. A. (1992) 'Employment patterns of mothers with a disabled young person', *Work, Employment & Society*, **6**, 1: 87–101.

Hirst, M. A., Jones, L., and Baldwin, S. (1990) 'Communication skills and research', in D. Robbins, and A. Walters (eds), *Department of Health Yearbook of Research and Development 1990*, London, HMSO.

Hirst, M. A., Parker, G., and Cozens, A. (1991) 'Disabled young people', in M. Oliver (ed.), *Social Work: Disabled People and Disabling Environments*, London, Jessica Kingsley Publishers.

Evaluation of Communication Aid Centres

In 1983, RADAR and the DHSS, including the Welsh Office, funded six Communication Aid Centres (CACs) in England and Wales for a five-year period.

Their original aims were:

◆ to undertake the assessment of clients for communication aids,
◆ to spread expertise to speech therapists and other relevant professions,
◆ to act as resource centres, and
◆ to undertake evaluation and research.

As little overall documentation of the centres had been published and no outside evaluation had taken place, the DHSS commissioned a study to be carried out by the Rheumatology and Rehabilitation Research Unit at Leeds and the Centre for Health Economics at York. The study aimed to determine:

(a) to what extent the original four main aims of the CACs were being met;
(b) the cost and effectiveness of communication aid provision;
(c) the satisfaction levels of clients, carers and professionals with regard to the service provided; and
(d) the scope of work carried out related to communication aid provision.

Method

The six CACs were studied together with four District Health Authority areas which did not have a CAC.

Background information was gathered, in all ten districts involved in communication aid provision, from key staff, who were interviewed at length in order to gain a current picture of communication aid provision.

Consultants and key administration staff were asked about their involvement in the service; and statistics on caseload were collected from district speech therapists and CAC managers.

Many aspects of the funding of the centres were monitored and their costs and effectiveness assessed.

Finally, details were collected about most clients who received the service, and many of them completed a questionnaire which incorporated a Quality of Life Measure.

Results

Over the one-year study period, a total of 430 clients covering all ages in the ten areas had received a communication aid service (268 males, 162 females, of whom 107 were aged 18 or under). Some people had more than one diagnosis: however, the main diagnoses were cerebral palsy (144), motor neurone disease (84), cerebro-

Cost-effectiveness

Consumer views

Quality of life

vascular accident (42), multiple sclerosis (23), laryngectomy (22) and learning disabilities (22).

Referrals to the communication aid service were mainly from speech therapists and consultants, although parents, occupational therapists, physiotherapists, social services and education authorities also referred a significant number. The service liaised with a number of outside bodies in order to obtain communication aids, including the Motor Neurone Disease Association, the Spastics Society and social services.

Funding of aids was the biggest problem encountered. There was no recognized funding route, rarely a specific budget for communication aids, and sometimes nobody claiming responsibility. However, the main sources of funding were found to be health authorities; charities; self/family/private; and social services.

Two hundred and four people were followed up during the study year: 127 had received their equipment and 77 were still waiting for it.

Quality of Life

Those people who had received their equipment were assessed for the impact that provision of communication aids had made on their lives, using a modified York Quality of Life measure. This examined changes in the clients' combined level of disability and distress, and also used a measure based on the client's own perception of changes in quality of life through use of a communication aid. One hundred and nine people completed the measures: 76 said that there was an improvement in the quality of life; 32 felt it was much better, and 54 felt it was slightly better.

Cost-Effectiveness

The research assessed the cost of CAC and non-CAC service delivery, including resource inputs paid for by the DHSS, District and/or Regional Health Authorities, local authorities, charities, business and other institutions.

The assumptions made in the costings make it difficult to give objective comparisons of average cost per person assessed between the CACs and the four health districts included for comparison. The costings for the CACs are particularly sensitive to the assumptions about the depreciation of the initial cost of the aids, and to the procedure used to allocate costs of linking therapists to each centre. In effect, CACs also provide services in addition to the assessment of clients and when due allowance is made for these functions the average cost per person assessed fell to £530 (low cost) per person for the CACs and £880 (low cost) per person for the Districts.

Although reservations have to be made about these calculations, they generally indicate that the specialized service can be run at costs per person assessed at or below non-specialist services in health districts.

CONCLUSION

CACs offer a valued specialist service for clients who have complex problems in communication, many of whom are physically disabled. They have been found to provide an efficient service, and to improve their clients' quality of life.

Researchers

Susan Hennessey, Brenda Leese, Keith Tolley, Ken Wright

Centre for Health Economics, University of York, Heslington, York YO1 5DD. (0904 433646)

Ann Chamberlain, Corinne Rowley, Janet Stowe

Rheumatology and Rehabilitation Unit, School of Medicine, University of Leeds, 36 Clarendon Road, Leeds LS2 9NZ. (0532 334936)

Publications

Leese, B., Tolley, K., Wright, K., Hennessey, S., Chamberlain, M. A., Stowe, J., and Rowley, C. (1992) 'Communication Aid Centres: Do they fulfil a need?', in A. Corden, E. Robertson, and K. Tolley (eds), *Meeting Needs in an Affluent Society*, Aldershot, Avebury. 164–177.

Tolley, K., Wright, K., Leese, B., Hennessey, S., and Stowe, J. A. (1991) 'Evaluation of Communication Aid Centres', *Communication Matters*, Spring, 17–18.

Adult Community Physiotherapy Project

The aim of the study was to evaluate the impact of a Community Physiotherapy Service by comparing this kind of intervention with existing care for adults and their carers. This involved describing the characteristics of the clients referred to the service and the service provided, comparing changes in the clients' lifestyle and health status attributable to their problems, comparing changes in their functional abilities, and describing differences in their use of health and social services.

The project was designed as a randomized controlled trial.

Consumer views

Outcomes

Semi-structured interviews were carried out with all patients by independent interviewers after referral to the study; three months after referral (or at the time of discharge from the Community Physiotherapy Service if it happened earlier); and finally, 12 months after referral. Data collected included demographic information, the use of informal helpers, home-helps or care assistants, health status (measured by the Nottingham Health Profile) and functional status (measured by the Barthel Index). All patients were given a record sheet to record all contacts with health or social services professionals, the place of contact and the length of contact time. They were also asked to record all admissions to hospital or residential home for respite-care. Service use was collected for 18 months following referral to the study.

In addition, the GPs' medical records were enhanced for each patient in the study, to allow the collection of data concerning the referral to the Community Physiotherapy Service, any contacts with the patient, any referrals to other agencies and any hospital admissions. The Community Physiotherapy records included the number of assessments, treatments and nature of treatments, and any referrals to other services.

PROGRESS

During the 12 months of the main study (April 1989–March 1990), 245 subjects were recruited. While a small number of GPs regularly referred appropriate patients to the study, the majority referred very few and some not at all. The reasons given by GPs for not referring patients include the extra work involved in obtaining informed consent from the patients and keeping data-sheets, a failure to appreciate the need for a controlled design (they wished to use the service but did not want to expose their patients to only a 50 per cent chance of receiving it, although the alternative was no chance) and a failure to develop an awareness of the potential of the service for their chronically sick and elderly patients.

In an unchanging environment, attempts would have been made to extend the length of the recruitment phase in order to approach the target number of subjects (400 trial and 400 control subjects). But by now, considerable changes were being made in the delivery of Community Health Services, which made this impractical.

The study was extended in order to follow up the first 100 referrals to the Community Physiotherapy Service, following the introduction of open access on March 9, 1990. The objectives of this phase are to compare the characteristics of the additional group with those of the subjects referred to the randomized controlled trial, in order to establish whether the sample in the trial is representative of those who would be referred to such a service, and to compare outcomes.

The data are being analysed and a report is planned for summer 1992.

Researchers

Barbara Gregson, Pam Dawson

Centre for Health Services Research, University of Newcastle upon Tyne, 21 Claremont Place, Newcastle upon Tyne NE2 4AA. (091 222 6000; FAX 091 222 6043)

Maintaining People with Chronic Non-Malignant Pain in the Community: Teaching Relaxation as a Coping Skill – Progress Report

PURPOSE

The aims of the study are to:

1) evaluate the effects of relaxation training with chronic non-malignant pain sufferers on their pain, mood, disability and health care use, both at the time of use and in the long term;

2) provide a simple treatment programme that could be used as a realistic clinical option by health professionals in their work.

BACKGROUND

Traditional medical techniques are often ineffective in relieving chronic non-malignant pain. Sufferers may be told that there is little that can be done medically to relieve their pain, and that they will have to learn to live with it. However, they are not always able to adapt to the pain or lead a normal life despite it. The effect pain has on their lives has been well documented. They often have disturbed sleep, feel exhausted, are usually taking analgesics with side effects such as upset stomach, heartburn and constipation. Physical symptoms are only part of chronic pain. Sufferers may become irritable, short-tempered, withdrawn and spend a lot of time alone, with little to distract them from their pain. They may not be able to work and loss of wages as well as damage to the family may result. Many studies report a link between chronic pain and depression.

Given this background, it would clearly be valuable to promote strategies which would complement any existing treatment, be easy to teach and use, and enable people to exert control over their pain. This could improve their ability to cope with the pain, reducing the impact it has on them, their families and the community.

Implications of the study

1. Quality of Care

The study will be of concern to all purchasers and providers, especially as the monitoring of quality becomes more a part of management in the health service. Clearly, health authorities are not currently meeting the health needs of those with chronic non-malignant pain. This research will evaluate one way of improving quality of care for this group of patients.

2. Delivery of Care

These patients have often been to several GPs and had multiple referrals to specialists. All these doctors have tried unsuccessfully to relieve the pain, and the patients, by default, have become responsible for their own care, often with little or no back-up from health care professionals. If nurses were able to teach relaxation, they would be in a position to support patients' own efforts at coping. Nurses are ideally placed to implement such a programme as they play a number of different roles, and have the opportunity to work with people as a practice nurse, district nurse, health visitor or hospital nurse.

3. Resources

The training package which is being developed has a potentially wide application, both in hospital and the community. It could be incorporated into basic and/or post-basic nurse training and be offered to patients as one of a wide range of skills. It needs no specialized equipment to implement it and would be a low cost, client-focused method of reducing the impact of pain. The cost of *not* providing treatment will be evaluated by assessing a control group, looking at health care use, number of medications used and the effects of pain on their daily lives.

Main study

The main study data-collection has taken a year and is nearing completion. The final report will be available in May 1993.

Researcher

C. J. Seers

Health Psychology Unit, Department of Psychiatry, Royal Free Hospital School of Medicine, Pond Street, London NW3 2QG. (071 794 0500 X 3712)

Analysis of the OPCS Disability Survey Data on Incontinence

The research was carried out through a combination of literature review and secondary analysis of data from the OPCS disability surveys. Its aims were:

Services
Extra costs

- to draw together existing evidence on incontinence in the six OPCS disability reports, and relate this to previous UK research on incontinence and incontinence services; and
- to carry out additional analysis of the data on incontinence gathered during the OPCS surveys, and produce reports covering: service provision for incontinence; incontinence-related expenditure; incontinence, education and employment; and the epidemiology of incontinence. The *first two* of these are now available.

Service Provision for Incontinence

Adults with impaired continence are highly likely also to have a range of other impairments and, consequently, a high degree of overall impairment/disability. Given this, the gaps revealed in service contacts and the provision of aids and equipment are disturbing. Those in the oldest age-group (75 and over) with the severest problems were most likely to have been in contact with community-based health professionals who could act as providers of, or routes to, assessment and appropriate intervention. However, a substantial proportion (a fifth) had no contact in the previous 12 months. The position among the most severely affected in younger age-groups was substantially worse.

Receipt of domiciliary services was at a very low level, even among the oldest and most severely incontinent people. In particular, services specifically aimed at incontinent people were minimal. There is also evidence to suggest that what little domiciliary help existed was directed to those living alone, in preference to those living with others.

These findings are reflected in the relatively high level of need for domiciliary services expressed by incontinent adults, particularly the most elderly.

There were substantial gaps in the use of incontinence aids, particularly amongst the older groups (65 and over); and these too were reflected in a relatively high level of expressed need for additional aids. Those currently buying (rather than being provided with), or not using incontinence pants and pads were likely to express a need for more of these items.

Contact with a community nurse was very important: those with similar degrees of incontinence who had contact with a community nurse were much more likely to be receiving services (even those which, overall, were very scarce) and incontinence aids.

Secondary analysis cannot tell us much about why incontinent people appear not to be receiving the services or aids one would expect them to need. But, obviously people will never receive help unless they are identified as being in need of it; and the role of the GP, in referring people on to the more specialist intervention or assessment that a hospital-based service or appropriately-trained community nurse can offer, is crucial.

Incontinence among children with disabilities is rather more likely to reflect the delayed achievement of control over the bladder or the bowels than it is among adults. Incontinent children identified in the OPCS survey were therefore more likely than incontinent adults to have no additional impairments, and had a lower overall level of disability. However, they were more severely disabled than average, among the children.

There was little evidence that GPs played any particular role in relation to disabled children's continence problems. Similarly, although both health visitors and community nurses had a slightly higher level of contact with incontinent children than with all disabled children, overall contact once children were beyond the age of five was limited. Fewer than half of the children in the two severest categories of incontinence had contact with any community-based nurse if they were aged five or over. Yet it is clearly important that incontinent children should be regularly assessed by relevant professionals, and helped towards appropriate intervention.

Few families received a domiciliary laundry or incontinence service, but many said they needed one. This increased with the age of the child. As with the adults, there are surprising and substantial gaps in the use of incontinence aids, particularly among those with the severest levels of incontinence.

For some disabled children, at least, incontinence may be a temporary problem, caused by delayed development of control, whether due to intellectual or physical causes. These children may be helped most by training programmes, rather than by the provision of aids. We do not know how many of the incontinent children surveyed were being actively trained, although very few were in regular contact with a psychologist who might initiate such a programme.

Continence, or adequately-managed incontinence, is one of the most important determinants of successful care in the community. Yet the analysis suggests that there has been little improvement in the provision of aids, equipment and services to incontinent children and adults since work carried out in the 1970s and early 1980s. This is despite considerable attempts to raise the profile of continence advice and awareness about incontinence.

Inevitably, these developments take time to become reflected in practice. The OPCS surveys were carried out some 5 to 6 years ago and there has been considerable continence-related activity since then, which may have resulted in improved practice. However, the literature suggests that there is still considerable confusion and debate about who is responsible for the supply of continence-related services, aids and equipment.

Incontinence-Related Expenditure

Despite difficulties with the data on costs, it is clear that incontinent, disabled adults do have expenditure, additional to that incurred by similarly disabled adults who are not incontinent, which is most likely to be on fuel, clothing and bedding, or laundry. Incontinent adults also spend more on items and services than similarly disabled, but continent adults.

Among disabled children, interpretation of the data was even more difficult. But here again, there is evidence to suggest that families with an incontinent disabled child are more likely to incur additional costs, and a higher level of costs, than families whose child is not incontinent.

Researchers

Gillian Parker and Julie Williams

Social Policy Research Unit, University of York, Heslington, York YO1 5DD. (0904 433608)

Publications

Parker, G., and Williams, J. (1991) 'Services aids and equipment for incontinent adults and children in private households', Secondary analysis of OPCS disability survey data on incontinence, Report 1, University of York, Social Policy Research Unit, Working Paper 774.

Parker, G., and Williams, J. (1991) 'Expenditure on incontinence for disabled adults and children in private households', Secondary analysis of OPCS disability survey data on incontinence, Report 2, University of York, Social Policy Research Unit, Working Paper 826.

Evaluation of Incontinence Training Packages

Three training packages, on the topic of incontinence, were developed as part of the Department of Health's initiative on Helping the Community to Care:

Information
Training
Nurses and
GPs

(1) A set of ten advisory leaflets for sufferers and carers.

(2) A set of four training packs to be used on one-day training courses for lay and paid carers in the community.

(3) A set of seven videos aimed at medical, nursing and paramedical practitioners and trainers.

The aims of the evaluation were:

▶ to assess the extent to which knowledge of the packages had spread to target audiences, and how far the packages had been taken up;

▶ to judge whether the packages had achieved their own stated goals; and

▶ to assess the value of the packages to those who had acquired them.

The leaflets were evaluated using a postal questionnaire sent to a random sample of recipients.

The training packs were evaluated by three case studies – one of a trainers' study-day and two of care staff study-days. This included the use of 'before' and 'after' questionnaires and a follow-up at three months to track changes in practice.

The videos were evaluated in two ways. First, a sample of relevant professionals, including GPs, in areas with high proportions of elderly patients, was surveyed by postal questionnaire to judge the spread of knowledge about the videos. Secondly, all known purchasers of the videos in Great Britain were surveyed by postal questionnaire to assess their use and views of the videos.

The Leaflets

The leaflets had reached many of those – particularly elderly sufferers and carers – for whom they were intended. For most, they were an effective source of information that was easy both to read and to understand. A small proportion of recipients, who were in particularly difficult situations, had problems reading and understanding the leaflets and saw themselves as needing individualized help. The majority felt that their knowledge and understanding had improved but few had made changes in the way they coped with incontinence, or had sought further help. This was especially true of the older and more disillusioned sufferers. However, those few who had made changes or sought help had experienced substantial improvements as a result.

The Training Packs

The training pack improved trainers' knowledge, coping and advisory skills, and their attitudes towards incontinence. However, those with little or no previous knowledge found that a single day's training was not enough to make them feel confident in offering training themselves in this topic. Few trainers actually went on to run training days, and those that did already had some experience in the area.

When used with care staff, on a training day run by the Age Concern continence adviser, the pack was found to be effective. Care staff improved their knowledge, understanding and attitudes towards sufferers. However, it was difficult for these changes to be maintained and for staff to influence practice once they returned to their place of work.

The study underlined the difficulty of offering updating training to long-established care staff, when their habitual ways of working with incontinence need to be challenged. It was clear that training should help them to change without leaving them feeling hopeless or annoyed at implied criticism.

The Videos

The videos did not seem to have reached their target groups. Most had never heard of, much less seen, the videos. This was particularly so with GPs, although more nurses were reached than any other professional group. Most of those surveyed did express an interest in the videos, suggesting that a well-researched and focused publicity drive might improve take-up.

Where videos had been obtained, they were mostly being used extensively and appropriately for the training of target groups. On the whole, fewer GPs and medical students were seeing them than other professional groups. Specialist nurses and doctors, by contrast, made extensive use of the videos in training a wide range of professional groups.

While most of those who had seen them considered the videos to be an adequate and comprehensive educational resource, fewer found them interesting to watch. Many considered the videos too expensive and a quarter found them too long.

Overall, the majority of those who had seen the videos thought that they would be effective in bringing about improvements in the care of incontinent people.

The evaulation demonstrated that there is a substantial need, in the community, for information and advice on incontinence. This was especially the case for sufferers and their informal carers. The leaflets clearly met this need, although there is probably some room for improvement of their readability and comprehensibility for older recipients. A large 'market' for the leaflets still exists, and one of the recommendations of the research was that they should remain available for carers and sufferers, as well as for community-based health workers to pass on to clients in their care.

The evaluation of the training packs raised questions not so much about the packs themselves, but rather about the contexts in which they were likely to be used. Training by itself does not result in improved practice unless all relevant staff can be trained and unless a supportive management infrastructure exists. Further, trainers themselves need to be expert or confident in the subject matter before they can encourage others.

As regards the videos, it was obvious that the original publicity campaign had not been successful in reaching the intended target groups, particularly GPs. Given the amount of promotional literature GPs already receive, additional mail-outs are unlikely to be effective. Publicity experts need to be consulted if take-up is to be improved substantially. However, it may be that videos are not the most appropriate form of educational material for GPs. Information on how GPs normally update their knowledge and about their preferred forms of material for updating is needed.

Researchers

Teresa Hagan and Gillian Parker

Social Policy Research Unit, University of York, Heslington, York YO1 5DD. (0904 433608)

Publications

Hagan, T. (1989) 'Evaluation of incontinence training packages', University of York, Social Policy Research Unit, Working Paper DHSS 550.

Hagan, T. (1989) 'Beyond plastic pants: improving care for incontinence sufferers (summary)', University of York, Social Policy Research Unit, Working Paper DHSS 560.

Hagan, T. (1989) 'More training required by care staff', *Caring Times*, September, 20–21.

Hagan, T. (1990) 'Nurses take the lead in continence work', *Nursing Standard*, **4**, 4: 24–28.

Research on the Current and Future Roles of Continence Advisers – Preliminary Findings

Attitudes toward incontinence and its management have changed radically over the past 20 years. Professionals have increasingly recognized it as a symptom which is sometimes curable and almost always amenable to improved management. Few would now dismiss it as an inevitable consequence of old age or mental disability. Part of the credit for these changes lies with continence advisers. Since 1981, their numbers have grown substantially and around three-quarters of all health districts now employ one.

Structure of service
Budgets
Training

The role of the continence adviser, however, is interpreted differently from place to place and from individual to individual. Some carry their own caseload; others do not. Some are based in hospital units or clinics; others in the community. Both catchment area and patient-group vary enormously: some advisers are restricted to a particular hospital or unit, others have a district-wide remit; some work only with elderly or psychiatric patients, others will see anyone. For some, the education and training of other professionals is the most important part of their work; for others, direct patient contact is more central. In addition, some commentators question whether advisers need to be nurses, while others see them very much as clinical nurse specialists in the Project 2000 mode. The Association for Continence Advice (ACA), established in 1981, offers a set of guidelines about the appropriate grading of an adviser's post, minimum training requirements, and the planning and establishing of a service. The extent to which these guidelines are implemented across the country, however, is unknown.

The research project is exploring variations in continence advisers' roles and canvassing opinions about options for future development. Information collected will include:

(1) essentially quantitative data about the number of continence advisers in post, their professional backgrounds and qualifications, the number of staff who work with them, caseload size, hours of work and so on;

(2) information about the structure within which continence advisers work. This covers issues such as budget-holding, supplies and equipment, the adviser's place in the administrative structure, the level of professional, administrative and technical support received, and relationships with social services departments, and with the private and voluntary sectors;

(3) details about continence advisers' current practice. Topics here include the range of activities pursued, the balance between direct clinical practice and educational and preventive work, and the extent of multi-disciplinary working.

The research will also explore how health authority and social services managers view continence advice, whether or not it is actually provided in their area.

Finally, information will be collected about past and future developments in continence advisers' work. This includes the ways in which individual continence advisers' posts were established; the use of research in developing good practice; the role of the clinical nurse specialist; the educational and training needs of advisers; the main problems to be overcome in developing continence advice, and a view of the future for continence advice nationally.

Although the research is still in the early stage, a literature review and the results of the pilot questionnaire indicate wide variations in the structure of posts and interpretation of the continence adviser role, and highlight a number of areas of concern to continence advisers.

Health Versus Social Care

In the proposals for the division of responsibility for health and social care in the two Government White Papers, 'Working for Patients' and 'Caring for People', it is not clear where continence fits in – that is, whether it is a health or a social issue. The future of a continence advice service depends on clarification of who is responsible for it.

Hospital Versus Community Services

Recent changes have resulted in a clearer demarcation between hospital and community services, and some advisers have found their opportunities to move between the two restricted. Particular problems may occur where patients are transferred from one sector to another – for example, on discharge from hospital, or from long-stay institutions into the community. Not only may the continuity and quality of care change, but also the availability of aids and disposables. The hospital–community split may mean that adequate liaison schemes are difficult to implement.

Teamwork

In 1988, the Department of Health recommended that each health authority should be responsible for setting up a multi-disciplinary continence service team, comprising a consultant having a special interest, a continence adviser and physiotherapist. Continence advisory services, however, have tended to develop in an individual, *ad hoc* way, with nurses taking the lead. These trends may have significant implications, not only for the prospects of inter-disciplinary working and for the way in which care is provided, but also for the way in which incontinence is seen as essentially a health concern.

Budgets

In many authorities, the appointment of an adviser seems to have been less a response to unmet need than to overspent budgets. This emphasis on budgetary control may overshadow opportunities for continence promotion and create tensions and resentment between the service and sufferers and carers. Although one of the adviser's most important tasks is to ensure that supplies are not provided inappropriately or unnecessarily, shortfalls can place him/her in the position of having to ration supplies to clients at levels which are not adequate to their needs.

Role Variations

The wide variations in interpretation of the continence adviser's role allow for flexibility and sensitivity to local conditions, but can lead to disagreement within the service and make it difficult to present a coherent image of the adviser's role to both professionals and the general public. Many advisers recognize the need for standard training and clarification of their role, in order to consolidate their professional identity; others fear that this will erode their professional autonomy.

Researcher

Penny Rhodes

Social Policy Research Unit, University of York, Heslington, York YO1 5DD.
(0904 433608)

An Investigation into the Effects of Case-Management after Severe Head Injury

THE STUDY

Rehabilitation
Outcome
Coordination

The provision of rehabilitation for victims of head injury has been found by a number of studies to be inadequate, partly as a result of patients slipping through the net of existing services. This project investigated the proposition that case-management would help to fill this gap by providing effective coordination, and would improve service input and patient outcome after severe head injury.

The effects of case-management on patients with head injuries from three hospitals and Districts which introduced it were compared with outcomes in three control hospitals and Districts which did not.

■ *Comparable trial groups*

Two groups of three hospitals were chosen, matched on the number and severity of admissions, the size and type of hospital, their geographical location and their facilities. The case manager was allocated to one group of hospitals whilst the other acted as control.

■ *Inclusion and exclusion criteria*

Patients admitted to the study from these hospitals after blunt head injury –

INCLUSIONS

— Age 16–60
— Post-Traumatic Amnesia >48 hours and/or coma 6 hours
— Patient or main carer resident in study District
— Informed consent from family

EXCLUSIONS

— Other disorders receiving hospital treatment including Central Nervous System disease, drug or alcohol abuse, psychiatric disturbance
— No fixed abode
— Follow-up unlikely

Patients in case-managed hospitals received normal services *plus* case-management, while those in control hospitals received normal services alone. An assessor, using an extensive range of tests, collected data at 0, 6, 12 and 24 months post-injury from both groups of patients to determine service provision and outcome. It was predicted that case-management would have little effect on service provision or outcome variables at a time when services are often provided, but would begin to show effects at 12–24 months post-injury, when service provision is absent, distress experienced by families is accelerating and the recruitment of statutory and voluntary community facilities poor.

Data collected from 56 case-managed (CM) and 70 control (C) patients have been analysed.

■ *Control Variables*

— Age, sex, cause of injury, alcohol intake at injury, and pre-morbid IQ, were similar in both groups.

— The CM group were more severely injured on entry to the study, having lower Glasgow Coma Scores and longer periods unconscious or in post-traumatic amnesia, and more tracheostomies. Subsequent analysis of service provision or outcome was adjusted for these differences, and the effect of hospital membership, by stratification or matching; these adjustments are reflected in the conclusions that follow.

RESULTS

Service Provision

● The duration of hospital stay was not shortened, or prolonged, by case-management. Case-management increased contact with hospital out-patient services, but the duration of contact did not differ between groups.
● After head injury of a given severity, case-management increased the chance of admission to a rehabilitation unit.
● Referral to clinical psychology or paramedical services (physio, occupational, and speech therapy and social work) occurred more often in the case-managed patients. The effect was more marked for clinical psychology, social work and speech therapy. If contact occurred, the duration of that contact was not increased by case-management.

Patient Outcome

There was no difference between the two groups of patients at 6, 12 and 24 months follow up in:

(a) residual physical and cognitive impairments;

(b) measures of personality, affect and social functioning;

(c) residual disability and handicap measured by the Barthel ADL (Activities of Daily Living) index, extended Glasgow Outcome Scale, Rappaport Disability Rating Scale, and Glasgow Assessment Schedule;

(d) distress reported by the family or relatives;

(e) hours of supervision or care as reported by the family;

(f) estimated potential for re-employment, actual return to work, or absence from work.

DISCUSSION

The model of 'external' case-management used here aims, by networking and negotiation, to put patients in touch with appropriate services. Studies have suggested that in mental health patients, this model can reduce in-patient care and lower overall costs of care[18], and result in more successful identification of service

---

[18] Mueller, J., and Hopp, M. (1983) 'A demonstration of the cost-benefits of case management service for discharged mental patients', *Psychiatry Quarterly*, **55**: 17–24.

needs[19]. In the frail elderly, lower costs and increased life expectancy resulted[20], and in patients with back injuries case-management led to reduced time off work, earlier discharge, and lower costs[21]. External case-management is also advocated in the United States for 'catastrophic' illness[22] although it has never been subjected to proper evaluation in these patients. Our study is the first to do this after severe head injury.

The study showed that after severe head injury, in North London and its environs, little formal rehabilitation is provided more than six months after injury in most cases. These findings confirm those in the West of Scotland; and this situation exists despite the fact that distress within families may increase with time.

The study also showed that case-management after severe head injury significantly increases the numbers of patients in contact with formal rehabilitation in hospital and the community. This effect was more marked for psychology, social work and speech therapy – professions to which referrals are, usually, rarely made.

Despite this increased contact with case-management, no difference in outcome was found in the two groups. It was expected that measures of physical and cognitive impairment would not be significantly changed by contact with rehabilitation. However, unexpectedly, we have also not been able to show that increased referral is followed by better functional ability within or outside the home, increased return to work, reduced family distress or reduced levels of supervision and care.

Our study shows that although case-management increases referral to rehabilitation services it does not increase hours of treatment. Similarly, provision of information to relatives did not have the predicted effect of reducing distress, despite 19 of 20 families at 24 months reporting that the case-management was 'very' or 'extremely' helpful.

Case-management therefore appears not to be of general use in the context of current service provision in the UK. If rehabilitation services after severe head injury become more sophisticated, coordinated continuity of treatment may be an inevitable part of management and make the role of an additional case manager redundant. Our clinical experience, however, leads us to believe that case-management is of use for selected patients – for example, those with severe residual deficit and no family back-up.

Acknowledgement

This study was funded by the Department of Health, the King's Fund and the Joint Research Board of St Bartholomew's Hospital.

Researchers

Dr Richard Greenwood and Dr Tom McMillan

Department of Neurological Sciences, St Bartholomew's Hospital, London EC1A 7BE. (071 601 7665)

[19] Perlmann, B. B., Melnick, G., and Kentera, A. (1985) 'Assessing the effectiveness of a case management programme', *Hospital and Community Psychiatry*, **36**: 405–407.
[20] Challis, J. D., Davis, B. (1986) *Case Management in Community Care*, Aldershot, Gower.
[21] Leavitt, S. S., Beyer, R. D., and Johnston, T. L. (1972) 'Monitoring the recovery process', *Industrial Medicine*, **41**: 25–30.
[22] Henderson, N. G., and Wallack, S. S. (1987) 'Evaluating case management for catastrophic illness', *Business in Health*, January, 7–11.

Publications

Murphy, L. D., McMillan, T. M., *et al.* (1990) 'Services for severely head injured patients in North London and environs', *Brain Injury*, **4**, 95–100.

Evaluation of the Quality and Costs of Residential Rehabilitation and Further Education Services provided by SENSE-in-the Midlands

This 21-month study will evaluate the quality and costs of rehabilitation and further education services provided by SENSE-in-the Midlands for people with dual sensory impairments and severe learning disabilities.

Indicators of service quality will be derived from:

◆ the direct observation of student and staff activity;
◆ monitoring of the student's use of time and social integration;
◆ longitudinal assessment of student development;
◆ parental satisfaction with service provision;
◆ monitoring of service use; and
◆ the evaluation of the social climate, and routines operating with care environments.

In addition, the costs of the packages of care delivered to individuals over a three-month period will be evaluated in a collaborative project with the Personal Social Services Research Unit, University of Kent at Canterbury.

The study will evaluate changes in these aspects of quality and costs for a cohort of 16 individuals prior to, and 4–7 months following the commencement of their placement at the SENSE facility. Organizational factors influencing staff turnover, retention and job satisfaction will also be investigated.

Information on students prior to their move has already been collected. The project will be completed by June 1992.

Sensory impairments
Learning disabilities

Researchers

Eric Emerson, Janet Cooper and Chris Hatton

Hester Adrian Research Centre, University of Manchester, Manchester M13 9PL.
(061 275 3340)

The Telecommunication Needs of People who are Deaf

This study had two main aims:

Social exclusion
Autonomy
Research methodology

- to explore severely deaf people's needs for access to telephone services and the impact on their lives of any restrictions they experienced; and
- to investigate the social and economic benefits of receiving different kinds of telecommunications service. These included ordinary telephones (usually with assistance from family and friends); the RNID (Royal National Institute for the Deaf) Telephone Exchange for the Deaf (TED) which relays conversations in text via an operator; and systems using terminals to transmit two-way conversations as text.

The immediate origins of the study lay in RNID's difficulty in meeting the costs of their relay system or expanding its very limited coverage. To make informed judgements about the future of TED, good information was needed on the role of the telephone in general in deaf people's lives. The study therefore identified severely deaf people's needs for the telephone and compared the benefits and costs of using the RNID relay and other telecommunications systems. It included only people who were severely deaf – unable to use ordinary 'phones even with amplification. This covered two main groups: people born deaf or deaf from early childhood, and those whose hearing loss had happened later in life. The first group mainly prefer to communicate in sign language, while the second are much more likely to retain speech and to rely on lip reading.

The study was carried out in 1989 and had three elements:

— an interview survey of around 100 subscribers to the RNID Exchange and 100 non-subscribers;
— follow-up interviews with 15 subscribers and 15 non-subscribers; and
— interviews in sign language with 20 deaf people, of whom 10 were subscribers to the RNID Exchange. These interviews were video-taped and later translated into English. They covered the same ground as the interviews conducted in speech.

FINDINGS

The first finding to emerge from this study was the dearth of information on conducting research with deaf people, who are often excluded from surveys because of communication problems. A significant part of the study's value lies in the research methods developed, which are potentially of use in enabling people who are deaf to be included in future research. The methods of communication developed in this study also have potential value in ensuring that deaf clients or customers are able to communicate their views fully to the providers of services.

The study demonstrated very clearly that deaf people felt disadvantaged in their access to the telephone. They deeply resented the dependence that their exclusion from ordinary telephone services created. Regardless of the telephone equipment they had, most respondents had to rely on relatives, friends, colleagues, neighbours and occasionally complete strangers. Most of the people interviewed wanted to use the telephone more than they were able to within the systems available at present, and to do so more easily and more cheaply. The restrictions they currently experienced affected their lives on a number of levels: contacts with friends and relatives; employment and promotion prospects; managing personal business affairs; dealing with emergencies such as accident and fire; access to help-lines; and contact with health and welfare services, and with lawyers and the courts.

The costs deaf people experience in using the telephone – ordinary or special – emerged as a concern. The time taken to use ordinary telephones through an intermediary increases the cost of calls. The RNID relay and text-telephones also take longer and cost more, while the equipment that is needed can be prohibitively expensive. (The Text Users Help Scheme introduced in 1989 provides some help with call charges.)

The potential benefits of a relay service were clearly demonstrated by the RNID Exchange. Subscribers reported that access to TED improved their quality of life. It had a significant impact on their use of the telephone for contacting friends and relatives and for managing personal business. It had also enabled some people to use the telephone independently in their work.

The RNID service was, nevertheless, seen as less than adequate. This was partly because it was linked to a very small number of subscribers (170 at the time of the study) and was heavily congested. Improvements to the RNID Exchange since the study will have resolved these difficulties. Some of the disadvantages mentioned were, however, inherent to relay systems – most obviously, the lack of privacy created by passing information via a third party. Text-telephones did not suffer from this restriction. The process of acquiring and using a text-telephone has much more in common with use of the ordinary phone than does being a TED subscriber. Access to text-phones was, however, very limited, and much lower than the demand for them. Cost was clearly a factor in this. A few respondents had been supplied with text-phones from their social services department under the provisions of The Chronically Sick and Disabled Persons Act, but this was exceptional.

The key distinction to emerge from the study was not, however, between TED subscribers and text-phone users. It was between those who used either of these 'special' systems (or both of them) and people who had access only to ordinary telephones or none at all. People with access to either TED or a text-phone were much better off than people with neither; those who used both TED and a text-phone were even more so.

Overall, then, the study found severely deaf people's access to and use of the telephone was very restricted. Their lives and those of close relatives were substantially affected by this. Technology and systems exist which can greatly improve the current situation, but cost appears to be a major factor preventing the wider use of these new systems. Deaf people, even those who are older, appear able and willing to cope with the new technology involved. Indeed many see it as inequitable that they are excluded from new developments in telephone technology.

Researchers

Sally Baldwin, Michael Hirst, Lesley Jones and Gloria Pullen

Social Policy Research Unit, University of York, Heslington, York YO1 5DD. (0904 433608)

Publications

Baldwin, S. M., Hirst, M. A., and Jones, L. (1992) 'Meeting the telecommunications needs of people who are deaf', in A. Corden, E. Robertson, and K. Tolley (eds), *Meeting Needs*, London, Routledge.

Baldwin, S. M., Hirst, M. A., Jones, L., and Pullen, G. (1990) 'Poor Connections: the telecommunications needs of people who are deaf', University of York, Social Policy Research Unit, Working Paper DHSS 677.

Baldwin, S. M., and Jones, L. (1990) 'Poor Connections', *New Statesman*, **3**, 125: 39.

Baldwin, S. M., Jones, L., Pullen, G., and Hirst, M. (1991) 'Plight of deaf telephone users', *Hearing Therapy*, **14** (April): 15–16.

Hirst, M. A., Baldwin, S. M., and Jones, L. (1991) 'Text telecommunication for people who are deaf: assessing the use of a text-relay service', *British Journal of Audiology*, **25**: 361–370.

Hirst, M. A., Jones, L., and Baldwin, S. M. (1990) 'Communications skills and research', in D. Robbins, and A. Walters (eds), *DH Yearbook of Research and Development 1990*, London, HMSO.

Jones, L. (1990) 'Changing places – relationships and hearing loss', in J. Jussen, and W. H. Claussen (eds), *Hilfen für Horgeschadigte Heute*, Munich, Ernst Rheinhardt Verlag.

Jones, L. (1990) 'Waiting for a phone call', *Community Care*, **823** (19 July): 27.

Video:

A Better Life, a subtitled video-tape version of the findings produced by Lesley Jones, co-produced by Gloria Pullen, who presented the findings in British sign language, Aspen Spafax Television (1990). Also available in text form. 'A Better Life: telecommunications needs of people who are deaf and use sign language' University of York, Social Policy Research Unit, Working Paper DHSS 654.

Services For and Social Care of Blind and Partially Sighted People – a Research Review

This study aimed to identify, list and review relevant recent and current social research concerning sight loss, and to advise on future research priorities.

Almost 70 recent research studies relevant to social care services for people with visual impairments were identified through a national postal survey and library searches. The studies were listed and the overall body of work was reviewed in the light of the policy and practice themes of *Caring for People* and the NHS and Community Care Act 1990. Priorities for future research are identified in this context.

Service planning
Coordination
Training

Findings

Information on 69 relevant projects was supplied by 31 organizations. Twenty-four studies were reported by academic or independent research bodies, 16 by statutory agencies (mainly social services departments), and 29 by voluntary organizations.

The Report on the review includes a directory of the individual projects identified. This is structured into eight main sections in terms of subject matter:

— service organization and strategy, client need, service initiatives;
— low vision/partial sight;
— mobility;
— training of specialist staff and assessment and training of visually-handicapped people;
— deaf–blind people;
— multi-handicapped and mentally-handicapped people;
— education;
— employment.

Each section is further split according to whether the studies were complete or in progress at the time of the survey. The eight main categories were selected to reflect the material submitted; over two-thirds of the entries are in the first four groups. There is a summary listing of the entries, an alphabetical index of project titles, and an index of the organizations responsible for the studies concerned. Individual entries contain abstracts of the studies, giving subject matter, aims and methods, and findings (where appropriate). There is further detail of the scope, timescale and costs of projects, contact names and addresses, and an indication of the availability of reports. The Report summarizes and draws together this body of research, following the sections of the directory.

Two major academic research centres, along with the Royal National Institute for the Blind, were responsible for most of the more substantial recent and current research falling within the criteria of the review; each reported a number of projects. A small number of other studies of some scale and national significance had been carried out in academic settings or independent research institutes. A handful of small voluntary bodies had also carried out valuable research with more than a local relevance.

On the other hand, the research reported by most local, service-providing agencies was rather piecemeal and of purely local concern. Individual studies were either highly specific or very general in terms of subject matter. Studies reported by social services departments and small voluntary organizations were often local numerical assessments of need, but differences of definition and in sampling-base make comparison or overall aggregation between local studies extremely difficult.

There was another basic difference in style and focus between the two main bodies of work. Most of the more formal or academic research reviewed gave little attention to the overall planning and organization of services, while much of the more operational work, typically carried out in a local authority or small voluntary agency context, tended to take existing definitions of need and approaches to meeting it as given. Although the themes of the White Paper *Caring for People* were not fundamentally new, in the field of visual impairment or elsewhere, they were not much in evidence as a backdrop to the research reported.

Apart from small-scale local work, mainly in the voluntary sector, there was little systematic qualitative research on the *care and support needs* felt by people with sight problems, and/or by their carers, nor any detailed exploration of their experience of services.

Very few reported studies involved *collaboration*, especially joint-working, between social and health services. This may reflect a lack of actual collaboration in services and care for people with visual impairments, particularly at frontline level. A particularly important gap was apparent in the crucial area of referral, assessment and subsequent provision of rehabilitative services and continuing support.

The initiative for research into the *social care needs* of multi-handicapped people and their carers and for service provision, has been taken by the voluntary sector – in particular the large national organizations. Some local authorities are now beginning to identify the extent and nature of need in their areas and to ensure that provision is made.

The organization and effectiveness of *training* for specialist workers and for visually-impaired people themselves, particularly in respect of mobility, has been a major focus of recent research in the visual handicap field. No local authorities reported involvement in any research concerning such training.

Future Research Priorities

Broad themes identified for future research include:

- identification of the population of people with visual handicaps – overall need and planning;
- monitoring and review of existing provision and resources;
- referral, assessment and review – identifying and meeting individual need;
- taking account of service users' views;
- inter-agency collaboration
- services for people with additional handicaps and special need;
- the needs of carers;
- staff development and training issues, including:
    - specialist training;
    - integration into mainstream provision;
    - identification and dissemination of good practice.

The Report recommends that priority should be given to a major study of the referral and assessment process. The views and experiences of service users, carers and the professionals directly involved, should be set alongside each other and compared with agencies' policy statements and plans. This would, necessarily, also illuminate some of the main issues concerning collaboration.

There is an associated need for a national research-based review of the nature, level and organization of SSD provision for people with sight problems. It should include an examination of how these services inter-relate with those provided by the health service and the independent sector.

Agencies' plans for change in the light of broader community care developments should be a key feature of these related studies. The Report stresses the training dimensions of many of the areas identified for further examination. There is also a continuing need for monitoring and evaluation of the specialist training courses, building upon recent critical studies.

Finally, the Report recommends a systematic attempt to identify new initiatives in both planning and frontline service delivery across the country. This should focus on collaborative activity across agency and sector boundaries, including work related to provision for deaf-blind people, those severely multi-handicapped, and elderly people with other social care needs as well as those resulting from sight problems.

Researcher

Robin Lovelock

Centre for Evaluative and Developmental Research, Department of Social Work Studies, University of Southampton, Highfield, Southampton SO9 5NH. (0703 592614/592565)

Publications

The full reference to the research report is:

Lovelock, R., and Edge, S. (1991) 'Research Review: Services For and Social Care of Blind and Partially Sighted People – Report to the Department of Health', Southampton, CEDR, Department of Social Work Studies, University of Southampton.

Lovelock, R. (in press) *Visual Impairment: Social Support – recent research in context*, Aldershot, Gower.

Task Analysis and Objective Measures of Mobility

The purpose of this research was to undertake a cognitive task analysis of mobility and orientation, and describe systematically the skills and abilities of experts in the field of visually impaired travel. Three groups of experts were used; they were experienced practitioners, tutors at the agencies which train new Rehabilitation Workers, and what we have called 'elite travellers'. These are the tiny minority of totally blind and partially sighted who have, to all intents and purposes, normal travel abilities. Many work in London or other large conurbations, and travel at will nationally or internationally. In contrast, we know from our research that 70 per cent of visually-impaired travellers go out less than once a week, and many of these will not go out at all.

Results

The results of our analysis are shown schematically in figure 6.1. It describes three main levels of skills, which serve four over-riding goals.

Figure 6.1: *Cognitive Task Analysis of Mobility and Orientation*

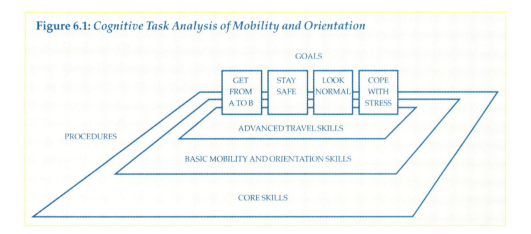

The bottom level comprises five very different types of skill which we call 'core skills'. They are the motor, perceptual, cognitive, social and emotional control skills without which travel would be impossible. Traditional mobility training concentrated almost exclusively on the first three of these, the classic package of skills. In contrast, travellers themselves are adamant that it is their additional proficiency in the other two categories of skill which enables them to travel at all. Without the skill to ask for help when needed, or the ability to cope with travel stress, travellers of all abilities say that their mobility training is effectively useless. Increasingly, Rehabilitation Workers are becoming aware of the need to help their clients improve their social skills, and cope better with stress; but they may not have the training to enable them to do this.

In an attempt to identify some ways in which their training might be improved, we have recently been exploring in more detail how the best – and the worst – travellers cope with travel stress. It may be that some emotional control skills can be taught by practitioners, as they have been to people in other stressful circumstances, such as visiting the dentist, taking examinations, coping with being a single parent or undertaking competitive sport. People in each of these situations have been helped to perform better by learning ways to cope with stress. Our hope is that such coping-skill training may also help visually-impaired travellers to improve their ability to travel.

The next level of skills describes the basic travel skills which will enable a person to undertake a simple 'round-the-block' journey. Many elderly clients will only reach this level of competence. They will only want to be able to visit the corner shop, or a neighbour. The mobility skills are about staying safely on the pavement; the orientation skills are about planning the journey, and staying in touch with one's position during travel. Each of these skills will draw on the lower, core skills as needed.

The advanced skills, *on the third level*, are used for road crossing, negotiating public transport, and dealing with urban problems such as escalators and revolving doors. Few travellers will need them, given the fact that most are elderly, and have little cause to visit city centres. On the other hand, for the younger client seeking work, these travel skills may be crucial. They, too, will draw on lower level skills.

The goals for travel – getting from A to B, staying safe, looking normal and coping with stress – were shared by all travellers, both totally blind and partially sighted, and experienced Mobility Officers. In addition, the rank order of these skills was essentially the same for Mobility Officers and partially sighted clients. This was an extremely encouraging finding, because rehabilitation goals are sometimes not shared by practitioners and service users.

Totally-blind clients' goals, however, were rather different, and differently ranked. They had an additional goal of not getting lost, and the ranking of their goals was different from Mobility Officers – coping with stress, not getting lost, getting from A to B, staying safe and looking normal. Subsequent probing revealed that the 'not getting lost' goal was, in reality, a stress-management tactic. Being lost, for a totally-blind traveller, is an extremely stressful situation. Thus, their goals during travel effectively reduce to the same four as other travellers, but stress-management rates most highly of all. For totally-blind clients in particular, travel stress is so unpleasant that they expend a lot of effort to keep it under control, and yet they are not currently being taught any techniques which might help. In our view, this mismatch between practitioner and client goals is most important.

CONCLUSION

This task analysis is the first comprehensive overview of the range of skills and abilities needed to travel successfully, and has enabled us to construct the first context-free skills-checklist for mobility and orientation. The core skills of motor, perceptual, cognitive, social and emotional control underpin all travel capabilities. Current training, however, virtually ignores the latter two skills. The relatively limited, yet widely used mobility and orientation skills needed for limited travel draw on these core skills, as do the more advanced road-crossing and urban travel skills needed by younger, employable clients.

Experienced practitioners and clients have very similar goals for travel – getting from A to B, staying safe, looking normal, and coping with travel stress. The relative importance of these goals during travel is very similar for Mobility Officers and partially-sighted clients. However, totally-blind clients seem badly served by current practice, which ignores the crucial importance of emotional control skills needed to cope with travel stress: they rate coping with travel stress as their most important consideration. We are investigating this area at present.

Researcher

W. D. A. Beggs

Blind Mobility Research Unit, Department of Psychology, University of Nottingham, University Park, Nottingham NG7 2RD. (0602 484848; FAX 0602 590339)

Publications

Beggs, W. D. A. (1992) 'A task analysis of visually impaired travel', *Journal of Applied Psychology*, BMRU 242.

Dodds, A. G., Howarth C. I., and Clark-Carter, D. D. (1982) 'The mental maps of the blind: The role of previous visual experience', *Journal of Visual Impairment & Blindness*, **76**, 1: 5–12, BMRU 80.

Training Style

Visual impairment Mobility

In order to investigate the *way* in which mobility and orientation training is conducted (rather than its content), we asked a sample of Mobility Officers to wear tape-recorders, and send us copies of the lessons which they conducted.

On the basis of material collected in this way, we attempted to answer a series of questions:

1. First, we looked at training episodes. Did the Mobility Officer simply 'instruct', and was the client required to submit to this instruction? Did the Mobility Officer facilitate the client's learning?

2. We looked at lesson management. Was the Mobility Officer authoritarian, or did the client have any say in the way things were conducted?

3. In addition, we examined the way in which the Mobility Officer dealt with errors, and how much s/he monopolized the conversation.

Findings

There were very significant differences in training and lesson management style within our sample. In training episodes, there was a clear bias towards an authoritarian approach, as measured by the ratio of telling to asking. Only one of our six had a 50/50 ratio of telling to asking; the rest had ratios between 90/10 and 70/30. In addition, these styles seemed to be very stable. They did not vary as training proceeded, nor did it seem to matter whether clients were totally blind, or had some useful vision. With regard to lesson management, Mobility Officers were again varied, but rather less authoritarian, particularly with partially-sighted clients. Their style, as before, remained stable over lessons.

These very directive styles may in theory produce two bad side-effects. First, by failing to generate any responsibility in the client for his or her own rehabilitation, they may help to make them helpless and dependent. Second, taking too much control over the learning process does little to help clients improve their awareness about the tasks involved in learning visually-impaired travel. We have attempted to establish whether these effects are produced in practice, using analogues for real-life mobility training.

Our first investigation was a qualitative one, using the staff at the South Regional Association for the Blind. They trained their Rehabilitation Officer students over a novel route, using either a telling or questioning style.

All of the students were successful in the travel itself, but we asked them how they felt about the two approaches. The telling style was:

★   thought patronizing, and made the learner feel dependent;

★   too passive, and thus could lead to loss of concentration;

★   characterized by overloading and interruptions;

★   not encouraging a feeling of self-confidence; but thought to have some relevance for basic techniques and facts.

In contrast, the questioning approach was seen as:

★ more active, enjoyable and challenging, and a positive experience;
★ encouraging an improvement in self-confidence.

Our second study used an orientation task. Two groups of undergraduates were taught the lay-out of the sea-front area of Paignton, with which none of them were familiar. One group were simply told the information; this is a very common technique for Mobility Officers to use. As well as being given information, the other group were frequently asked questions, and were corrected if they made errors. The teaching time for each group was the same. Both groups were then tested on their knowledge of the geography of the area. There were very significant differences. The use of questions seemed to have helped students build up a clearer, more detailed cognitive map of the area.

Our third attempt used a complex motor task, three-ball juggling, as an analogue for mobility skill itself. Children in two schools were tested for self-esteem, and high and low self-esteem groups identified. At one school, we taught the groups to juggle using an approach very biased towards questioning. It was designed to help them to focus their attention on the task and errors in its performance. They were also given control over the lesson goals. At the second school, the high and low self-esteem groups were taught to juggle in a very directive way, external feedback was provided, and the goals for each lesson were imposed by us. We measured confidence to juggle with three balls before and after each lesson, and after four lessons, we tested each group for performance on this task. The results were very interesting, and we are currently trying to replicate them.

Both high self-esteem groups performed well, and their confidence grew steadily. The low self-esteem group who were taught using the questioning and self-set goal technique also did well, and had an equally impressive growth in confidence. However, the low self-esteem group who were taught by a more directive, authoritarian method performed badly, and their confidence soon began to decline.

The evidence seems to suggest that many Rehabilitation Workers and Mobility Officers use a very over-controlling approach to training, particularly with totally-blind clients. Training style, however, is learnt and can be changed. It seems likely that by using a less authoritarian training style – specifically by using appropriate questioning techniques – they may be able to affect both the learning and confidence of their clients.

Researcher

W. D. A. Beggs

Blind Mobility Research Unit, University of Nottingham, Department of Psychology, University Park, Nottingham NG7 2RD. (0602 484848; FAX 0602 590339)

Publications

Beggs, W. D. A. (1985) 'Giving blind people access to the world', *Social Work Today*, **17**, 7: 14–16, 18–23, (BMRU 145).

Beggs, W. D. A. (1986) 'Developing independence and responsibility in performers', *Coaching Focus*, **4**: 5–6, (BMRU 187).

Beggs, W. D. A. (1987) 'Mobility training today, II: Differences in approach', *British Journal of Visual Impairment*, **V**: 13–16, (BMRU 153).

Beggs, W. D. A. (1988) 'Different approaches to training the low vision client', in N. Neustadt-Noy, S. Merin, and Y. Schiff (eds), *Orientation and Mobility of the Visually Impaired*, Jerusalem, Heiliger, (BMRU 165).

Beggs, W. D. A. (1988) 'Training style', in N. Neustadt-Noy, S. Merin, and Y. Schiff (eds), *Orientation and mobility of the visually Impaired*, Jerusalem, Heiliger, (BMRU 164).

Beggs, W. D. A. (1990) *A question of style*, Leeds, National Coaching Foundation.

Assessing Clients' Training Potential

Summary

The work described below has enabled us to fulfil a number of important objectives.

- It provides a working definition of adjustment which can form the basis for discussion.

- It provides empirical support for the concept of hopelessness–depression which has recently been predicted on theoretical grounds as being a distinct sub-type of clinical depression.

- It has enabled workers to evaluate objectively rehabilitation outcome in the psychological domain.

- It provides researchers with a prototype model of the adjustment process which can be tested, unlike existing models of adjustment.

- It enables the assessment team to identify clients who can benefit from counselling or psychotherapy before being given skill training.

Visual impairment

Independence

Depression

Understanding 'Adjustment'

Rehabilitation workers are required to assess their clients on a wide range of abilities and performance before they can begin to implement skill training. Assessing current performance is relatively straightforward, but assessing psychological factors is something which rehabilitation staff are not trained to do, and their appraisals of a client's psychological state tend to remain at an intuitive level. Two of the most commonly experienced difficulties are assessing levels of **confidence** and **motivation**, and these factors are crucial to the outcome of any independence training. In a recent study, it was found that over 40 per cent of orientation and mobility instructors experienced difficulties with their clients which fell under these two headings.

The commonly-used term *'adjustment'* is equally ambiguous and complex. When a normally-sighted person loses a significant amount of vision there is an emotional response which can be overwhelming. Extreme anxiety and deep depression are typical responses, and clinical depression has been observed in almost 50 per cent of individuals as long as four years after sight loss.

Losing something necessary but formerly taken for granted is depressing; and recent evidence suggests that depression can also be caused by the ways in which people think about events and how these events relate to them. Another line of research suggests that depression can result from learning to be helpless, and sight-loss renders people helpless almost at a stroke. There are therefore both common sense and theoretical reasons for expecting a person who suddenly loses their sight to show depression.

Anxiety can also be understood at both levels. Finding oneself unable to do anything causes immediate anxiety, and sudden helplessness is not something to which people immediately adjust. The prospect of remaining dependent on others engenders fears for the future; and ignorance of what blind people can achieve and acceptance of the stereotype of the blind person as helpless increases anxiety. In addition, the act of registration stigmatizes the individual and encourages the adoption of a negative role. As a consequence of these beliefs and perceptions, depression, anxiety and loss of self-esteem are commonly found among those who lose their sight.

Mainstream psychological thinking suggests that it might be possible to develop a testable model of the adjustment process. Before this can be done, however, a working definition of adjustment is needed which does justice to the range of psychological factors involved in the early response to onset of sight loss. Adjustment has to take place on a number of levels simultaneously; that is why sudden loss of sight is so catastrophic. Perceptual, behavioural, cognitive and emotional adjustments are all required, and these can be overwhelming when presented as simultaneous demands.

Adjustment is sometimes regarded as the ultimate product of rehabilitation, but it may also be seen as a process. Regarding adjustment both as a process and a product forces one to consider what psychological mechanisms might underlie the product. At the theoretical and practical levels, the process view is appropriate: at the final evaluative level, the product view is appropriate. But until a multi-dimensional model of adjustment is developed, rehabilitation specialists will be unable to determine how to facilitate adjustment and how to evaluate their effectiveness in fostering it.

The Research

For the purposes of our research, we considered that emotional and cognitive factors needed to be understood better. From an extensive reading of the literature, we conceptualized adjustment in terms of seven possible psychological factors. The first two are anxiety and depression, and we measured these by means of a general health questionnaire. The third is self-esteem, and this was measured by means of an existing questionnaire. The fourth is self-efficacy, which is simply how strongly the person believes they can succeed at various life tasks. The fifth is locus of control, a concept closely related to self-efficacy, but more global: we looked at locus of control for recovery. The fifth is acceptance of blindness, and an existing questionnaire on acceptance of disability was adapted for use with visually-impaired people. The sixth is attitudes to blindness, and an existing 20-item questionnaire was used. Lastly, we measured people's attributional styles; that is to say, how they accounted for successes and failures.

We administered the resulting 140 items to an initial sample of 50 blind people attending a residential rehabilitation centre and analysed the results. This analysis enabled us to reduce the number of questions to 55; we then administered the shortened questionnaire to 350 clients over the course of two years.

> **Analysis of the results showed that the concept of adjustment could be understood in terms of five principal components. The first is hopelessness–depression; the second is acceptance; the third is self-efficacy; the fourth is anxiety, and the fifth is attitudes to blindness**.

This analysis enables us to understand how the original seven aspects of adjustment may be understood. The next stage in the work will be to develop a testable model of how the factors interact with one another. This has important implications for the ways in which rehabilitation is delivered. Meanwhile, we have administered the questionnaire to 80 clients before and after rehabilitation, in order to see if the questionnaire can pick up any psychological changes. Results clearly show that the greatest changes occur in clients' self-esteem, acceptance of blindness, self-efficacy and anxiety/depression. This means that existing rehabilitation practices can now be evaluated more objectively, and that specific rehabilitation objectives can be measured.

The model need not be restricted to visual loss: it is equally appropriate to the psychological processes underlying adjustment to the loss of any function, either sensory or motor.

Researcher

Dr A. G. Dodds

Blind Mobility Research Unit, University of Nottingham, Department of Psychology, University Park, Nottingham NG7 2RD. (0602 484848; FAX 0602 590339)

Publications

Dodds, A. G. (1988) *Mobility Training for Visually Handicapped People: A Person-Centred Approach*, London, Croom-Helm, (BMRU 193).

Dodds, A. G. (1991) 'The psychology of rehabilitation', *British Journal of Visual Impairment*, **9**, 2: 38–40, (BMRU 241).

Dodds, A. G., Bailey, P., Pearson, A., and Yates, L. (1991) 'Psychological factors in acquired visual impairment: The development of a scale of adjustment', *Journal of Visual Impairment & Blindness*, **85**, 7: 306–310, (BMRU 237).

Motion Vision as an Independent Channel

PROGRESS REPORT

Measuring Impairment

The movement aspect of vision is not generally regarded as being different from its other functions. There is, however, some evidence that people can lose motion vision **specifically**. The kind of tests that people are given when their eyesight starts to fail take very little account of motion as a separate function, and the assumption is that a deterioration in central vision will imply a similar deterioration in all other aspects. Therefore it is possible that some people with very poor sight, as measured by the existing tests, may have a level of motion vision which is potentially of greater use to them. On the other hand, there may be people with quite good sight in the conventional sense, who nevertheless unknowingly have impaired motion vision which makes certain motion-dependent activities such as driving, crossing the road and walking on crowded pavements more difficult or even dangerous than normal.

We decided to try to measure the characteristics of motion vision in normally-sighted people to provide a standard against which defective performances might be judged. It is important to understand that what is being discussed here is not the ability to make a judgement about whether an object is or is not moving, but the underlying response of the visual system to large coherent changes in the total input field. This aspect of vision is below the conscious level and therefore it is necessary to use special equipment to measure it. We chose standing balance as the task because it has already been well established that this takes place below the conscious level, and that the response can be measured fairly easily. The apparatus used in the first set of experiments was a modified and updated version of a device called the 'swinging room', used by David Lee of Edinburgh some 20 years ago to explore the visual aspects of balance.

Our findings so far indicate quite clearly that for most people, any part of the eye can extract the motion information needed to keep balanced. This raises some interesting theoretical questions, and certainly challenges the current view that the periphery in some way specializes in movement information. Its most immediate practical use is as a simple but reliable measure of motion vision as a separate channel. The next planned stage is to measure people with partial sight in the existing apparatus in order to compare them with the normal performances found above. We have also designed a simplified, portable version of the apparatus that could be used in clinics, to investigate the degree of motion impairment in individual cases and collect more information about normal performances from a wider section of the community. A future possible use might be a feedback version of the clinical apparatus, to enable people with very poor central vision to develop their motion acuity in much the same way that bio-feedback allows people to control their heart-rates.

Researchers

A. J. R. Doyle, M. Lee, P. Bailey, A. Pearson and H. Flannigan

Blind Mobility Research Unit, Department of Psychology, University of Nottingham, University Park, Nottingham NG7 2RD. (0602 484848; FAX 0602 590339)

Spatial Problems in the Congenitally Blind

Background

Total, congenital blindness is comparatively rare, yet it occurs sufficiently frequently to pose a problem for mobility instructors. In particular, children suffering from retinopathy of prematurity, (ROP – formerly known as retrolental fibroplasia,) have been identified by many practitioners as having additional spatial problems compared with children whose congenital blindness is caused by other conditions. In a previous study, the authors found that congenitally-blind children exhibited a much poorer performance on spatial tasks than did children who became blind later, although the study did not examine ROP children as a special group.

The research literature on the effects of ROP has been inconclusive. Whereas some workers have found that IQ does not differ between ROP and non-ROP children, other workers have found that ROP children scored lower than non-ROP children. However, it has been pointed out that low IQ and prematurity are themselves related by definition, although one would expect this relationship to disappear over time.

There is no firm research evidence to show that ROP children suffer from greater spatial difficulties than do non-ROP children; but practitioners often believe that they do, and cite examples of congenitally-blind children who appear to have considerable difficulty in understanding layout, position in a spatial array, and similar tasks. Teachers even refer to such individuals as 'typical retrolentals', which suggests that they may indeed be picking up real deficits.

The purpose of the study was to examine this assumption, and to try to relate any findings to cognitive factors which might be expected to have some bearing on spatial task performance.

Performance on spatial tasks depends, *prima facie*, on memory. Memory can be thought of as being of two types: static or dynamic. Static memory involves literal recall of presented material; dynamic memory involves transforming literally-stored information. With respect to orientation, static memory can provide information about a single perspective on a scene. However, when moving about, without the benefit of vision, dynamic memory is involved in updating spatial position as it changes. In addition, there is good reason to believe that intelligence, however it is conceived, may be a factor in the ability to carry out an orientation task successfully.

The Study

It was with the above factors in mind that we conducted a study of the ability of two groups of congenitally-blind students to carry out a simple orientation task. The study sample consisted of 40 totally congenitally-blind students, 20 ROP and 20 non-ROP, drawn from five schools for the blind. Ages ranged from 9 to 19 years, with a mean of 15.0 years for the ROP group and 13.8 years for the non-ROP group.

Visual impairment
Children
Mobility training

Children were tested for knowledge of the cardinal points of the compass, and those showing an incomplete understanding of these were considered to be unsuitable as one of the tasks required such an understanding.

Five tasks in all were presented. The first consisted of the subset of orientation questions from the Standford–Binet IQ test. Twelve spatial reasoning problems were presented in increasing order of difficulty, and the number of correct answers was expressed as a proportion of the total number of questions. The second consisted of the Forward Digit Span from the Weschler Intelligence Scale for Children (WISC-R). A list of digits was read out in increasing order of difficulty, and scores were expressed as proportions. The third was the Backward Digit Span from the WISC-R. A list of digits was read out in increasing order of difficulty and the child was required to repeat them in reverse order. The fourth was the Similarities task from the WISC-R. The task consists of twelve conceptual questions about the relationship between two objects, for example, a pair of scissors and a copper pan, and the child has to say how they are similar. The fifth task was a modified Orientation task developed by the authors in a previous study. In this task, the student is taken on a short route consisting of a number of right-angled turns, and is required to indicate his/her position in relation to the initial starting-point by pointing, using a pointer-board.

Results

Scores on each of these tasks were inter-correlated to examine possible relationships between them. The hypothesis that performance on the Orientation task would be a function of cause of blindness was not supported, the ROP children performing as well as the non-ROP children. What was surprising, however, was that performance on the Similarities task correlated significantly with performance on the Orientation task in both groups, whereas performance on none of the other tasks did. These findings require further consideration.

Spatial memory tasks such as the Orientation task presented here depend upon short-term working-memory and the ability to reorganize spatial material. One would therefore predict that performance on digit forward and backward tasks, and on a mental, spatial problem-solving task would correlate with performance on the Orientation tasks. By the same token, one would not predict that a non-spatial task which did not depend upon working memory would in any way correlate with an Orientation task. How can such a pattern of results be explained?

The results can be understood with reference to the fact that performance on a real-life Orientation task is assisted by previous environmental experiences: performance on the Similarities task would also be expected to be assisted by previous environmental experiences. Poor spatial performance and poor understanding of the world therefore jointly result from inadequate perceptual experiences in the world. This interpretation fits well with the observation that parents of congenitally-blind children often over-protect them.

Over-protection can occur if the parents of a blind infant either neglect to stimulate it, or actively prevent it from exploring its environment. In such cases children are kept immobile, avoiding the spatial problems created in moving about. By the same token, these children are prevented from exploring other aspects of the physical world which would help them to understand how it is constructed. Their spatial and conceptual deficits may be traced back to the same source.

These findings suggest two conclusions. First, exploration of the environment needs to be encouraged through early mobility. Second, teachers should not automatically assume that ROP children require special treatment for spatial

deficits. Indeed, the findings suggest that any congenitally-blind children may be handicapped by lack of early experiences, and that non-ROP children requiring special attention may be overlooked if the teacher concentrates her efforts on the ROP child.

Researcher

Dr A. G. Dodds

Blind Mobility Research Unit, Department of Psychology, University of Nottingham, University Park, Nottingham NG7 2RD. (0602 484848; FAX 0602 590339)

Publications

Dodds, A. G. (1983) 'Mental rotation and visual imagery', *Journal of Visual Impairment & Blindness*, **77**, 1: 16–18, (BMRU 81).

Dodds, A. G. (1986) 'Spatial awareness training', in N. Neustadt-Noy, S. Merin, and Y. Schiff (eds), *Orientation and Mobility of the Visually Impaired*, Jerusalem, Heiliger, (BMRU 167).

Dodds, A. G., Hellawell, D. J., and Lee, M. D. (1991) 'Congenitally blind children with and without retrolental fibroplasia: Do they perform differently?', *Journal of Visual Impairment & Blindness*, **85**, 5: 225–227, (BMRU 227).

Dodds, A. G., Howarth, C. I., and Clark-Carter, D. D. (1982) 'The mental maps of the blind: The role of previous visual experience', *Journal of Visual Impairment & Blindness*, **76**, 1: 5–12, (BMRU 80).

Supplement

Research Relating to HIV, AIDS and Substance Misuse

DH-Funded Community Care Research Projects Relating to HIV, AIDS and Substance Misuse, 1988–1992

Living with AIDS
The experiences of, and attitudes towards, the care received by those with HIV infection and AIDS.
Researchers: Ms K. McCann, Ms E. Wadsworth
Institute for Social Studies in Medical Care, 14 South Hill Park, London NW3 2SB (071 794 7793)

HIV Infection, AIDS and Community Nursing
The study provided a national profile of the extent and nature of community nursing staff's HIV- and AIDS-related work in England and Scotland, their beliefs and knowledge regarding HIV infection and AIDS.
Researchers: Dr S. Bond, Mr J. Bond
Health Care Research Unit, University of Newcastle, 21 Claremont Place, Newcastle upon Tyne NE2 4AA (091 222 7045)

Economics of Alcohol Abuse
A critical review of the uses made of data on alcohol consumption, to evaluate how existing and new sources of data may be used more effectively.
Researcher: Dr C. Godfrey
Centre for Health Economics (CHE), University of York, Heslington, York YO1 5DD (0904 430000)

HIV, ARC and AIDS: The Need for Social Care and the Development of Provision
The social care needs of people with HIV/ARC/AIDS and their carers, the development of relevant social care provision, and the financial input of HIV/ARC/AIDS.
Researchers: Professor D. Robinson, Professor G. Smith (Hull), Professor A. Maynard (York)
CHE/Institute of Health Studies, University of Hull, Hull HU6 7RX (0482 465966)

Social Services Resources and AIDS/Developing AIDS Policies in Local Authorities
The development of policy and its resource implications in local authorities in South London.
Researchers: Mr A. Bebbington, Dr R. Feldman, Dr P. Galter
South Bank University, Castle House, 2 Walworth Road, London SE1 1DW

The Monitoring and Evaluation of the Landmark Centre
Includes an assessment of the influence on services from other agencies of this initiative by Lambeth AIDS Action.
Researchers: Mr A. Bebbington, Ms P. Warren
Personal Social Services Research Unit, Cornwallis Building, University of Kent, Canterbury CT2 7NF (0227 764000)

National Evaluation of Syringe-Exchange Schemes and HIV Risk Behaviour of Clients and a Comparison Group
Assessed the development of syringe-exchange schemes – their ability to reach and retain injecting drug-users, service delivery and service organization – and examined short and long-term changes in HIV risk-related behaviour.
Researcher: Professor G. V. Stimson
Centre for Research on Drugs and Health Behaviour, 200 Seagrave Road, London SW6 1RQ (081 846 6565)

HIV and AIDS: Needs for Social Services and the Development of Provision
The range and cost of HIV/AIDS-generated demands for social care, the management and coordination of that care, and SSDs' development of provision.
Researcher: Profesor D. Robinson
Institute for Health Studies, University of Hull, Hull HU6 7RX (0482 465966)

Evaluation of Central London AIDS Prevention Outreach Project
Investigated ways of reaching and reducing HIV-related risk behaviours in hard-to-reach populations such as drug-injectors, prostitutes and homeless young people.
Researchers: Mr R. Hartnoll, Dr J. Holland, Dr. T. Rhodes
Birkbeck College, University of London, 16 Gower Street, London WC1E 6DP (071 631 6512)

Development of AIDS Services by DHAs: The Organizational Response to AIDS
Comparative analysis of four DHAs' responses to AIDS, covering the whole spectrum of service provision.
Researcher: Professor A. Pettigrew
Centre for Corporate Strategy and Change, University of Warwick, Coventry CV4 7AL (0203 523523)

The Role of GPs in the Treatment of Drug Misuse
Quantified the extent of GPs' involvement in the treatment of drug-misusers, and identified factors influencing their response to such patients.
Researcher: Mr A. Glanz
Addiction Research Unit, Institute of Psychiatry, De Crespigny Park, Denmark Hill, London SE5 8AF (071 703 5411)

Assessing Drug Treatment at Satellite Clinics of a Regional Drug Dependence Unit
The impact on local agencies of clinics offering both visiting specialist staff and local generic staff, and community drugs teams.
Researcher: Dr J. Strang
North Western Regional Drug Research Unit, University of Manchester, Prestwich Hospital, Bury New Road, Manchester M25 7BL (061 798 0544)

Evaluation of the Centrally-Funded Initiative on Services for Drug-Misusers
Described and analysed the service projects supported through the CFI.
Researcher: Dr S. MacGregor
Birkbeck College, University of London, 16 Gower Street, London WC1E 6DP (071 631 6222)

Managing the Nursing Care of People with AIDS in the Community – An Evaluation of Workshops
Aimed to prepare senior community nursing staff for the management of AIDS patients in the community, and identified key areas of education, practice and policy.

Researcher: Ms B. M. Robottom

English National Board for Nursing, Midwifery and Health Visiting, Victory House, 170 Tottenham Court Road, London W1E 4YZ (071 388 3131)

Monitoring Injecting-Equipment Exchange Schemes

Monitored the implementation of 13 pilot schemes – how they were established, service delivery and their ability to reach and retain clients – and changes in their clients' behaviour.

Researcher: Dr G. V. Stimson

Department of Sociology, Goldsmiths' College, University of London SE14 6NW (081 692 7171)

Costing of Personal Social Services Expected to be used by People with AIDS

Researcher: Professor B. Davies

Personal Social Services Research Unit, Cornwallis Building, University of Kent, Canterbury CT2 7NF (0227 764000)

AIDS, HIV Infection and General Practice

Examined the GP consultation rate of people with HIV-related infections and AIDS.

Researcher: Mr C. Foy

Health Care Research Unit, University of Newcastle, 21 Claremont Place, Newcastle upon Tyne NE2 4AA (091 222 7045)

Survey of Pharmacy Sales of Needles and Syringes

Investigated the involvement of community pharmacists in needle and syringe supply, to assess the extent to which needle-sharing leads to the spread of HIV.

Researcher: Mr A. Glanz

Addiction Research Unit, Institute of Psychiatry, De Crespigny Park, Denmark Hill, London SE5 8AF (071 703 5411)

A Study of Help-Seeking and Service Utilization by Problem Drug-Takers

Explored the reasons why people seek or do not seek help with problems related to their drug use, and the subsequent interaction between agencies and clients.

Researcher: Mr R. Hartnoll

Birkbeck College, University of London, Malet Street, London WC1E 7HX (071 631 6371)

Evaluation of the London Lighthouse

Aims to evaluate the London Lighthouse, an innovative provider of services to people affected by AIDS.

Researcher: Dr E. Stern

Tavistock Institute, The Tavistock Centre, Belsize Lane, London NW3 5BA (071 435 7111)

AIDS – Referral and Community Nursing Care

The coordination and planning of referral systems, case-management, networking and service delivery for patients with HIV disease, including models of good practice.

Researcher: Professor C. A. Butterworth

Department of Nursing, University of Manchester, Oxford Road, Manchester M20 9PT (061 275 5346)

Community Services for People with HIV infection

The costs and appropriateness of current community care provision for heterosexuals, injecting drug-users, homosexuals and bisexuals with HIV infection, living in Greater London.

Researcher: Professor D. Miller

St Mary's Hospital Medical School, Norfolk Place, London W2 1PG (071 725 1673)

Treatment Outcomes of Opiate Drug Misusers in General Practice and Hospital Clinic Settings

Assesses the impact of specialist support to GPs in the treatment of drug misusers and in reducing HIV-risk behaviour.

Researcher: Dr J. Edeh

St George's Hospital Medical School, Department of Mental Helath Sciences, Cranmer Terrace, London SW17 0RE (081 672 9944)

The Implications for Service Delivery of Coping Strategies Adopted by Illicit-Drug Users not in Treatment

Examines the ways in which injecting drug-users not in touch with existing services devise coping strategies to control drug use and HIV-related risk behaviour, and how these may be incorporated into service provision.

Researcher: Dr R. Power

Charing Cross and Westminster Medical School, 200 Seagrave Road, London SW6 1RQ (081 846 6565)

The Daily Lives and Smoking Behaviour of Working-Class Women with Children

Identifies similarities and differences in lifestyle, social support, health attitudes and coping strategies between maternal smokers and non-smokers, as well as factors associated with sustained cessation of smoking among mothers caring for young children.

Researcher: Professor H. M. Graham

Department of Applied Social Studies, University of Warwick, Coventry CV4 7AL (0203 523164)

The Future Role of Drug Advisory Committees

Examines the role of regional and local drug advisory structures in the context of legislative change, and concern over drug misuse and the spread of HIV infection.

Researcher: Mr R. Howard

14 The Colonnades, 107 Wilton Way, London E8 1BH (081 895 3165)

Living with AIDS

Explores the ways in which people's lives are affected by AIDS.

Researcher: Dr A. Richardson

Social and Community Planning Research, 35 Northampton Square, London EC1V 0AX (071 250 1524)

Women, Risk and AIDS

Analysis of data on the sexual knowledge, understanding and practice of young women – both in general, and in relation to HIV and AIDS.

Researcher: Dr J. Holland

Social Science Research Unit, Institute of Education, 55–59 Gordon Square, London WC1H 0NT (071 636 1500)

Need Assessment for Alcohol Service Provision in Community Care

Development of a method to assess the need for community alcohol services.

Researcher: Ms C. Godfrey

Centre for Health Economics, University of York, Heslington, York YO1 5DD (0904 430000)

Index

Printed in the United Kingdom for HMSO
Dd295547 2/96 C10 4533 13795